YOUTH SUBSTANCE ABUSE and Co-occurring Disorders

YOUTH SUBSTANCE ABUSE and
Co-occurring Disorders

Edited by

Yifrah Kaminer, M.D., M.B.A.

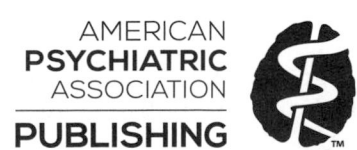

AMERICAN
PSYCHIATRIC
ASSOCIATION
PUBLISHING

Note: The authors have worked to ensure that all information in this book is accurate at the time of publication and consistent with general psychiatric and medical standards, and that information concerning drug dosages, schedules, and routes of administration is accurate at the time of publication and consistent with standards set by the U.S. Food and Drug Administration and the general medical community. As medical research and practice continue to advance, however, therapeutic standards may change. Moreover, specific situations may require a specific therapeutic response not included in this book. For these reasons and because human and mechanical errors sometimes occur, we recommend that readers follow the advice of physicians directly involved in their care or the care of a member of their family.

Books published by American Psychiatric Association Publishing represent the findings, conclusions, and views of the individual authors and do not necessarily represent the policies and opinions of American Psychiatric Association Publishing or the American Psychiatric Association.

If you wish to buy 50 or more copies of the same title, please go to www.appi.org/specialdiscounts for more information.

Copyright © 2016 American Psychiatric Association
ALL RIGHTS RESERVED

Manufactured in the United States of America on acid-free paper
19 18 17 16 15   5 4 3 2 1
First Edition

Typeset in Palatino LT Std and Trade Gothic LT Std.

American Psychiatric Association Publishing
1000 Wilson Boulevard
Arlington, VA 22209-3901
www.appi.org

Library of Congress Cataloging-in-Publication Data

Youth substance abuse and co-occurring disorders / edited by Yifrah Kaminer.—
First edition.
    p. ; cm.
    Includes bibliographical references and index.
    ISBN 978-1-58562-497-3 (pbk. : alk. paper)
    I. Kaminer, Yifrah, 1951- , editor. II. American Psychiatric Association.

    [DNLM: 1. Substance-Related Disorders—complications. 2. Substance-Related Disorders—therapy. 3. Adolescent. 4. Child. 5. Comorbidity. 6. Mental Disorders—complications. 7. Mental Disorders—therapy. WM 270]
    RJ506.D78
    618.92'86—dc23

                                                                        2015019660

British Library Cataloguing in Publication Data
A CIP record is available from the British Library.

CONTENTS

Yifrah Kaminer, M.D., M.B.A.

Ralph E. Tarter, Ph.D.
Michelle S. Horner, D.O.

Marc Fishman, M.D.

Yifrah Kaminer, M.D., M.B.A.
Ken C. Winters, Ph.D.
John Kelly, Ph.D.

Oscar G. Bukstein, M.D., M.P.H.

CONTRIBUTORS

Kara S. Bagot, M.D.
Fellow, Albert J. Solnit Integrated Training Program in Adult, Child, and Adolescent Psychiatry, Yale University School of Medicine Child Study Center, New Haven, Connecticut

Jessica H. Baker, Ph.D.
Assistant Professor, Department of Psychiatry, University of North Carolina at Chapel Hill, Chapel Hill, North Carolina

Jessica J. Black, Ph.D.
Postdoctoral Research Scholar, Department of Psychiatry and Graduate School of Public Health, University of Pittsburgh, Pittsburgh, Pennsylvania

Oscar G. Bukstein, M.D., M.P.H.
Medical Director, DePelchin Children's Center; Clinical Professor of Psychiatry, University of Texas Health Science Center–Houston, Baylor College of Medicine, Houston, Texas

Cynthia M. Bulik, Ph.D.
Distinguished Professor of Eating Disorders, Department of Psychiatry, University of North Carolina at Chapel Hill, Chapel Hill, North Carolina; Professor, Department of Medical Epidemiology and Biostatistics, Karolinska Institutet, Stockholm, Sweden

Tammy Chung, Ph.D.
Associate Professor, Departments of Psychiatry and Epidemiology, University of Pittsburgh, Pittsburgh, Pennsylvania

Duncan B. Clark, M.D., Ph.D.
Associate Professor, Department of Psychiatry, University of Pittsburgh, Pittsburgh, Pennsylvania

John F. Curry, Ph.D., ABPP
Professor, Department of Psychiatry and Behavioral Sciences and
Department of Psychology and Neuroscience, Duke University,
Durham, North Carolina

Jeffrey L. Derevensky, Ph.D.
Professor, Department of Psychiatry and Department of Educational
and Counselling Psychology, and Director, International Centre for
Youth Gambling Problems and High-Risk Behaviors, McGill University, Montreal, Quebec, Canada

Anne Duffy, M.D., M.Sc., FRCPC
Campus Alberta Innovates Program (CAIP), Research Chair in Youth
Mental Health, and Professor, Department of Psychiatry, University of
Calgary, Mathison Centre for Mental Health Research and Education,
Calgary, Alberta, Canada

Christianne Esposito-Smythers, Ph.D.
Associate Professor, Department of Psychology, George Mason
University, Fairfax, Virginia

Marc Fishman, M.D.
Assistant Professor, Department of Psychiatry, Johns Hopkins Univer-
sity School of Medicine; Medical Director, Maryland Treatment Centers,
Baltimore, Maryland

Julian D. Ford, Ph.D.
Professor, Department of Psychiatry, University of Connecticut Health
Center, Farmington, Connecticut

Josephine M. Hawke, Ph.D.
Assistant Professor, Department of Psychiatry, University of Connecticut Health Center, Farmington, Connecticut

Jacqueline Hersh, Ph.D.
Postdoctoral Fellow, Department of Psychology, Harvard University,
Cambridge, Massachusetts

Michelle S. Horner, D.O.
Assistant Professor, Department of Psychiatry and Behavioral Sciences,
Johns Hopkins School of Medicine, Baltimore, Maryland

Yifrah Kaminer, M.D., M.B.A.
Professor of Psychiatry and Pediatrics, University of Connecticut
Health Center, Farmington, Connecticut

John Kelly, Ph.D.
Elizabeth R. Spalin Associate Professor of Psychiatry, Harvard Medical
School; Director, Recovery Research Institute, Massachusetts
General Hospital, Boston, Massachusetts

Kyla Machell, M.A.
Graduate Student in Clinical Psychology, Department of Psychology,
George Mason University, Fairfax, Virginia

Lauren M. Metzger, LCSWA
Clinical Instructor, Department of Psychiatry, University of North
Carolina at Chapel Hill, Chapel Hill, North Carolina

Robert Milin, M.D., FRCPC
Head, Division of Addiction and Mental Health, and Associate Professor, Department of Psychiatry, University of Ottawa; Clinical Scientist,
Institute of Mental Health Research; Director, Adolescent Day Treatment Unit, Youth Psychiatry Program, Royal Ottawa Mental Health
Centre, Ottawa, Ontario, Canada

Maryam Nemati, M.A., CCC
Research Associate, Mood Disorders Centre of Ottawa, Ottawa,
Ontario, Canada

Alexandra Perloe, M.A.
Graduate Student in Clinical Psychology, Department of Psychology,
George Mason University, Fairfax, Virginia

Marc N. Potenza, M.D., Ph.D.
Professor, Departments of Psychiatry, Child Study, and Neurobiology,
Yale University, New Haven, Connecticut

Bethany Rallis, Ed.M.
Graduate Student in Clinical Psychology, Department of Psychology,
George Mason University, Fairfax, Virginia

Ralph E. Tarter, Ph.D.
Professor, Center for Education and Drug Abuse Research, School of
Pharmacy, University of Pittsburgh, Pittsburgh, Pennsylvania

Timothy E. Wilens, M.D.
Chief of Child and Adolescent Psychiatry, Director, Center for Addiction Medicine, and Director, Substance Abuse Services in Pediatric
Psychopharmacology, Massachusetts General Hospital; Associate Professor of Psychiatry, Harvard Medical School, Boston, Massachusetts

Ken C. Winters, Ph.D.
Professor of Psychiatry, University of Minnesota Medical School,
Minneapolis, Minnesota

Yvonne H.C. Yau, M.Sc.
Ph.D. Candidate, Department of Neurology and Neurosurgery,
McGill University, Montreal, Quebec, Canada

Courtney A. Zulauf, B.A.
Doctoral Student, Department of Psychology, University of Illinois
at Chicago, Chicago, Illinois

Disclosure of Competing Interests

The following contributors to this book have indicated a financial interest in or other affiliation with a commercial supporter, a manufacturer of a commercial product, a provider of a commercial service, a nongovernmental organization, and/or a government agency, as listed below:

Cynthia M. Bulik, Ph.D.—*Consultant:* Shire Pharmaceuticals; *Royalties:* Pearson.

John F. Curry, Ph.D., ABPP—*Research support:* Pfizer for a naturalistic follow-up study on the safety of sertraline in youth, Forest Research Institute for a clinical trial of vilazodone for adolescent major depressive disorder; *Member:* Integrated Psychotherapy Consortium, which provides training in cognitive behavior therapy through the REACH Institute.

Marc Fishman, M.D.—*Research support:* US WorldMeds.

Julian D. Ford, Ph.D.—*Co-owner:* Advanced Trauma Solutions, Inc.

Robert Milin, M.D., FRCPC—*Speaker's honorarium:* Bristol-Myers Squibb Canada

Marc N. Potenza, M.D., Ph.D.—*Consultation and advisement:* Boehringer Ingelheim, Lundbeck, Ironwood, Shire, INSYS; *Consultation and financial interests:* Somaxon; *Research support:* National Institutes of Health, Veteran's Administration, Mohegan Sun Casino, National Center for Responsible Gaming and its affiliated Institute for Research on Gambling Disorders, Forest Laboratories, Ortho-McNeil, Oy-Control/Biotie, Glaxo-SmithKline, Pfizer, Psyadon Pharmaceuticals. The author has participated in surveys, mailings, or telephone consultations related to drug addiction, impulse control disorders, or other health topics; has consulted for law offices and the federal public defender's office on issues related to impulse control disorders; provides clinical care in the Connecticut Department of Mental Health and Addiction Services Problem Gambling Services Program; has performed grant reviews for the National Institutes of Health and other agencies; has guest-edited journal sections; has given academic lectures in grand rounds, CME events, and other clinical or scientific venues; and has generated books or book chapters for publishers of mental health texts.

Timothy E. Wilens, M.D.—*Grant support:* NIH (NIDA), Pfizer, Shire; *Consultant:* Bay Cover Human Services, Euthymics/Neurovance, Major/Minor League Baseball, US National Football League/ERM Associates, NIH (NIDA), Shire, Theravance, TRIS; *Author: Straight Talk About Psychiatric Medications for Kids; Co-editor: ADHD in Children and Adults* and *Comprehensive Clinical Psychiatry.*

The following contributors to this book have indicated no competing interests to disclose during the year preceding manuscript submission:

Kara S. Bagot, M.D.
Jessica H. Baker, Ph.D.
Jessica J. Black, Ph.D.
Oscar G. Bukstein, M.D., M.P.H.
Tammy Chung, Ph.D.
Duncan B. Clark, M.D., Ph.D.
Jeffrey L. Derevensky, Ph.D.
Anne Duffy, M.D., M.Sc., FRCPC
Christianne Esposito-Smythers, Ph.D.
Jacqueline Hersh, Ph.D.
Michelle S. Horner, D.O.
Yifrah Kaminer, M.D., M.B.A.
John Kelly, Ph.D
Kyla Machell, M.A
Alexandra Perloe, M.A.
Ralph E. Tarter, Ph.D.
Ken C. Winters, Ph.D.
Yvonne H. C. Yau, M.Sc.
Courtney A. Zulauf, B.A.

PREFACE

There is a continuing worldwide public health challenge: adolescents with substance use disorders (SUDs). Heterogeneity with respect to severity of substance use and the association of comorbid psychiatric disorders is characteristic of this population according to clinical consensus. Indeed, it is the rule rather than the exception that the majority (70%–80%) of adolescents with the diagnosis of SUD manifest comorbid psychopathology, known also as co-occurring disorders or *dual diagnosis*—that is, the presence of one or more comorbid psychiatric disorders in addition to SUD (Bukstein et al. 1989). Psychiatric disorders in childhood, including disruptive behavior and mood and anxiety disorders, increase risk for the development of SUD in adolescence. Etiological mechanisms have not been methodically researched; however, a number of possible relationships exist between SUD and psychopathology. Psychopathology may precede SUD in the majority of cases. It may also develop as a consequence of a preexisting SUD or may influence the severity of SUD. Psychopathology may be unrelated or may arise from a common vulnerability.

The objective of this book is to address theory and practice pertaining to understanding and treating psychiatric comorbidity in adolescents with SUDs. Some of the most prominent investigators in the field have contributed scholarly chapters to this volume. Given the growing interest in clinical research and the advancement of treatment, it is important to note that future directions in clinical research are emphasized in each and every chapter. The authors are hoping that this book will enhance and inspire continued clinical and research investment in the dual-diagnosis domain. For instance, although comorbidity is a key correlate of treatment outcome among adolescents in treatment for SUDs, most studies examine comorbidity as a static patient characteristic that affects drug use severity and outcomes. The stability or lability of psychiatric diagnostic status among substance-using adolescents has not been systematically investigated. Additional research on this aspect of the diagnostic status of substance-using youths is warranted.

Improved understanding of the relationship between SUD and psychiatric comorbidity among youth, including how the respective courses of SUD and psychiatric disorders are related, how changes occur across different types of disorders, and how trajectories of change affect the clinical course of recovery from SUD, is essential. Finally, clinical trials for specific treatment modalities for SUDs should include youths with psychiatric comorbidity, but they should also examine specific interventions for specific comorbid conditions, for example, attention-deficit/hyperactivity disorder, depression, and anxiety disorders. This book should stimulate further discussion and advancement of the field, with the ultimate result of better care and more effective services and intervention modalities for these youth.

All but chapters 13 and 14 include in the titles the terms substance use disorder or disorders. Chapters 13 and 14 are included in this edition because they represent important emerging non-substance-related addictive disorders; both gambling disorder and Internet gaming disorder are represented in DSM-5 (American Psychiatric Association 2013). In both chapters, there is a limited review of co-occurring disorders because the literature is still lagging behind in publications on substance-related disorders.

Chapters 5–14 include DSM-5 criteria for the reviewed respective disorders. This allows readers to compare these criteria with previous editions of DSM. Finally, it remains to be seen whether the DSM-5 diagnostic criteria for substance-related and addictive disorders will meet the needs of adolescents better than DSM-IV (American Psychiatric Association 1994) diagnostic criteria, which also included the abuse and dependence categories. Some criticisms about the limitations of the new diagnostic formulation for youth have already emerged (Kaminer and Winters 2015). These include questioning the utility and justification for the low two-symptom threshold for SUD (out of 11 potential symptoms) and the inclusion and definition (or lack of) of symptoms such as tolerance, withdrawal, hazardous use, and craving.

The applied approach of this book will serve the needs of clinicians, clinical researchers, and students in the fields of mental health, public health, and medicine (particularly in pediatrics, family medicine, and child and adolescent psychiatry).

As the editor of this volume, I wish to acknowledge current support from the National Institute on Drug Abuse and the National Institute on Alcohol Abuse and Alcoholism.

Yifrah Kaminer, M.D., M.B.A.

References

American Psychiatric Association: Diagnostic and Statistical Manual of Mental Disorders, 4th Edition. Washington, DC, American Psychiatric Association, 1994

American Psychiatric Association: Diagnostic and Statistical Manual of Mental Disorders, 5th Edition. Arlington, VA, American Psychiatric Association, 2013

Bukstein O, Brent DA, Kaminer Y: Comorbidity of substance abuse and other psychiatric disorders in adolescents. Am J Psychiatry, 146:1131–1141, 19892669535

Kaminer Y, Winters K: DSM-5 adolescent substance use disorders: lost in translation? J Am Acad Child Adolesc Psych 54(5):350–351, 2015 25901770

CHAPTER 1

Developmental Pathways to Substance Use Disorder and Co-occurring Psychiatric Disorders in Adolescents

Ralph E. Tarter, Ph.D.
Michelle S. Horner, D.O.

Substance use disorder (SUD) in adolescents typically is preceded by and co-occurs with other psychiatric disorders. The large number of disorders in DSM-5 (American Psychiatric Association 2013) potentially combine to form thousands of diagnostic configurations. Individuals displaying a particular combination of disorders are widely thought to constitute a particular subgroup of SUD. Emerging cross-disciplinary research indicates, however, that deficient psychological self-regulation during childhood and adolescence, manifested in varying severity, antedates SUD and co-occurring psychiatric disorders. Furthermore, prefrontal cortex dysfunction underlies poor psychological self-regulation and heightens risk for SUD and co-occurring disorders. Thus, rather than representing specific SUD subtypes, the myriad

This research was supported by grants P50 DA05605, K05 DA031248, and K12 DA000357.

1

combinations instead reflect variants of one core disorder. In this chapter, we review the empirical literature documenting evidence that heritable prefrontal cortex dysfunction underlies SUD vulnerability, which is overtly expressed as psychological dysregulation. In addition, we describe a measurement schema to guide research aimed at delineating the ontogenetic pathways linking SUD vulnerability to SUD outcome. Importantly, this schema is also informative for SUD prevention and treatment. Last, we examine the key factors that span the period from fetal development through adolescence that bias ontogeny toward SUD.

At the outset, it is important to note that findings from postmortem (Benes et al. 1994; Marsh et al. 2008) and neuroimaging (Lenroot and Giedd 2006; Toga et al. 2006) research indicate that synaptic connections are formed and eliminated throughout life. During the protracted period of neuromaturation, which extends for three decades after birth, neural circuitry is genetically programmed and fine-tuned by numerous factors, including experience, the environment, and sex hormones. Concomitant with puberty onset and continuing through adolescence, gonadal hormones sculpt the structural organization of the brain (Giedd et al. 2006; Sisk and Zehr 2005) in conjunction with profound remodeling of neural circuitry manifesting as progressive cell growth, axonal sprouting and dendritic arborization, and regressive apoptosis and synaptic pruning. Up to 40% of redundant and irrelevant synapses are pruned, resulting morphologically in thinning of the cerebral cortex corresponding with enhanced cognitive and intellectual competence (Sowell et al. 2003, 2004).

Pubertal changes in neuromaturation are associated with amplified motivation for reward and sensation seeking, evinced in many youths as substance use (Forbes and Dahl 2010). Because substance use experimentation is normative during adolescence (Johnston et al. 2012), many youths are exposed to potentially neurotoxic substances, which can exacerbate vulnerabilities, during a sensitive period of neurodevelopment. Thus, the period spanning puberty onset to adult brain maturation sets the stage for substance use experimentation and progression to SUD. When a person reaches age 30, the modal lifetime period of risk for developing SUD has passed, coinciding with completion of prefrontal cortex maturation (Giedd et al. 1999; Sowell et al. 2004).

Notably, frontal cortex gray matter organization covaries with severity of externalizing behavior and risk for substance abuse (Weiland et al. 2014). Moreover, disruption of prefrontal cortex in youths at high risk for developing SUD (e.g., offspring of addicted parents) has been observed using neuroimaging (Benegal et al. 2007; Eldreth et al. 2004; McNamee et al. 2008; Schweinsburg et al. 2004), electrophysiological (Bauer and Hesselbrock, 1993, 2001; Buss et al. 2003; Finn and Justus 1999; Habeych et al. 2005), psychophysiological (Iacono et al. 2008), and neuropsychological (Iacono et al. 2008; Ivanov et al. 2008) methods of measurement. Significantly, frontal cortex gray matter is more strongly correlated in monozygotic than dizygotic twins (Thompson et al. 2001), and maturation of frontal cortex is strongly influenced by genetics (Peper et al. 2007). Almost all the variance related to executive cognitive capacities that are subserved by neural systems in the anterior cortex is heritable (Friedman et al. 2008). Many studies demonstrate that the executive cognitive processes, listed in Table 1–1, are integrally related to risk for developing SUD.

Executive cognitive capacities, externalizing behavior, and internalizing disturbances constitute a unidimensional trait: neurobehavioral disinhibition (Mezzich et al. 2007). The score on this trait predicts the development of SUD between childhood and adulthood (Tarter et al. 2004) and covaries with frontal cortex hypoactivation during performance of an inhibitory task (McNamee et al. 2008). The empirical literature thus indicates that the vulnerability to SUD consists of a heritable neuromaturational disorder having primarily prefrontal cortex localization that is overtly manifested as psychological dysregulation (Tarter et al. 2012a).

It is also noteworthy that the clinical outcome, SUD, is similarly a continuous variable. Although specified as 10 categories in DSM-5, distinguished by specific drug (e.g., phencyclidine, tobacco) or drug class (e.g., inhalants, sedatives), these putative categories are strongly correlated and are indicators of a unidimensional trait (Kirisci et al. 2006). Indeed, almost 100% of genetic risk is shared among the various SUDs (Kendler et al. 2003; Tsuang et al. 1998). Hence, rather than discrete disorders, the various SUDs are variants of one disorder. As we discuss in the section "Connecting SUD Liability to Clinical Outcome," unidimensionality of both the liability and clinical disorder has important ramifications for understanding the co-occurrence of SUD with other psychiatric disorders. At this juncture, it is important to note that although the particular SUD variant manifested is contingent on many factors, the severity of externalizing the disorder during childhood is especially salient (Krueger et al. 2002). Specifically, low externalizing disorder severity, reflecting a low propensity to violate societal norms, portends SUD consequent to legal drugs (for adults), whereas high externalizing symptom severity predicts SUDs consequent to using "hard" illegal drugs.

TABLE 1–1.	Executive cognitive functions

Attention control and concentration

Organization of action plan for goal-directed behavior

Anticipation of consequences of decisions and behavior (foresight)

Problem-solving flexibility

Self-monitoring of ongoing behavior

Modulation of emotions appropriate to external circumstances

Cognitive control of impulses

Timely termination of goal-directed behavior

Developmental Patterning of SUD

Epidemiological findings reveal that the peak prevalence of cannabis use disorder occurs at ages 18–19 years (Wagner and Anthony 2007). In effect, cannabis use disorder most frequently manifests soon after physical and sexual maturation is completed and during ongoing neuromaturation. Figure 1–1, adapted from Vanyukov et al. (2003a, 2003b), depicts a developmental framework for researching SUD etiology. Consistent with the NIH Roadmap (Collins et al. 2014; Woolf 2008; Zerhouni 2003), this framework informs intervention practice linked to etiology (Tarter et al. 2012b).

A large array of characteristics spanning all levels of biobehavioral organization is associated with the risk for SUD. Magnitude of expression of each biobehavioral characteristic ($V_1 \ldots V_n$) results from the interaction of many genes and multiple environments. The aggregate of scores on all characteristics constitutes the individual's SUD *liability phenotype* (V_R). Importantly, the liability phenotype is a vector; namely, it has force impacting the course of future development. Accordingly, the liability phenotype at each particular stage of development influences risk as well as momentum (rate) for developing SUD.

The overall liability phenotype is uniquely configured within each individual because of the large number of constituent characteristics and their wide range of severity. Thus, individuals evincing the same magnitude of SUD risk—namely, the same score on the measure of the liability phenotype—are qualitatively different. Accordingly, prevention and treatment must have an idiographic focus to account for the uniqueness of each individual. Thorough evaluation of the characteristics that make up the liability phenotype affords the opportunity to tailor intervention to an individual's strengths and liabilities. As shown in

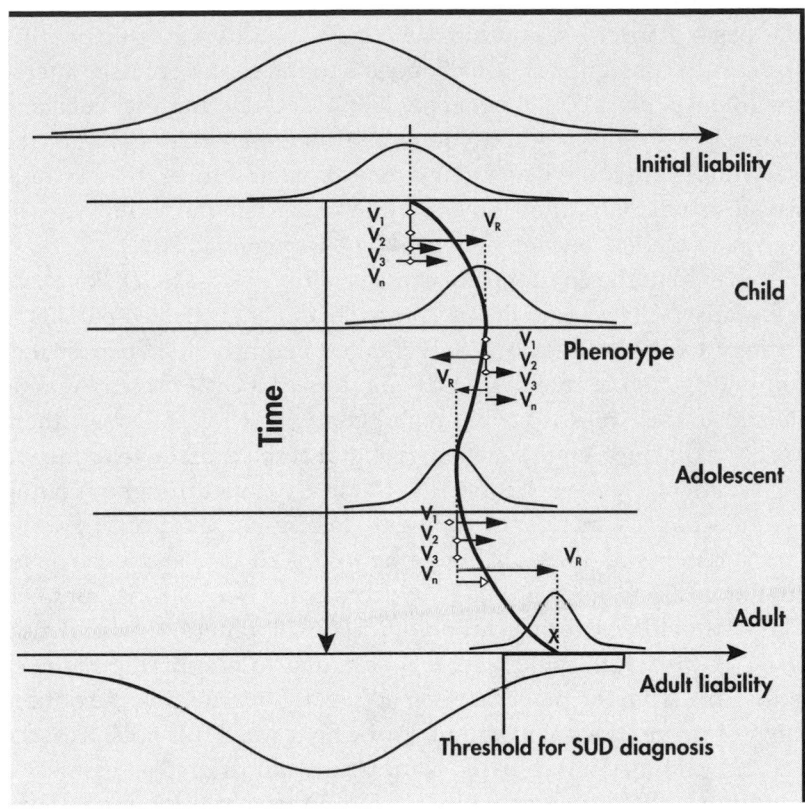

FIGURE 1–1. Developmental pathway to substance use disorder.

See text for discussion. SUD=substance use disorder.

Source. Adapted from Vanyukov et al. 2003a, 2003b.

Figure 1–1, the overarching objective of treatment is to deflect the individual from the affected to the nonaffected segment of the population, whereas prevention is aimed at shifting the person closer to the low end (left tail) of the liability scale.

Connecting the V_R scores (SUD liability phenotype) graphs the individual's trajectory toward or away from SUD outcome. As illustrated in Figure 1–1, the trajectory is not likely to be linear, consequent to biological and psychological changes occurring in the context of continuously changing multiple environments. For example, precocious sexual maturation is overtly manifested as a growth spurt along with the appearance of secondary sex characteristics (e.g., facial hair in boys, breast development in girls). Early-onset sexual maturation thus produces a physical mismatch with same-age peers and is a social stimulus for older peers. Forming friendships with older youths may enhance SUD risk because consumption usually begins in the context of peer interactions (Bahr et al. 2005; Ennett et al. 2006). Considering that substance consumption beginning at a young age increases SUD risk and that older youths are more likely to use abusable substances, the timing of onset of sexual maturation is therefore an important individual variable that can accelerate development of SUD (Horner et al. 2013).

A change in the environment can also alter risk for SUD. For example, because SUD commonly leads to social decline, affected parents relocating to an economically disadvantaged neighborhood expose their children to a higher rate of illegal behaviors and easier access to abusable substances. Youths having high genetic risk for SUD may, therefore, also have high environmental risk that accelerates development of SUD. In effect, changes occurring in the individual throughout ontogeny and changes in the environment determine severity of liability characteristics and overall liability phenotype so as to shape the developmental trajectory toward or away from SUD. Because magnitude of SUD risk fluctuates during chronological development, temporal monitoring of the liability phenotype is essential to identifying high-risk youths and, from the practical perspective, to determining the optimal timing of prevention intervention. Working toward this goal, Kirisci et al. (2012) validated a Web-based computer-administered assessment of the transmissible (intergenerational) component of SUD liability having age-specific content and norms for individuals at ages 10–12, 12–14, 16, 19, and 22 years.

Connecting SUD Liability to Clinical Outcome

Almost two decades elapse before the conclusion of adolescence. Many factors during this protracted period can amplify or attenuate heritable risk for SUD. Thus, intervention informed by etiology requires understanding the components of SUD liability during ontogeny.

At the outset, it is important to note that although numerous studies have shown that heritability accounts for a significant portion of variance associated with SUD risk, it is not possible to determine genetic susceptibility at the individual level. It is feasible, however, to evaluate transmissible risk—namely, the biobehavioral characteristics that have intergenerational continuity between parents and their biological children. Significantly, for example, over 40% of variance associated with the risk for cannabis use disorder has been reported to be transmissible—that is, conveyed to children via conjointly genetic and parenting influences (Hopfer et al. 2003).

A series of investigations conducted at the Center for Education and Drug Abuse Research also demonstrates that a set of psychological characteristics (encompassing both internalizing and externalizing features) have intergenerational continuity and compose a unidimensional trait. This trait has been termed the *transmissible liability index* (TLI) (Vanyukov et al. 2009). Between 75% (Vanyukov et al. 2009) and 85% (Hicks et al. 2012) of TLI variance is heritable. Moreover, genetic factors account entirely for the association between childhood TLI score and diagnosis of SUD in adulthood (Vanyukov et al. 2015). In effect, the TLI captures the intergenerational (and in large part genetic) aspect of SUD risk overtly evinced as deficient psychological self-regulation.

A main challenge in etiology research involves identifying the factors during specific periods of ontogeny that bias the genetic risk for SUD to SUD outcome. The following section reviews factors to consider at each stage of development.

Prenatal Stage

Passive drug exposure during gestation has long-term deleterious effects on fetal development (Behnke et al. 2013). Prenatal nicotine exposure, for example, increases the likelihood of nicotine (Cornelius et al. 2007) and polydrug (Goldschmidt et al. 2012) abuse. The New England Family Study tracked mother-infant dyads for 40 years and demonstrated that nicotine dependence in female offspring is predicted by the mother's smoking and stress hormone levels (Stroud et al. 2014). Maternal stress also predicts externalizing behavior in children (Choe et al. 2013; Huizink et al. 2003), which is well known to heighten risk for substance abuse and SUD. Stress can emanate from many sources in substance-abusing women (e.g., low social support, violent or absent partner, economic adversity) and portends neurobehavioral disinhibition in their adolescent children (Fisher et al. 2011), which is well known to presage SUD (for a review, see Tarter et al. 2012a).

Infancy

Stress during infancy alters frontal cortex functioning (Hanson et al. 2010), which, as noted in the introduction of this chapter, is integral to psychological self-regulation. Dysregulated infants augment parental stress, thereby hampering caregiving that in extreme circumstances may result in frustration-induced maltreatment. Experiencing abuse or neglect early in life disrupts brain development (Whittle et al. 2013) and increases the risk for SUD (Dunn et al. 2002). Supporting caregivers with home visitation by nurses has been shown to reduce the child's risk for a range of adverse outcomes (Olds 2002; Olds et al. 1998).

A dysfunctional caregiver-infant relationship impedes the infant's prospects for secure attachment to the mother, which, in turn, amplifies risk for conduct problems in middle childhood, substance use in adolescence, and progression to SUD (Bahr et al. 2005; Kostelecky 2005; Oxford et al. 2001). It has been suggested that interventions to potentiate infant-mother attachment ought to begin during pregnancy (Figueiredo and Costa 2009; Mikhail et al. 1995), which may be of even greater importance for women using drugs. Considering that the pregnancy is often unplanned in addicted women (Heil et al. 2011) and that some substance-abusing women are less prepared to raise a child (Velez and Jansson 2008), a strong case can be made for attachment-focused SUD prevention beginning during gestation. Inculcating secure infant-mother attachment has been shown to be beneficial to children who are at high risk for developing various problems (Cooper et al. 2005; Dozier et al. 2008), including children who have been maltreated (Stronach et al. 2013) or who have drug-dependent mothers (Cassidy et al. 2010). Relatedly, it is noteworthy that breast-feeding promotes mother-infant bonding as well as neuromaturation and physical growth in the infant (Isaacs et al. 2010; Jansen et al. 2008). A lactation nurse, therefore, may be a valuable interventionist to lower SUD risk by promoting breast-feeding, thereby inculcating a strong mother-infant bond.

Toddlerhood

Psychological dysregulation is evinced as a difficult temperament during toddlerhood (Martel and Nigg 2006). The main features include intense emotion reactivity, elevated behavior activity level, irregular rhythms (sleep, eating), and low social conviviality. Difficult temperament in 2-year-old children predicts the psychological characteristics that constitute transmissible risk at ages 10–12 for SUD, which, in turn, predicts SUD a decade later (Horner et al., in press). In addition, it has been shown that low inhibitory control in 3-year-old boys predicts SUD up to two decades later (Caspi et al. 1996). The dearth of research focusing on this developmental period notwithstanding, the available evidence suggests that SUD liability at this stage manifests as a combination of emotional and behavioral dysregulation.

Middle Childhood

Difficult temperament in 7-year-old children portends a wide spectrum of psychiatric disorders during adolescence, including anxiety, depression, and antisociality, which frequently precede or co-occur with SUD. In addition, attention-deficit/hyperactivity disorder (ADHD), conduct disorder, anxiety disorders, and depressive disorders often co-occur with and presage SUD (Bukstein and Horner 2010; Maziade et al. 1990). Moreover, deviations in psychological traits reflecting internalizing and externalizing propensities are more common or severe among high-risk youths as well as children who subsequently qualify for SUD (Tarter et al. 2012a). Thus, rather than a particular disorder or psychological dimension predisposing to SUD, the vulnerability appears to comprise, instead, an overall presentation consisting of both emotion and behavioral dysregulation.

Adolescence

Hormonal, psychological, neurological, and social factors during adolescence interact in myriad ways to promote substance use onset, which, in a subset of youths, leads to SUD before adulthood. As social role performance progresses toward adopting adult behaviors, consumption of abusable drugs may likewise be perceived as normative. Stress during the transition to adolescence may also lead to consumption, prompted by popular belief that abusable substances (e.g., alcohol, marijuana) have anxiolytic properties. An upsurge in gonadal hormones during adolescence potentiates behaviors that predispose to substance abuse (Forbes and Dahl 2010). Relatedly, onset of puberty produces significant body changes that may activate or exacerbate low self-esteem, including social challenges and negative appraisal of physical attractiveness (e.g., acne, menstrual pain, dental disconfiguration) that may impact mood and promote substance use. Puberty also facilitates the emulation of behaviors that are normative for adults, including alcohol use (Bahr et al. 2005). Substance use among psychologically dysregulated youths is additionally catalyzed by friendships with similarly dysregulated youths, thereby increasing access to abusable substances. Although much emphasis has been directed at use of illegal drugs, which include alcohol and tobacco use by youths, adolescents who consume legal hypercaffeinated ("energy") beverages are at elevated risk of transitioning to illegal drugs (Arria et al. 2010). In addition, adolescence is marked by heightened sensitivity to positive rewards and attenuated sensitivity to punishment (Spear 2010). Thus, drug reward may catalyze habitual consumption, which, in turn, leads to chronic tolerance and other neu-roadaptational changes that exacerbate the risk for social maladjust-ment and emotional disorder (Koob 2009; Koob and Kreek 2007). Considering that the threshold for diagnosis of SUD is low, requiring any 2 from a panel of 11 symptoms in DSM-5, it is quite easy to qualify for a use disorder.

Understanding the Origins and Patterns of Psychiatric Disorders Occurring With SUD

Elucidating the etiological pathway from predisposing liability to SUD outcome requires taking into account circumstances surrounding the onset of drug exposure. Substance dependence can emanate, for exam-ple, from a lifestyle marked by nonadherence to social mores and laws. Because all abusable substances, except caffeine, are illegal for youths, consumption is de facto norm violating. Not surprisingly, therefore, de-viance proneness is frequently reported in substance users and shown to amplify risk for SUD.

Another pathway to drug dependence begins with using prescribed medications such as amphetamines or opiates under medical supervi-sion. In contrast to the deviance proneness pathway to SUD, this trajec-tory is marked by compliance with societal norms. Currently, SUD risk associated with using prescribed medications that have abuse potential remains poorly understood. For example, youths with ADHD are com-monly treated with stimulant medication, which can be addictive. Stim-ulant treatment started during childhood appears to be protective against developing SUD in adulthood (Biederman et al. 2008; Wilens et al. 2003), whereas initiation of stimulant treatment during adolescence may increase SUD risk (Dalsgaard et al. 2014; Mannuzza et al. 2008). Al-though controversial (Volkow and Swanson 2008), these findings un-derscore the importance of brain maturational stage in relation to enhanced sensitivity to drug reward during adolescence (Spear 2010).

As discussed in the introduction of this chapter, the SUDs in DSM-5 are strongly correlated and scalable as a continuous trait. Consequently, a huge assortment of co-occurring SUDs is possible. Arbitrary distinc-tions (e.g., legal vs. illegal) and distinct pharmacological and metabolic properties of different substances notwithstanding, genetic and pheno-typic risk is largely shared across SUDs (Kendler et al. 2003; Tsuang et al. 1998). Furthermore, because internalizing and externalizing trait scores are strongly correlated (Tarter et al. 2008), high scores on both dimensions manifest as childhood co-occurring psychiatric disorders related to ADHD, conduct disorder, anxiety disorder, and depression. Notably, within the prefrontal region, the inferior frontal cortex subserves emotion and behavior regulation (Tabibnia et al. 2011, 2014). In effect, poor emotion modulation (internalizing dimension) and behavioral undercontrol (externalizing dimension) have underpinnings in a common neurological substrate (for reviews, see Li and Sinha 2008 and Muraven and Baumeister 2000). Considering that inferior frontal cortex connects directly to brain structures integral to behavior control (e.g., globus pallidus, motor cortex, thalamus) (Aron 2011) and emotion modulation (e.g., amygdala) (Ochsner and Gross 2005), it is plausible to speculate that disruptions of specific circuitry underlie the propensity to develop a particular configuration of SUD and co-occurring psychiatric disorder. Significantly, drug craving is also associated with lower gray matter in inferior frontal cortex (Tabibnia et al. 2011). Last, research having a developmental focus provides insights into the etiology of psychiatric disorders co-occurring with SUD. In particular, difficult temperament, conjointly featured by behavior undercontrol and poor emotion modulation in middle childhood, portends internalizing and/or externalizing psychiatric disorders in adolescence (Hill et al. 2000; Maziade et al. 1990). Difficult temperament, as discussed in the subsections "Toddlerhood" and "Middle Childhood," predisposes youths to SUD. Thus, although many studies have been conducted with the aim of organizing the vast array of co-occurring SUD and psychiatric disorder patterns into mutually exclusive categories or "types," replicable and clinically useful results have not been forthcoming from this line of research. This is expected in view of the findings obtained in genetic, neurological, and psychological research. Whether the defining criterion is temporal order of diagnosis (e.g., SUD as first disorder followed by another psychiatric disorder), genetic contribution to etiology, or statistically derived clusters, the derived groups or types are not mutually exclusive but rather overlap, illustrating that the huge variety of co-occurring psychiatric disorders and SUD are actually variants of one disorder.

Understanding the myriad permutations of psychiatric disorders co-occurring with SUD in adolescents needs to be anchored to predisposing liability. As discussed in the section "Connecting SUD Liability to Clinical Outcome," the liability phenotype is evinced as psychological dysregulation, consisting of both behavior under impaired or compromised control and poor modulation of emotions. Hence, severe expression on these aspects of liability, manifested as externalizing and internalizing disturbance, may amplify in severity to qualify for the homologous psychiatric disorder. Thus, severe externalizing behavior may manifest as ADHD and/or conduct disorder, whereas severe internalizing propensity manifests as anxiety and/or depression prior to first drug use. Because internalizing and externalizing traits are not orthogonal but rather are strongly correlated, a high score on both dimensions is common, which manifests as psychiatric disorder encompassing both dimensions (e.g., ADHD and anxiety). Notably, a child can shift from subdiagnostic to affected status contingent on quality of interactions with the environment. For example, a child with externalizing behavior may qualify subsequently for conduct disorder when the child's parenting is ineffective or the friendship cluster promotes socially nonnormative behavior. However, the high-risk youngster can revert to the nonaffected range following treatment (e.g., stimulant medication for ADHD) or changes in the environment (forming new friendships, joining a prosocial organization).

Habitual substance use alters the individual's internal physiological and social milieu. Inasmuch as abusable substances are both reinforcers and stressors, repetitive consumption exacts "wear and tear" on the individual, termed *allostatic load* (McEwen and Stellar 1993). High allostatic load, defined as "the price the body pays for being forced to adapt to adverse psychosocial and physical conditions" (McEwen 2000, p. 110), potentiates substance-induced psychological dysregulation, which, upon surpassing diagnostic threshold, manifests as psychiatric disorder co-occurring with SUD. In turn, the comorbid disorder causes or amplifies social maladjustment, leading to further substance abuse. As discussed by Koob (2009), habitual substance use fosters psychiatric disturbance, which leads to further substance use and ultimately to brain changes that shift motivation for consumption toward averting (e.g., withdrawal syndrome) or attenuating (e.g., depression) an aversive subjective state.

Psychiatric disorder thus presages as well as emerges consequent to substance abuse. Moreover, acute psychiatric disorders may be intertwined with personality disorder, thereby further complicating the configuration of psychopathology co-occurring with SUD. Antisocial personality disorder (most frequently in males) (Fu et al. 2002; Regier et al. 1990) and borderline personality disorder (most frequently in females) (Trull et al. 2000; van den Bosch et al. 2001) often co-occur with SUD. Thus, personality disorder, an outgrowth of difficult temperament in early childhood, is characterized by deficient psychological self-regulation manifesting from prefrontal cortex dysfunction.

Summary and Future Directions

In this chapter, we briefly examined the etiology of SUD in relation to co-occurring psychiatric disorders. The main conclusion is that disorders co-occurring with SUD are characterized by psychological dysregulation evinced in early childhood that is rooted in prefrontal cortex dysfunction. Thus, the various co-occurring disorders do not characterize distinct groups of youths; rather, the manifold permutations are variants of one disorder.

Future etiology research should be directed toward elucidating how suboptimal acquisition of psychological self-dysregulation from infancy onward biases development toward low adherence to mores and laws, including substance use segueing to SUD. From the prevention perspective, it remains to be determined whether interventions that improve neuropsychological processes subserved by frontal-limbic circuitry avert or delay substance use onset, thereby lowering SUD risk. For example, physical exercise in children with ADHD (which commonly presages SUD and shares significant genetic variance with SUD) improves neurocognitive capacities and emotion regulation (Pontifex et al. 2013). Whether prevention targeted at inculcating values and habits associated with a healthy lifestyle (e.g., healthy diet, orodental health, regular sleep-wake cycle) potentiates psychological self-regulation, which, in turn, lowers SUD risk, remains to be investigated.

KEY POINTS

- Substance use disorder and co-occurring psychiatric disorder emanate from suboptimal acquisition of psychological regulation during childhood and adolescence.

- Psychological dysregulation consisting of low executive cognitive capacities, poor modulation of emotions, and behavior undercontrol are the main features of transmissible (intergenerational) risk for substance use disorder (SUD).

- Psychological dysregulation manifests from dysfunction of neural circuitry in frontal cortex, striatum, and limbic system.

- Psychological dysregulation, via interaction with multiple facets of the social and physical environment during childhood, biases the youngster toward onset of substance use at a young age as one aspect of social deviancy and nonnormative socialization.

- The diagnostic presentation consisting of SUD and co-occurring psychiatric disorder, including personality disorder, reflects the relative salience of behavioral and emotional components of psychological dysregulation.

References

American Psychiatric Association: Diagnostic and Statistical Manual of Mental Disorders, 5th Edition. Arlington, VA, American Psychiatric Association, 2013

Aron AR: From reactive to proactive and selective control: developing a richer model for stopping inappropriate responses. Biol Psychol 69(12):e55–e68, 2011 20932513

Arria AM, Caldeira KM, Kasperski SJ, et al: Increased alcohol consumption, nonmedical prescription drug use, and illicit drug use are associated with energy drink consumption among college students. J Addict Med 4(2):74–80, 2010 20729975

Bahr SJ, Hoffmann JP, Yang X: Parental and peer influences on the risk of adolescent drug use. J Prim Prev 26(6):529–551, 2005 16228115

Bauer LO, Hesselbrock VM: EEG, autonomic and subjective correlates of the risk for alcoholism. J Stud Alcohol 54(5):577–589, 1993 8412148

Bauer LO, Hesselbrock VM: CSD/BEM localization of P300 sources in adolescents "at-risk": evidence of frontal cortex dysfunction in conduct disorder. Biol Psychiatry 50(8):600–608, 2001 11690595

Behnke M, Smith VC, Committee on Substance Abuse, et al: Prenatal substance abuse: short- and long-term effects on the exposed fetus. Pediatrics 131(3):e1009–e1024, 2013 23439891

Benegal V, Antony G, Venkatasubramanian G, et al: Gray matter volume abnormalities and externalizing symptoms in subjects at high risk for alcohol dependence. Addict Biol 12(1):122–132, 2007 17407506

Benes FM, Turtle M, Khan Y, et al: Myelination of a key relay zone in the hippocampal formation occurs in the human brain during childhood, adolescence, and adulthood. Arch Gen Psychiatry 51(6):477–484, 1994 8192550

Biederman J, Monuteaux MC, Spencer T, et al: Stimulant therapy and risk for subsequent substance use disorders in male adults with ADHD: a naturalistic controlled 10-year follow-up study. Am J Psychiatry 165(5):597–603, 2008 18316421

Bukstein OG, Horner MS: Management of the adolescent with substance use disorders and comorbid psychopathology. Child Adolesc Psychiatr Clin N Am 19(3):609–623, 2010 20682224

Buss KA, Schumacher JR, Dolski I, et al: Right frontal brain activity, cortisol, and withdrawal behavior in 6-month-old infants. Behav Neurosci 117(1):11–20, 2003 12619903

Caspi A, Moffitt TE, Newman DL, et al: Behavioral observations at age 3 years predict adult psychiatric disorders: longitudinal evidence from a birth cohort. Arch Gen Psychiatry 53(11):1033–1039, 1996 8911226

Cassidy J, Ziv Y, Stupica B, et al: Enhancing attachment security in the infants of women in a jail-diversion program. Attach Hum Dev 12(4):333–353, 2010 20582844

Choe DE, Olson SL, Sameroff AJ: Effects of early maternal distress and parenting on the development of children's self-regulation and externalizing behavior. Dev Psychopathol 25(2):437–453, 2013 23627955

Collins FS, Wilder EL, Zerhouni E: Funding transdisciplinary research. NIH Roadmap/Common Fund at 10 years. Science 345(6194):274–276, 2014 25035478

Cooper G, Hoffman KT, Powell B, et al: The circle of security intervention: differential diagnosis and differential treatment, in Enhancing Early Attachments: Theory, Research, Intervention, and Policy. Edited by Berlin LJ, Ziv Y, Amaya-Jackson LM, et al. New York, Guilford, 2005, pp 127–151

Cornelius MD, Goldschmidt L, DeGenna N, et al: Smoking during teenage pregnancies: effects on behavioral problems in offspring. Nicotine Tob Res 9(7):739–750, 2007 17577803

Dalsgaard S, Mortensen PB, Frydenberg M, et al: ADHD, stimulant treatment in childhood and subsequent substance abuse in adulthood—a naturalistic long-term follow-up study. Addict Behav 39(1):325–328, 2014 24090624

Dozier M, Stovall-McClough KC, Albus KE: Attachment and psychopathology in adulthood, in Handbook of Attachment: Theory, Research and Clinical Application, 2nd Edition. Edited by Cassidy J, Shaver PR. New York, Guilford, 2008, pp 718–744

Dunn MG, Tarter RE, Mezzich AC, et al: Origins and consequences of child neglect in substance abuse families. Clin Psychol Rev 22(7):1063–1090, 2002 12238246

Eldreth DA, Matochik JA, Cadet J-L, et al: Abnormal brain activity in prefrontal brain regions in abstinent marijuana users. Neuroimage 23(3):914–920, 2004 15528091

Ennett ST, Bauman KE, Hussong A, et al: The peer context of adolescent substance use: findings from social network analysis. J Res Adolesc 16(2):159–186, 2006

Figueiredo B, Costa R: Mother's stress, mood and emotional involvement with the infant: 3 months before and 3 months after childbirth. Arch Womens Ment Health 12(3):143–153, 2009 19259772

Finn PR, Justus A: Reduced EEG alpha power in the male and female offspring of alcoholics. Alcohol Clin Exp Res 23(2):256–262, 1999 10069554

Fisher PA, Lester BM, DeGarmo DS, et al: The combined effects of prenatal drug exposure and early adversity on neurobehavioral disinhibition in childhood and adolescence. Dev Psychopathol 23(3):777–788, 2011 21756431

Forbes EE, Dahl RE: Pubertal development and behavior: hormonal activation of social and motivational tendencies. Brain Cogn 72(1):66–72, 2010 19942334

Friedman NP, Miyake A, Young SE, et al: Individual differences in executive functions are almost entirely genetic in origin. J Exp Psychol Gen 137(2):201–225, 2008 18473654

Fu Q, Heath AC, Bucholz KK, et al: Shared genetic risk of major depression, alcohol dependence, and marijuana dependence: contribution of antisocial personality disorder in men. Arch Gen Psychiatry 59(12):1125–1132, 2002 12470129

Giedd JN, Blumenthal J, Jeffries NO, et al: Brain development during childhood and adolescence: a longitudinal MRI study. Nat Neurosci 2(10):861–863, 1999 10491603

Giedd JN, Clasen LS, Lenroot R, et al: Puberty-related influences on brain development. Mol Cell Endocrinol 254–255:154–162, 2006 16765510

Goldschmidt L, Cornelius MD, Day NL: Prenatal cigarette smoke exposure and early initiation of multiple substance use. Nicotine Tob Res 14(6):694–702, 2012 22180590

Habeych ME, Sclabassi RJ, Charles PJ, et al: Association among parental substance use disorder, p300 amplitude, and neurobehavioral disinhibition in preteen boys at high risk for substance use disorder. Psychol Addict Behav 19(2):123–130, 2005 16011382

Hanson JL, Chung MK, Avants BB, et al: Early stress is associated with alterations in the orbitofrontal cortex: a tensor-based morphometry investigation of brain structure and behavioral risk. J Neurosci 30(22):7466–7472, 2010 20519521

Heil SH, Jones HE, Arria A, et al: Unintended pregnancy in opioid-abusing women. J Subst Abuse Treat 40(2):199–202, 2011 21036512

Hicks BM, Iacono WG, McGue M: Index of the transmissible common liability to addiction: heritability and prospective associations with substance abuse and related outcomes. Drug Alcohol Depend 123 (suppl 1):S18–S23, 2012 22245078

Hill SY, Shen S, Lowers L, et al: Factors predicting the onset of adolescent drinking in families at high risk for developing alcoholism. Biol Psychiatry 48(4):265–275, 2000 10960157

Hopfer CJ, Crowley TJ, Hewitt JK: Review of twin and adoption studies of adolescent substance use. J Am Acad Child Adolesc Psychiatry 42(6):710–719, 2003 12921479

Horner MS, Tarter R, Kirisci L, et al: Modeling the association between sexual maturation, transmissible risk, and peer relationships during childhood and adolescence on development of substance use disorder in young adulthood. Am J Addict 22(5):474–480, 2013 23952893

Horner M, Reynolds M, Braxter B, et al: Temperament disturbances in infancy progress to substance use disorder 20 years later. Pers Individ Diff (in press)

Huizink AC, Robles de Medina PG, Mulder EJ, et al: Stress during pregnancy is associated with developmental outcome in infancy. J Child Psychol Psychiatry 44(6):810–818, 2003 12959490

Iacono WG, Malone SM, McGue M: Behavioral disinhibition and the development of early onset addiction: common and specific influences. Annu Rev Clin Psychol 4:325–348, 2008 18370620

Isaacs EB, Fischl BR, Quinn BT, et al: Impact of breast milk on intelligence quotient, brain size, and white matter development. Pediatr Res 67(4):357–362, 2010 20035247

Ivanov I, Schulz KP, London ED, et al: Inhibitory control deficits in childhood and risk for substance use disorders: a review. Am J Drug Alcohol Abuse 34(3):239–258, 2008 18428067

Jansen JC, Weerth D, Riksen-Walraven JM: Breastfeeding and the mother–infant relationship—a review. Dev Rev 28(4):503–521, 2008

Johnston L, O'Malley P, Bachman J, et al: Monitoring the Future: National Results on Adolescent Drug Use: Overview of Key Findings, 2011. Ann Arbor, MI, Institute for Social Research, 2012

Kendler KS, Jacobson KC, Prescott CA, et al: Specificity of genetic and environmental risk factors for use and abuse/dependence of cannabis, cocaine, hallucinogens, sedatives, stimulants, and opiates in male twins. Am J Psychiatry 160(4):687–695, 2003 12668357

Kirisci L, Tarter RE, Vanyukov M, et al: Application of item response theory to quantify substance use disorder severity. Addict Behav 31(6):1035–1049, 2006 16647219

Kirisci L, Tarter R, Reynolds M, et al: Computer adaptive testing of liability to addiction: identifying individuals at risk. Drug Alcohol Depend 123 (suppl 1):S79–S86, 2012 22391133

Koob GF: Dynamics of neuronal circuits in addiction: reward, antireward, and emotional memory. Pharmacopsychiatry 42(suppl 1):S32–S41, 2009 19434554

Koob G, Kreek MJ: Stress, dysregulation of drug reward pathways, and the transition to drug dependence. Am J Psychiatry 164(8):1149–1159, 2007 17671276

Kostelecky KL: Parental attachment, academic achievement, life events and their relationship to alcohol and drug use during adolescence. J Adolesc 28(5):665–669, 2005 16203200

Krueger RF, Hicks BM, Patrick CJ, et al: Etiologic connections among substance dependence, antisocial behavior, and personality: modeling the externalizing spectrum. J Abnorm Psychol 111(3):411–424, 2002 12150417

Lenroot RK, Giedd JN: Brain development in children and adolescents: insights from anatomical magnetic resonance imaging. Neurosci Biobehav Rev 30(6):718–729, 2006 16887188

Li CS, Sinha R: Inhibitory control and emotional stress regulation: neuroimaging evidence for frontal-limbic dysfunction in psycho-stimulant addiction. Neurosci Biobehav Rev 32(3):581–597, 2008 18164058

Mannuzza S, Klein RG, Truong NL, et al: Age of methylphenidate treatment initiation in children with ADHD and later substance abuse: prospective follow-up into adulthood. Am J Psychiatry 165(5):604–609, 2008 18381904

Marsh R, Gerber AJ, Peterson BS: Neuroimaging studies of normal brain development and their relevance for understanding childhood neuropsychiatric disorders. J Am Acad Child Adolesc Psychiatry 47(11):1233–1251, 2008 18833009

Martel MM, Nigg JT: Child ADHD and personality/temperament traits of reactive and effortful control, resiliency, and emotionality. J Child Psychol Psychiatry 47(11):1175–1183, 2006 17076757

Maziade M, Caron C, Côté R, et al: Psychiatric status of adolescents who had extreme temperaments at age 7. Am J Psychiatry 147(11):1531–1536, 1990 2221169

McEwen BS: Allostasis and allostatic load: implications for neuropsychopharmacology. Neuropsychopharmacology 22(2):108–124, 2000 10649824

McEwen BS, Stellar E: Stress and the individual: mechanisms leading to disease. Arch Intern Med 153(18):2093–2101, 1993 8379800

McNamee RI, Dunfee K, Luna B, et al: Brain activation, response inhibition, and increased risk for substance use disorder. Alcohol Clin Exp Res 32(3):405–413, 2008 18302723

Mezzich AC, Tarter RE, Feske U, et al: Assessment of risk for substance use disorder consequent to consumption of illegal drugs: psychometric validation of the neurobehavior disinhibition trait. Psychol Addict Behav 21(4):508–515, 2007 18072833

Mikhail MS, Youchah J, DeVore N, et al: Decreased maternal-fetal attachment in methadone-maintained pregnant women: a preliminary study. J Assoc Acad Minor Phys 6(3):112–114, 1995 7663100

Muraven M, Baumeister RF: Self-regulation and depletion of limited resources: does self-control resemble a muscle? Psychol Bull 126(2):247–259, 2000 10748642

Ochsner KN, Gross JJ: The cognitive control of emotion. Trends Cogn Sci 9(5):242–249, 2005 15866151

Olds DL: Prenatal and infancy home visiting by nurses: from randomized trials to community replication. Prev Sci 3(3):153–172, 2002 12387552

Olds D, Henderson CR Jr, Cole R, et al: Long-term effects of nurse home visitation on children's criminal and antisocial behavior: 15-year follow-up of a randomized controlled trial. JAMA 280(14):1238–1244, 1998 9786373

Oxford ML, Harachi TW, Catalano RF, et al: Preadolescent predictors of substance initiation: a test of both the direct and mediated effect of family social control factors on deviant peer associations and substance initiation. Am J Drug Alcohol Abuse 27(4):599–616, 2001 11727879

Peper JS, Brouwer RM, Boomsma DI, et al: Genetic influences on human brain structure: a review of brain imaging studies in twins. Hum Brain Mapp 28(6):464–473, 2007 17415783

Pontifex MB, Saliba BJ, Raine LB, et al: Exercise improves behavioral, neurocognitive, and scholastic performance in children with attention-deficit/hyperactivity disorder. J Pediatr 162(3):543–551, 2013 23084704

Regier DA, Farmer ME, Rae LB, et al: Comorbidity of mental disorders with alcohol and other drug abuse: results from the Epidemiologic Catchment Area (ECA) study. JAMA 264(19):2511–2518, 1990 2232018

Schweinsburg AD, Paulus MP, Barlett VC, et al: An FMRI study of response inhibition in youths with a family history of alcoholism. Ann N Y Acad Sci 1021:391–394, 2004 15251915

Sisk CL, Zehr JL: Pubertal hormones organize the adolescent brain and behavior. Front Neuroendocrinol 26(3–4):163–174, 2005 16309736

Sowell ER, Peterson BS, Thompson PM, et al: Mapping cortical change across the human life span. Nat Neurosci 6(3):309–315, 2003 12548289

Sowell ER, Thompson PM, Toga AW: Mapping changes in the human cortex throughout the span of life. Neuroscientist 10(4):372–392, 2004 15271264

Spear L: The Behavioral Neuroscience of Adolescence. New York, WW Norton, 2010

Stronach EP, Toth SL, Rogosch F, et al: Preventive interventions and sustained attachment security in maltreated children. Dev Psychopathol 25(4 Pt 1):919–930, 2013 24229539

Stroud LR, Papandonatos GD, Shenassa E, et al: Prenatal glucocorticoids and maternal smoking during pregnancy independently program adult nicotine dependence in daughters: a 40-year prospective study. Biol Psychiatry 75(1):47–55, 2014 24034414

Tabibnia G, Monteross JR, Baicy K, et al: Different forms of self-control share a neurocognitive substrate. J Neurosci 31(13):4805–4810, 2011 21451018

Tabibnia G, Creswell JD, Kraynak T, et al: Common prefrontal regions activate during self-control of craving, emotion, and motor impulses in smokers. Clin Psychol Sci 2(5):611–619, 2014 25485181

Tarter R, Kirisci L, Habeych M, et al: Neurobehavior disinhibition in childhood predisposes boys to substance use disorder by young adulthood: direct and mediated etiologic pathways. Drug Alcohol Depend 73(2):121–132, 2004 14725951

Tarter R, Kirisici L, Ridenour T, et al: Prediction of cannabis use disorder between childhood and young adulthood using the Child Behavior Checklist. J Psychopathol Behav Assess 30(4):272–278, 2008

Tarter R, Horner M, Ridenour T: Developmental perspective of substance use disorder etiology, in APA Addiction Syndrome Handbook. Edited by Shaffer HJ. Washington, DC, American Psychological Association, 2012a, pp 261–287

Tarter R, Kirisci L, Ridenour T, et al: Application of person-centered medicine in addiction. Int J Pers Cent Med 2(2):240–249, 2012b 23243492

Thompson PM, Cannon TD, Narr KL, et al: Genetic influences on brain structure. Nat Neurosci 4(12):1253–1258, 2001 11694885

Toga AW, Thompson PM, Sowell ER: Mapping brain maturation. Trends Neurosci 29(3):148–159, 2006 16472876

Trull TJ, Sher KJ, Minks-Brown C, et al: Borderline personality disorder and substance use disorders: a review and integration. Clin Psychol Rev 20(2):235–253, 2000 10721499

Tsuang MT, Lyons MJ, Meyer JM, et al: Co-occurrence of abuse of different drugs in men: the role of drug-specific and shared vulnerabilities. Arch Gen Psychiatry 55(11):967–972, 1998 9819064

van den Bosch LMC, Verheul R, van den Brink W, et al: Substance abuse in borderline personality disorder: clinical and etiological correlates. J Person Disord 15(5):416–424, 2001 11723876

Vanyukov MM, Tarter RE, Kirisci L, et al: Liability to substance use disorders, 1: common mechanisms and manifestations. Neurosci Biobehav Rev 27(6):507–515, 2003a 14599432

Vanyukov MM, Kirisci L, Tarter RE, et al: Liability to substance use disorders, 2: a measurement approach. Neurosci Biobehav Rev 27(6):517–526, 2003b 14599433

Vanyukov MM, Kirisci L, Moss L, et al: Measurement of the risk for substance use disorders: phenotypic and genetic analysis of an index of common liability. Behav Genet 39(3):233–244, 2009 19377872

Vanyukov M, Kim K, Irons D, et al: Genetic relationship between the addiction diagnosis in adults and their childhood measure of addiction liability. Behav Genet 45(1):1–11, 2015 25502189

Velez M, Jansson LM: The opioid dependent mother and newborn dyad: non-pharmacologic care. J Addict Med 2(3):113–120, 2008 19727440

Volkow ND, Swanson JM: Does childhood treatment of ADHD with stimulant medication affect substance abuse in adulthood? Am J Psychiatry 165(5):553–555, 2008 18450933

Wagner FA, Anthony JC: Male-female differences in the risk of progression from first use to dependence upon cannabis, cocaine, and alcohol. Drug Alcohol Depend 86(2–3):191–198, 2007 17029825

Weiland BJ, Korycinski ST, Soules M, et al: Substance abuse risk in emerging adults associated with smaller frontal gray matter volumes and higher externalizing behaviors. Drug Alcohol Depend 137:68–75, 2014 24513182

Whittle S, Dennison M, Vijayakumar N, et al: Childhood maltreatment and psychopathology affect brain development during adolescence. J Am Acad Child Adolesc Psychiatry 52(9):940–952e1, 2013 23972696

Wilens TE, Faraone SV, Biederman J, et al: Does stimulant therapy of attention-deficit/hyperactivity disorder beget later substance abuse? A meta-analytic review of the literature. Pediatrics 111(1):179–185, 2003 12509574

Woolf SH: The meaning of translational research and why it matters. JAMA 299(2):211–213, 2008 18182604

Zerhouni E: Medicine. The NIH Roadmap. Science 302(5642):63–72, 2003 14526066

CHAPTER 2

Relationship Between Substance Use Disorders and Psychiatric Comorbidity

Implications for Integrated Health Services

Marc Fishman, M.D.

Adolescent substance use disorders (SUDs) commonly co-occur with other psychiatric disorders (Kuepper et al. 2011). These comorbid disorders present considerable public health and clinical challenges associated with increased severity, and poorer response to treatment, especially when treatment focuses exclusively on one disorder but not the other.

The nature of the association between co-occurring disorders (CODs) and SUDs has been explained by a variety of hypotheses. Other psychiatric symptoms or disorders may develop as a consequence of or alter the course of SUDs. Likewise, SUDs may develop as a consequence of or alter the course of other psychiatric disorders. SUDs and CODs might originate from a common vulnerability or may be mutually exclusive but coincidentally manifested (Meyer 1986). In either case, they tend to be mutually exacerbating and sustaining. The differentiation between substance abuse–originated and mental health–originated symptomatology is challenging. Symptoms of co-occurring disorders have considerable functional impact and often persist even in situations in which substance use remits or decreases (Subramaniam et al. 2007). Consequently, designing interventions for CODs may require enhanced, or combined, or integrated behavioral health programming. Although the evidence base for co-occurring treatment of youth is limited compared with that for adults, it is growing. For example, there is mounting expectation that identifying and treating co-occurring psychiatric disorders in youths with SUDs would improve outcomes of both conditions. However, as indicated in the chapters in this book that are devoted to specific psychiatric disorders, the findings are not always definite and do not follow simplistic etiological pathways such as the disease model or the self-medication model.

Barriers to Integration of Treatment Services

There are many areas of broad overlap among the various disciplines that provide services to youths with CODs. Furthermore, there is some natural commonality of skill sets among providers who specialize in SUDs and other mental health problems. However, currently, the differences seem to be more prominent than the points of integration.

Despite calls for integration and the increasing marketing of programs as "co-occurring capable," the historic bias that treatment is emphasized as primarily either for SUD or COD, not both, remains intact, and the choice of treatment is often likely to be the result of an accident of the portal of service presentation rather than a thoughtful consideration of an integrated approach. The sometimes unspoken default view remains that one category of disorder is explained away as a secondary manifestation of the other, which is seen as underlying and primary, again as a function of the bias of which door the patient walks through, which disorder seems more obvious, or which is easier to address in a particular context (easier to prescribe a medication, easier to talk about drug abstinence, easier to focus on delinquency and disruptive behavior, easier to get reimbursement, etc.).

Depending on their comfort level, providers often shy away from problems in the "other" arena. Referral patterns tend to proceed by the labeled categories of one arena or the other. Confusion about the goals of treatment, lack of thoughtful formulation, and too little coherence of treatment are common, both in the pharmacological and psychosocial modalities. There are few sustainable models for longitudinal care delivery, and both research and practice have focused on time-limited discrete episodes of care. Both funding and provider care models favor acute care delivery rather than continuing care, longitudinal recovery management, early intervention to reduce severity, or even linking of acute episodes of care into a longitudinal course.

The pressures to respond to crises, as well as the reimbursement patterns that drive acute care, also muddy diagnosis and service delivery, such as when youths present emergently with a jumbled picture of escalating symptoms of SUD and COD. Typical confusions in this context can include the difficulties distinguishing intentional suicidal overdose from accidental extreme intoxication; or the erratic, explosive lability that may be persistent in the context of severe substance use from the episodic symptoms suggestive of bipolar disorder; or the episodic oppositional threats of self-harm or aggression reflecting family conflict over substance use–related behaviors from the persistent negativism or despair suggesting a suicidal depressive disorder. It is obviously hard to make a nuanced formulation in the emergency department. Also, in a psychiatric hospitalization lasting only several days, it is unreasonable to expect anything more than the formulaic diagnoses and reflex prescriptions that are all too common.

Variability in public sector funding models (both through the block grant and through Medicaid) leads to wide variations in the kinds of services covered and incentivized in different states, and sometimes even within the same state. Funding tends to be categorically distinct either for SUD or psychiatric treatment, which does not promote optimal access or integration of care. Payers tend to categorize with excessive rigidity, even finding it convenient to deny treatment in the "wrong" category as inappropriate to the service level or covered benefit at hand. Many community treatment programs, especially those with traditional expertise in SUD treatment, are smaller and do not have the financial sophistication and economies of scale to manage multiple payers, blended and braided funding streams, complex reimbursement schemes such as capitation, episode-of-care cost contracting, risk sharing, pay for performance, or electronic health record requirements.

Managed care strategies have restricted access for services both on the patient demand side (through cost sharing such as deductibles and co-pays, utilization review, care "management" or restriction, and disproportionate limitations on higher-intensity services such as intensive outpatient, inpatient, and residential treatments) and on the provider supply side (with carve-outs and utilization review subcontracts). In combination, these market forces have narrowed the available continuum of services. Most of the subspecialty carve-out and behavioral health administrative services strategies that have ostensibly been implemented to reduce costs and so-called unnecessary care have resulted in unlinking or isolating both SUD and psychiatric services from general medical care and often both from each other, in direct contradiction to the principles of integration.

Integrated Care for Mental Health and SUD: Progress Toward Models That Work

One of the clear imperatives for progress toward addressing the barriers currently preventing integrated mental health and SUD care is the establishment of broader experience and deeper expertise in the integrated treatment of youths with CODs. There is a need to articulate and disseminate approaches to and models of integrated treatment that will eventually coalesce into a standard of care. This goal requires expert consensus, followed gradually by empirical testing. Various approaches currently in use or under development and refinement offer glimpses of models of care that have potential for moving the field forward.

Diagnostic Approaches

The question of psychiatric diagnostic precision for CODs in the face of SUDs is frequently vexing to practitioners. Certainly, precision can be improved through thorough and thoughtful assessment. Factors that should be considered include family history, chronological onset of symptoms in relation to substance use, persistence of symptoms through periods of no substance use or decreased substance use, and past response to medication trials. However, given the lack of diagnostic biomarkers for psychiatric illness in general, the overlap with symptoms of SUDs, and the waxing/waning course of symptoms, precision may often be hard to come by. Some practitioners have suggested waiting a standard amount of time until a patient has persistent symptoms following abstinence from (or substantially decreased use of) substances, such as 2 weeks or 4 weeks or 6 weeks, but this advice does not help to provide guidance for the patient whose presentation suggests a compelling treatable co-occurring condition prior to that arbitrary threshold or for the patient for whom the attainment of abstinence and/or return for treatment is unlikely because of the reciprocally exacerbating and sustaining interaction between SUD and COD.

An important consideration is whether one should err on the side of specificity or sensitivity—that is, whether one should undertreat or overtreat. Inevitably, each clinician will do one and/or the other. An approach that favors specificity—that is, delaying initiation of treatment until the confound of possible substance-induced states can be eliminated or reduced—will reduce patients' exposure to unnecessary treatments, side effects, and treatment burdens but will miss treating patients who could have benefited from earlier or withheld treatment. An approach that favors sensitivity—that is, initiating treatment for what seem to be compelling symptoms or syndromes despite the confound of possible substance-induced states—will capture more treatable cases and accelerate improvement in some patients but will also expose patients to possibly unnecessary treatments when they might have remitted "spontaneously" with abstinence and/or time.

Instead, it is probably more practical and helpful to develop an intentional stance for one's own personal practice approach, whether it is more aggressive or more conservative. With the explicit recognition that we in the field do not yet have the diagnostic precision we might someday aspire to, we have to proceed with an "empirical" treatment approach that acknowledges and accounts for error or bias in the absence of a gold standard.

In either case, diagnosis should proceed not by cross-sectional symptom checklists alone but rather with a broader view of how symptoms may cohere longitudinally into syndromes. Injudicious focus on cross-sectional symptoms can give an incomplete picture, leading to overdiagnosis or misdiagnosis, for example, jumping prematurely to the conclusion of a diagnosis of attention-deficit/hyperactivity disorder (ADHD) in a substance-involved youth with symptoms of attention disturbance or to the conclusion of bipolar disorder unspecified for a youth with symptoms of mood lability and explosiveness. In both of these scenarios, substance use and its behavioral correlates may play a prominent role and can often color the presentation and obscure the diagnosis of major depression, which should always be high on the differential of mood or attention problems in substance-involved youth.

The DSM-5 (American Psychiatric Association 2013) approach to the diagnosis of SUDs may prove to be an advance because of its inclusion of a dimensional grading of severity based on numerical counts of SUD criteria:

- Mild: 2 or 3 of the 11 symptoms
- Moderate: 4 or 5 symptoms
- Severe: 6 or more symptoms

This approach may provide some guidance to clinicians about how much consideration or priority should be given to the SUD in diagnostic considerations for CODs, as well as providing a basis for research on mediation of outcomes. However, some have argued that the lower threshold of needing only 2 of 11 criteria for an SUD diagnosis, even with the "mild" modifier, might lead to a disproportionate overprioritizing of SUDs at the expense of COD treatment. Another concern has been that families and youths might be too easily driven away from services if they feel stigmatized by the adult-style label of "addiction" at earlier stages of severity (Kaminer and Winters 2012).

There is much overlap in the risk factors that precede both SUDs and CODs. There are also enduring preexisting vulnerabilities that can be expressed concurrently in both SUDs and CODs. An emerging body of work on impairment of affective regulation highlights the importance of temperament, maturational trajectory, and a developmental perspective. Emotional and/or behavioral dyscontrol identified in early childhood is frequently cited as a common antecedent marker (possibly even a causal pathway) for later development of both SUDs and other emotional and/or behavioral disorders (Brook et al. 1998; Hawkins et al. 1992).

One particularly important example along these lines is illustrated in the descriptions of persistent traits of irritability, anger, and lability encompassed in the concept of severe mood dysregulation (Leibenluft 2011). When followed longitudinally, many of the children and early adolescents identified under this rubric go on to develop SUDs and then constitute an intriguing subgroup of youths with comorbidities. Many but not all of them declare their conditions over time as major depression and other affective disorders (although very few of them turn out to have bipolar disorder). Some have persistent vulnerabilities in affective regulation that are difficult to label. The conditions of some improve or even resolve with maturation. These findings support the idea that dimensional traits (including irritability, reactivity, impulsivity, and disinhibition) are themselves important developmental constructs that can enrich more conventional categorical diagnoses. The findings also suggest that the current diagnostic catalog is still evolving and is sometimes inadequate (Leibenluft 2011).

The leap from severe mood dysregulation as an investigational concept focused on dimensional traits of impairment of affective regulation to a categorical diagnosis in DSM-5 as disruptive mood dysregulation disorder (Roy et al. 2014) may have been premature, outstripping the state of actual knowledge. In any case, whether or not a clear, homogeneous, and longitudinally coherent diagnostic category is confirmed, this approach, by providing a broader vocabulary for the identification and classification of CODs and focusing attention on the developmental trajectory of an important symptom cluster, will likely move the field forward. In the future, researchers may be able to map and differentiate the various pathways that lead to different combinations of disorders and, even more ambitiously, to use these pathways to craft specific interventions.

Overall, the likelihood of diagnostic accuracy is improved by taking a hypothesis-driven approach, frequently retesting the hypothesis, and being open to changing the hypothesis with new information.

Psychiatric Pharmacotherapy

A small but growing body of literature supports the approach of proceeding with integrated treatment for youths who are actively engaged in substance use with COD, including therapy that addresses specific cognitive-behavioral skills related to the psychiatric problem, counseling that specifically addresses substance use and recovery skills, urine testing, and pharmacotherapy specific to the psychiatric disorder (Belendiuk and Riggs 2014). Questions of safety addressed by the work done thus far have continued to reassure clinicians that judicious use of medications does not confer substantial added risk (Riggs 2014), including for those youths actively using intoxicating substances (Kaminer et al. 2010). Agents that have been examined specifically include fluoxetine (Cornelius et al. 2005; Riggs et al. 2007), osmotic-release methylphenidate (Riggs et al. 2011; Tamm et al. 2013), lithium (Geller et al. 1998), atomoxetine (Thurstone et al. 2010), bupropion (Riggs et al. 2014) and pemoline (Riggs et al. 2004).

Work by Riggs et al. (2007) shows us that in youth with major depression and SUDs who are actively using substances, treatment with fluoxetine (and presumably therefore other antidepressants) is safe and efficacious for depression outcomes in an integrated rather than sequential approach. Similarly, work by Riggs et al. (2011) shows us that in youth with ADHD and SUDs who are actively using, employing the same integrated approach, treatment with osmotic-release methylphenidate, is safe. And although it did not significantly separate from placebo on the primary ADHD outcome, it showed promise on some of the secondary outcomes. Interestingly, in neither of those studies did active medication versus placebo produce superior substance use outcomes in the intent to treat analyses.

What was perhaps most remarkable in both of those studies is that when the pooled data were reanalyzed not by randomly assigned condition (medication vs. placebo) but rather by whether patients had substantial reduction over the course of the trial in symptoms of the co-occurring depression or ADHD, there was a significant and clinically meaningful correlation with improvement in substance use outcomes. In other words, if the concurrent psychiatric illness improved, whether through medication, psychotherapy, or both, then the substance use disorder improved. And reciprocally, if the concurrent psychiatric illness did not improve, then the substance use disorder did not improve. If this finding generalizes, then we should expect that when the SUDs and CODs improve, they are likely to improve together because of active synergistic treatment of both simultaneously. However, if we do not address one of the co-occurring conditions or are stymied in getting an effective response, we should not be surprised when the other also does not respond.

Although the existing evidence is limited, emerging consensus supports aggressive but thoughtful and judicious use of pharmacotherapies for CODs in youths with SUDs, avoiding oversimplistic heaping of one symptom-driven medication on top of another and avoiding excessive polypharmacy except when necessary. Many other questions remain, including choice of medication and optimal dosing strategies in the face of active substance use and/or relapse vulnerability. This is certainly an area in which further advances can be expected.

Relapse Prevention Medication

Another area of active inquiry and newly emerging knowledge is the use of pharmacotherapies as direct antiaddiction treatments to reduce use, facilitate abstinence, and/or prevent relapse (Belendiuk and Riggs 2014). This has been an area of considerable excitement in adult treatment, and medications are in use or under development for numerous target substances and with numerous potential mechanisms. These medications include agonists, antagonists, reward modulators, enzymatic agents that promote metabolic degradation or enhance production of toxic punishing metabolites, vaccines, and stress response modulators. However, relatively little exploration has been done of primary antiaddiction medication in youth. The little work that has been done has mostly involved opioid addiction (Pecoraro et al. 2013). A single-site randomized controlled trial (RCT) showed an advantage of extended detoxification (4 weeks) with buprenorphine compared to clonidine in adolescents with opioid dependence (Marsch et al. 2005). A multisite RCT showed effectiveness of buprenorphine treatment compared with no medication for youths with opioid addiction over

12 weeks (Woody et al. 2008). Several secondary analyses from this study have also explored safety, mediators, and moderators (Subramaniam et al. 2011; Warden et al. 2012). A case series has suggested the feasibility and possible effectiveness of extended-release naltrexone over 4 months for youths with opioid addiction (Fishman et al. 2010). Other retrospective, nonrandomized preliminary work (Fishman et al. 2011; Matson et al. 2014; Pugatch et al. 2014) has also suggested the benefits of buprenorphine and/or extended-release naltrexone in standard community treatment conditions, and additional trials are under way. For patients with cannabis dependence, an RCT has shown the effectiveness of N-acetylcysteine in enhancing the effectiveness of intensive outpatient treatment (counseling plus contingency management) over 12 weeks (Gray et al. 2012).

Although very promising, this work has led to as many questions as answers. Questions include the following: If the effectiveness of anti-addiction medications is confirmed for youth, who are the optimal candidates? If more than one medication is available (e.g., buprenorphine and extended-release naltrexone), what are the appropriate selection strategies? What is the optimal duration of treatment? What are the optimal psychosocial interventions to support these medications and optimize synergy in an integrated multimodality package? What are the delivery systems that could make such approaches broadly feasible? What are the appropriate responses to diversion and misuse of those medications that have intrinsic reinforcing properties (buprenorphine for opioid addiction or prescription stimulants for cocaine)? Nevertheless, despite all the unanswered questions, it seems likely that use of medication will be an expanding scope of practice that broadens the treatment toolbox.

Treatment of opioid use disorders in youth provides a model for service delivery, because this is an arena in which there are established medication treatments and growing demand for them. The involvement of addiction psychiatry or addiction medicine physicians in prescribing relapse prevention medications creates an implicit role for the treatment of other CODs, as well as the opportunity for the use of other medications. Engagement of patients with opioid use disorder through medications that they may be motivated to obtain can promote action orientation in at least that one domain, with implications for generalization to engagement in other domains. Furthermore, dissemination of antiaddiction pharmacotherapy may lead to greater involvement of physicians and patient access to concurrent pharmacotherapy for CODs.

Integration of the Treatment Team

One of the common models for achieving better integration of care is delivery of both SUD and COD treatment by a single integrated treatment team. This confers the logistical advantage of one-stop shopping to patients and families, thereby reducing treatment burden. It improves communication among providers, both because of formal organizational communication forums (rounds, team meetings) and because of informal workplace discussions (curbside consults, hallway staff discussions). An integrated treatment team eliminates redundancy but more importantly reduces the opportunity for cross-purposing or misinterpretation of treatment instructions or confusion over treatment messages ("splitting"). It allows for consistent coordination of treatment goals and priorities. It is generally associated with more coherent orchestration or "quarterbacking" of an overall treatment plan and the collaborative deployment of the different members of the multidisciplinary team. Integration can also lead to better utilization management, increased efficiency, and better cost management.

Integration and Development of the Workforce

To implement an integrated treatment team, a professional workforce is needed with the requisite training and skills. Although psychiatrists must be trained, mobilized, and focused on new approaches to integrated practice, there will never be enough psychiatrists to deliver all the care that is needed. Psychiatric resources can be leveraged through the development and integration of the workforce. Providers that refine and systematize such models will likely be more successful than those that maintain traditional rigid disciplinary categories and roles.

Some professional organizations and states have begun to develop and articulate standards for a new professional discipline of adolescent (or perhaps youth and young adult)-oriented COD therapists (and/or counselors, because this distinction is often regional and not uniform). This new discipline will require the development of training curricula, degree programs, and practice competencies. Some states have begun to develop and implement special certification and/or licensure for a new specialty discipline of COD counseling. Some states have created an enhanced reimbursement structure for COD treatment in the public sector to systematize and institutionalize COD practices and to incentivize the creation of a workforce and specialty delivery system.

This new discipline will also certainly involve cross-training of the existing workforce in the current disciplines of mental health therapy and substance abuse counseling. Some states have already started to develop shortened pathways to dual licensure or certification in the second discipline for clinicians who already have the other. Other states have developed add-on certifications or added qualifications in COD from one or both nonintegrated disciplines. However, in either case, over time the differences (and similarities) between this new emerging discipline and the older, separated historical disciplines need to be articulated.

Some models of workforce integration emphasize cross-training of COD therapists to augment the role of the psychiatrist by teaching these therapists to work outside their traditional boundaries. Although not trained as licensed independent practitioners with prescriptive authority, such broadly trained and supervised COD therapists can act as physician "extenders" by broad incorporation of some of the traditionally "psychiatric" components of the treatment as part of their explicit scope and focus. Prepackaged COD algorithms and treatment manuals that include both SUD and COD materials can be useful tools for cross-training and implementation of such approaches to leveraging psychiatric resources. Another tool is clinical supervision of these therapists by psychiatrists, so that psychiatric thinking and methods become embedded in therapists' clinical practice.

The key is to train therapists to shift away from their previously typical behavior of compartmentalizing and avoiding psychiatric management issues in COD cases ("talk to your doctor about that...") to an explicit and assertive focus on tracking psychiatric management issues, seeing these as fully within their scope. Although initially developed for medical clinicians working with adults treated with relapse prevention medications, components of approaches such as BRENDA (biopsychosocial evaluation, report to patient, empathic understanding, needs collaboratively identified, direct advice, assess reaction; Volpicelli et al. 2001) and medical management (Lee et al. 2010) can be adapted for use by nonmedical clinicians with youths treated with psychiatric medications. Therapists can be trained to be quite competent at tracking and documenting symptoms; weighing diagnostic considerations; and monitoring medication compliance, response, and side effects. Rather than conceptualizing medication treatments and psychosocial treatments as distinct, this model conceptualizes "medication management" as an explicit component and goal of psychosocial treatment and vice versa. Similar approaches have been used successfully in adult clinics for chronically mentally ill adult populations and by assertive community treatment teams.

Furthermore, the ongoing monitoring and direction of the work of these therapists in specialty COD positions should routinely be seen as a natural expectation of the case leadership by the psychiatrist. Unfortunately, this model is not reflected in the practice of most psychotherapy delivered to patients under general psychiatric care, in which psychiatrist and psychotherapist may loosely coordinate care but are not integrated in a stronger sense. In fact, in some practice settings the psychiatrist's role is even marginalized to that of a prescriptive technician for medication only.

Two of the most important characteristics of this ideal integration are a well-understood toolbox of standard treatments and a routine expectation of standard goals of treatment. When an orthopedist prescribes physical therapy with the specific goal of "increased range of motion" and/or "increased strength" for a particular orthopedic condition involving a particular joint (e.g., adhesive capsulitis of the shoulder), every well-trained physical therapist knows what to do, and every well-trained orthopedist knows what to expect for the patient and how to monitor progress. Although there may be variations in the local details of technique and equipment, there is considerable uniformity and a shared *standard of care.* Similarly, the psychiatrist should be expected to direct the care in a close collaboration, not only knowing what happens in the therapy but also leading it and taking responsibility for it.

Delivery and Management of Treatment

Treatment Matching and Placement Strategies

The concept that SUD services for youth must be at least co-occurring capable, and better yet co-occurring enhanced, is fortunately growing increasingly common. However, the actual realization of such integrated care in community treatment remains slow, the resources in most communities remain scant, and the difficulties faced in appropriately matching and placing youths in services remain prominent. The American Society of Addiction Medicine (ASAM) Patient Placement Criteria (MeeLee et al. 2013) have become the U.S. national (and, increasingly, the international) standard for treatment matching, placement decisions, and utilization management for SUDs. The criteria include a section that addresses SUDs and CODs in youth (Fishman 2014; Fishman et al. 2011).

Although there has been relatively little empirical testing of the adolescent ASAM criteria, a growing body of work verifies that assessment-based stratification of severity can yield stable prognostic staging predictions and that placement based on such stratification can predict treatment response. These findings apply to the ASAM criteria for adults in particular (Gastfriend 2003; Gastfriend and McLellan 1997; MeeLee et al. 2013) and apply in more general terms for adolescents (Dasinger et al. 2004; Stevens et al. 2006).

As the ASAM criteria and similar standards become increasingly embedded in regulation and more widely adopted, an increasing incentive for adoption of integrated COD care is created because of 1) the implicit focus on attention to mental health problems and needs in the multidimensional assessment of the ASAM criteria and 2) the explicit prescription of mental health interventions in the context of SUD treatment and placement.

The ASAM criteria create a road map for how CODs impact treatment matching and placement service needs for patients with SUDs. In the ASAM criteria's multidimensional assessment schema of six assessment dimensions, the third dimension—Emotional, Behavioral, or Cognitive Conditions and Complications—relates most specifically to CODs. This dimension's five subdomains, 1) dangerousness/lethality, 2) interference with addiction recovery efforts, 3) social functioning, 4) ability for self-care, and 5) course of illness, described next, help the user think through the ways in which service needs for patients with CODs interrelate to the more traditional service needs and service delivery settings for those with SUDs. This approach is particularly useful because it emphasizes the assessment of severity of symptomatic functional impairment rather than any specific categorical diagnosis.

Subdomain 1, dangerousness/lethality, refers to the extent of risk of imminent harm to self or others. Assessment considerations may include suicidality, assaultiveness, risk of victimization, and exposure to the elements. Treatment decisions in this subdomain focus on safety and protection from dangerous consequences and may include such interventions as residential containment or high-intensity family monitoring between outpatient sessions.

Subdomain 2, interference with addiction recovery efforts, refers to the extent to which psychological and behavioral symptoms are a distraction from treatment participation or engagement. Examples include difficulty attending to treatment sessions because of problems with concentration; difficulty in completing recovery assignments or absorbing treatment materials because of problems with concentration/attention, memory, or comprehension; inability to attend treatment consistently because of running away; inability to participate in treatment because of disruptive behavior; and distraction caused by preoccupying worries.

Subdomain 3, social functioning, refers to the extent to which emotional, behavioral, and cognitive problems cause impairments in meeting responsibilities in major social arenas such as family, school, work, and personal relationships. Examples of assessment considerations in this subdomain include problems managing peer or family conflict, legal and conduct problems, problems with truancy or school performance, ungovernability at home, and narrowing of social repertoire and isolation.

Subdomain 4, ability for self-care, refers to the extent to which the adolescent has problems in managing activities of daily living and personal care. Assessment considerations in this subdomain include behaviors associated with patterns of victimization, high-risk or indiscriminate sexual behaviors, disorganization that interferes with emerging independent living skills, poor self-regulation (or poor cooperation with external regulation) of daily routine, and problems with hygiene or nutrition.

Subdomain 5, course of illness, refers to an interpretation of the adolescent's present situation and symptoms in the context of his or her history and response to treatment, with a goal of predicting future course and relative stability. For example, the history may suggest that a mood disorder decompensates rapidly with medication noncompliance, suggesting a higher instability and severity than if the historical deterioration occurred more slowly and suggesting the need for a more urgent and/or more intensive treatment response. Other examples include an adolescent who has tended to run away soon after an episode of family conflict or an adolescent who tends to relapse to substance use following recurrence of depression or anxiety symptoms.

One of the goals of the ASAM criteria is to articulate an idealized treatment continuum of services to provide for the needs of youths with SUD and COD. Such a continuum takes into account that young patients could move flexibly through different specific services, up and down various intensities, across different levels of care, all while longitudinal monitoring and continuity of coordination are maintained, in contrast to the currently prevalent system of discrete unconnected episodes of discontinuous care. This vision can accommodate acute crisis care as well as longer-term, even indefinite, maintenance and monitoring. The specific levels of care itemized in the ASAM criteria are finite, certainly not encompassing all the innovative programmatic possibilities that have been described or even that already exist; however, even the "limited" continuum of treatment settings described in the criteria is not yet available in most communities. The reality of limited availability of services is a major problem, but the ASAM criteria represent the gold standard to aspire to.

Organizational and Financial Incentives for Integrated Care

Presumably, some of the next wave of advances will be driven by factors that incentivize integration at organizational and institutional levels. Several unfolding trends in the health care delivery landscape have the potential to be positive in this regard. Recent health care reforms, including federal legislation, emerging regulatory interpretation and implementation, and state and local regulatory changes, have been aligning to create cautious optimism among observers. The term *integration* has become something of a banner and topical buzzword, sometimes promoted as a panacea for every imaginable problem in health care. However, the term also seems to be applied increasingly with real and thoughtful meaning in some potentially useful applications.

The Mental Health Parity and Addiction Equity Act of 2008 (referred to hereafter simply as "Parity") requires that insurance plans provide coverage for behavioral health care services that is equivalent to (i.e., no more restrictive than) the coverage for medical and surgical conditions. This act has raised considerably the national prominence of behavioral health care—for both mental health and substance abuse. It has also increasingly framed the conversation to consider these both as parts of a single spectrum. Most important, Parity is expected to ease many of the long-standing disproportionate restrictions on behavioral health care compared to somatic health care, including co-pays, coinsurance, and out-of-pocket maximums; limitations on quantitative services coverage, such as limits on the number of inpatient days or outpatient visits; use of care management tools; criteria for medical necessity determinations; and coverage for out-of-network providers. The hope is that with implementation of the act, service capacity, demand, and utilization will increase.

Other major trends arise out of the Affordable Care Act of 2010 (ACA). Some of the ways in which the ACA is forecasted to increase access and thereby demand include Medicaid expansion, broadening of coverage through the health care exchanges, requirements for employer-based coverage, and elimination of exclusions for preexisting conditions.

Another trend is the integration of mental health and substance abuse regulatory and policy authorities at the level of state and local governments. Some have expressed concern that the agendas of substance abuse treatment providers and specialty services will be swallowed up into the much larger pool of mental health, becoming an "afterthought." Others describe this integration as a long overdue expression of an enduring trend to eliminate artificial factional divisions in the behavioral health field, analogous to the previous mergers of drug abuse agencies with alcoholism agencies, also unthinkable to some at the time. In either case, merger or swallowing, common policy and regulatory authorities will dissolve some of the barriers and promote some forms of integration.

As mental health and substance abuse services become increasingly counted as part of the same coverage package, the more likely they are to be delivered together. More care, in many cases, will mean more integrated care, especially in larger health care delivery systems in which scalability is critical. Such systems are more likely to capture data systematically, allowing providers to explore the utilization patterns (Chi et al. 2006) and outcomes of integrated care in better detail, document its benefits, and pursue its advantages. Such systems are also more likely to be capable of following and motivated to follow the incentives that may emerge out of any scalable efficiencies from integrated care.

To the extent that payers and large delivery systems and municipal governments see substance abuse and mental health services as subtly different shades of essentially the same services category, they will incentivize delivery of services that are labeled "co-occurring." This may have the advantage of incentivizing efficient *and* effective integration; however, the primary systemic incentive will more likely be the pursuit of the elimination of "duplicative" services as a cost-saving measure rather than long-term improvement of outcomes, and this may have the side effect of new restrictions on utilization of services that are not actually duplicative. Although some models may do better with services that simultaneously address both realms of substance abuse and mental health in the same unit of service, other models of integration will emphasize closely coordinated concurrent services in both realms that remain somewhat distinct in their emphases. In either case, there will likely be pressures on total dose of services, under the banner of efficiency and integration, in advance of any evidence that better integration actually lowers any need for total dose. We need to be careful that providers and patients do not end up with integration that is more efficient (meaning less expense and less care) but less effective.

Another trend is the increasing call for the integration of behavioral health care into general health care. This trend grows partly out of the promotion of access by the ACA and Parity. The more demand there is for behavioral health care as one of many components of broader health care and the more the structure of its coverage and reimbursement and delivery resembles that of health care in general, the more likely it is that its delivery will be incorporated into general health care settings, such as large health plans, health maintenance organizations, federally qualified health centers, and hospital-based health care systems. The trend also grows out of the awareness that there may be increasingly tangible economic incentives. Cost offsets and savings from investments in behavioral health care for the society at large are relatively straightforward and clear; however, the value and timing of distal cost offsets versus the proximal investments of organizations that make the actual investment (insurance company, health system, etc.) have been vexingly difficult to pin down. What gives newer and more pressing impetus to this older idea are recent changes to reimbursement for hospitals, penalizing for readmissions soon after discharge. Suddenly, there is salience in linking acute medical crises to the chronic conditions that drive them through predictable reexacerbations. Substance use and psychiatric illness have long been known to be very prominent among linked chronic conditions, but now this will matter to the business office in a way it never did before. Behavioral health care has been seen as a rounding error in the overall health care budget, but the hidden multiplier will, it is hoped, become more explicit.

Hospitals and large delivery systems will be strongly incentivized to deliver behavioral health services, targeting both potentially preventable cases of acute medical consequences and existing high utilizers, not so much as a way of doing the right thing but rather as a way of controlling costs. The institutions will do this by developing new internal capacity, developing partnerships, or both. In either case, this new demand from hospitals and large health care delivery systems will probably do a lot to shape the marketplace. Also, the services encouraged by this trend will be increasingly "medicalized"; that is, they will become more amenable to medical system delivery and will emphasize medical interventions. This change will promote integration of substance abuse and mental health services both because the specialist behavioral health physicians called on to lead are more likely to lead in that direction and because the historical specialty substance abuse delivery system, which has previously been unfriendly to medical system delivery, will to some extent be left behind.

An unintended consequence of these trends, however, may also be that substance abuse services become incorporated into general health care delivery primarily through addiction medicine, with less emphasis on CODs and less integration with psychiatry (which has also historically been somewhat marginalized from general health care delivery). Another cynical possibility is that the expectations of pharmacotherapy, as an example of a more medical-style intervention, will outstrip the real effectiveness of medications and leave more nuanced psychosocial intervention behind in the new delivery landscape.

Other organizational incentives include the increasing prominence of quality indicators and outcome measurement in shaping care delivery. Because there is more pressure to document results, through electronic health records, pay-for-performance contracting, the adoption of standard data-driven quality metrics, and pressure for public dissemination of comparative outcomes, the presumed benefits of integrated treatment are likely to be more easily demonstrated, and therefore, integrated treatment is more likely to be widely adopted.

Changes in reimbursement favor integration. Previously, substance abuse treatment providers often could not find room in line-item block-grant budgets for new mental health services and therefore had no incentive to invest. As public sector substance abuse services have shifted away from block-grant budgets based on programs, treatment slots, and cost reimbursement to fee-for-service arrangements, substance abuse treatment providers have been incentivized to promote utilization and to adopt more sophisticated financial management based on diversified multipayer braided funding streams. This change has been conducive to the provision of more mental health care from substance abuse treatment providers. This trend will progress even further as fee-for-service reimbursement gives way to other innovative models, such as case rates, capitation, cost sharing, and others in which integrated services can create value (Sterling et al. 2010).

Overcoming Barriers and Next Steps: A Call to Action

The puzzle of integrated treatment for the future includes several critical pieces that, we hope, will help overcome the most significant barriers to integration: clinical practice approaches, workforce development, capacity expansion, realignment of economic incentives, and improved linkages to the natural touchpoints of adolescent life to improve engagement. The following subsections present these critical elements and the next steps that need to be taken.

Clinical Practice Approaches

The most important piece to the puzzle is the refinement of emerging clinical practice approaches, in an effort to overcome the barriers of divided, shortsighted, haphazard, uncoordinated, episodic, and crisis-driven care. The successful treatment of individual patients will serve as guideposts that cumulatively drive the other aspects of integrated care delivery.

The following is a summary of some of the clinical principles of co-occurring treatment integration that are emerging from practice, research, and expert consensus:

- Simultaneous (concurrent) rather than sequential treatment of SUDs and other psychiatric disorders.
- Delivery of care by a single integrated team. When this is not practical, care by separate specialists should be coordinated with frequent communication, common goals, and shared decision making. This integration or coordination should usually be anchored by the primary leadership of the most senior specialist, ideally the addiction psychiatrist, or whoever has the most experience to direct and orchestrate the efforts of the various clinicians involved and services across time.
- Use of standard psychiatric medications for co-occurring psychiatric conditions despite ongoing active substance use, informed by the experience that this is generally safe.
- Adoption of a longitudinal view, with a view to engagement of patients and families over the long term.
- Emphasis on active, even assertive, engagement of the patient and family as a primary goal and responsibility of the treatment team, in contrast to the older, more passive approach of "they'll come when they're ready."
- Expectation of incremental progress, with nonlinear and even non-unidirectional movement through the stages of change, often with a remitting and relapsing course (e.g., three steps forward and one step back) as the rule rather than the exception.
- Adoption of the perspective that although abstinence is the gold standard and goal of treatment, reductions in use short of abstinence are associated with functional improvement and should be appreciated as partial steps toward recovery. A very difficult balancing act for therapists and parents alike is the simultaneous celebration of partial success and lack of satisfaction with incomplete success.
- Expectation that behavior change in youths will often not come from insight and introspection. Rehearsal of new behavior changes will often precede insight in a change process that may be counterintuitive to adults and therapists. Although the lightning-bolt epiphany

or the "aha" moment may be desired by the therapist, it may not be the typical mechanism of adolescent learning.

• Use of antiaddiction medications (anticraving or relapse prevention medication or medication-assisted treatment) as additional evidence for effectiveness in youth confirmed.

Workforce Development

Workforce development is another critical piece of the puzzle. We in the field need to leverage existing resources and develop new ones by training the next generation of psychiatrists who have a full range of skills in the treatment of these patients. Psychiatry, the discipline with the broadest and deepest view, will need to take a primary leadership role. This requires that the psychiatrist have both expertise and a willingness to assume leadership, including the sense of ownership and accountability that comes with that. The psychiatrist should know enough about the details of available counseling, psychotherapy, and behavioral treatments to prescribe them thoughtfully; make good treatment-matching decisions; and supervise a multidisciplinary team in implementing co-occurring–enhanced treatment interventions.

We also need to train a next generation of counselors and therapists to have broader and deeper knowledge of both SUDs and CODs and to educate them in the state-of-the-art treatment developments in the field. Our efforts to grow a technically competent workforce will require investment in both the development of a robust professional discipline of adolescent/youth–oriented integrated treatment specialists and an enticing career pathway for them to pursue.

Expanding Capacity

Expanding treatment capacity is in some sense the simplest of the necessary next steps. Increased capacity will, it is hoped, come with a convergence of several trends. As treatment programs increasingly recognize the need to become co-occurring enhanced, they will develop new expertise, incorporate psychiatrists (or at least link closely with them), and, importantly, incorporate psychiatric leadership. As psychiatrists recognize the need to integrate treatment, they will develop new expertise and form collaborations with therapists, counselors, and programs that have sophistication in treating COD. On the demand side, the market will increasingly drive the expansion of capacity as consumers increasingly call for integrated treatment. These trends are illustrated by several common observations. There is already a widespread tendency for programs to advertise themselves as "co-occurring" whether or not they actually deliver integrated treatment. It is also all too common for regional specialists to hear families ask where they can find practitioners or programs that will address "both sets of problems" at the same time, despairing that there is no local availability. Presumably, the pent-up demand is huge.

Economic Incentives

The alignment of economic forces to incentivize integration of treatment is already at least partially under way, and if hopes are realized, it will increase. We in the field may have arrived at a particularly historically opportune moment. The multiple trends summarized earlier in this chapter, including reimbursement changes that incentivize the salience of SUDs as drivers of readmission, Parity's casting of SUD and COD treatment together as behavioral health treatment, and increases in coverage under the ACA that drive demand, will likely all encourage treatment integration.

This is an exciting time in which changes in the health care landscape may favor progress. We need to be mindful, however, to document outcomes in the real world to advocate for what really works. As experts and specialty providers, we need to learn to create cost-effectiveness for health care delivery systems that transcends simple cost savings to the realization of value through better outcomes.

Involvement of Primary Care and Other Natural Touchpoints

Our specialty system for treatment of SUDs and CODs is fairly isolated from the other systems through which youth receive services. We in the field need to improve the reach of integrated SUD and COD services by learning to deliver them where youths are. These settings include primary care, schools, juvenile justice arenas, child welfare and foster care systems, and other youth-serving agencies.

From the perspective of these systems, which are outside our specialty (or subspecialty), the distinctions between SUD and COD problems and treatment already appear small, and the need for integration is obvious. Attempts to collaborate more seamlessly with these other systems will pressure us to make our services more integrated in order to better meet the needs of these stakeholders.

Summary and Future Directions

A great need clearly exists for further exploration and empirical testing of a wide range of interventions and treatment-matching hypotheses. Treatment in the real world encompasses more heterogeneous patient populations with more complex multimorbidity than in research settings with artificial contexts of small caseloads, grant-enriched resources, and relatively homogeneous populations.

The following are some important questions for research and for exploration in practical clinical practice:

- How does the presence of SUD affect selection of pharmacological agents and medication treatment strategies from among those commonly used for youth?
- What are the strategies for optimizing benefit of psychosocial treatments in the real world (e.g., dose including intensity and frequency, group vs. individual, content, focus on specific disorders vs. more generalized attention to overlapping symptoms vs. mix and match, minimizing treatment burden, maximizing engagement and adherence under real-world reimbursement conditions including public sector settings)?
- What are the optimal durations of treatment for both pharmacological and psychosocial treatments?
- What are the strategies for optimizing synergy between pharmacological and psychosocial treatments (e.g., choice of particular treatments, staging, sequencing, dosing)?
- What is the effectiveness of medications with potential combined effects (e.g., serotonin-norepinephrine reuptake inhibitors or bupropion for depression plus ADHD) and of combinations of medications (e.g., stimulants plus antidepressants)?
- What is the effectiveness of some of the common but untested pharmacological strategies in current clinical practice in youths with SUDs and CODs, such as use of lower-dose neuroleptics for mood lability or antidepressant augmentation, use of medications with sedating side effects (e.g., trazodone, quetiapine, mirtazapine) for insomnia, or use of mood stabilizers for nonspecific impulsiveness or disinhibition?
- What are the impacts of level of care, and how should best practices account for staging and sequencing, as well as movement across levels over time?
- Are there specific pharmacotherapy strategies that might take advantage of specific anti-SUD properties (bupropion because of dopaminergic repletion, stimulants for ADHD plus methamphetamine/cocaine addiction, combinations with buprenorphine or naltrexone for opioid addiction)?
- What are the developmentally informed adaptations of delivery of relapse-prevention medications that will maximize benefit in youth?

- What are the realistic ways to expand the involvement of primary medical care with more effective and practical support from specialty care, using Screening, Brief Intervention, and Referral to Treatment (SBIRT) or other models for referral portals of entry and/or as longitudinal monitoring and management touchpoints?
- What are the ways to practically empower families to navigate and get better results from the complex specialty care system?
- How can we in the field test and validate treatment matching and placement criteria, both in their current forms and in more reliable, more precise future iterations?
- What are the economic models that will best incentivize sustainable integration of care?

Although the knowledge base for treatment of CODs in youth is in its early stages and treatments are still generally modest in their outcomes, the growing body of research increasingly encourages optimism about effective interventions. Also, although there is a paucity of developmentally informed co-occurring enhanced treatment services and there are many barriers to access for the co-occurring services that do exist, there is increasing recognition of these barriers as well as focus on strategies to overcome them. Broad principles for approaches to integrated treatment with improved effectiveness are evolving, supported by emerging evidence and expert consensus that should provide guidance for clinical practice. The testing of these principles, as well as the many other questions that remain, should inform a much needed, robust agenda of exploration for the future.

We need to channel further energies and resources into this important subspecialty to enrich the field through research that informs evidence-based practice. We need to learn how to use outcomes tracking in standard community practice to enrich the field through practical experience that informs practice-based evidence.

We have come a long way, *and* we have a long way to go.

KEY POINTS

- Psychiatric comorbidity or co-occurring disorders (CODs) in youth with substance use disorders (SUDs) should be considered the rule rather than the exception, and integrated approaches that identify and treat both SUDs and CODs together and simultaneously will improve outcomes of both conditions.

- Clinical practice is improving with emphasis on and greater knowledge about the use of psychiatric medications combined with empirically supported psychosocial interventions, the use of relapse prevention medications, and the longitudinal engagement of patients and families.

- Workforce development is essential, with emphasis on the training of both psychiatrist and therapist specialists with a broadened scope of competence in both SUDs and CODs.

- There is a critical need for expansion of co-occurring treatment capacity.

- There are many encouraging current opportunities for overcoming barriers to integration, including developing approaches to treatment matching and emerging health care organizational and financial incentives.

References

American Psychiatric Association: Diagnostic and Statistical Manual of Mental Disorders, 5th Edition. Arlington, VA, American Psychiatric Association, 2013

Belendiuk KA, Riggs P: Treatment of adolescent substance use disorders. Curr Treat Options Psychiatry 1(2):175–188, 2014 24855595

Brook JS, Cohen P, Brook DW: Longitudinal study of co-occurring psychiatric disorders and substance use. J Am Acad Child Adolesc Psychiatry 37(3):322–330, 1998 9519638

Chi FW, Sterling S, Weisner C: Adolescents with co-occurring substance use and mental conditions in a private managed care health plan: prevalence, patient characteristics, and treatment initiation and engagement. Am J Addict 15 (suppl 1):67–79, 2006 17182422

Cornelius JR, Clark DB, Bukstein OG, et al: Acute phase and five-year follow-up study of fluoxetine in adolescents with major depression and a comorbid substance use disorder: a review. Addict Behav 30(9):1824–1833, 2005 16102905

Dasinger LK, Shane PA, Martinovich Z: Assessing the effectiveness of community-based substance abuse treatment for adolescents. J Psychoactive Drugs 36(1):27–33, 2004 15152707

Fishman M: Placement criteria and treatment planning for adolescents with substance use disorders, in Clinical Manual of Adolescent Substance Abuse Treatment. Edited by Kaminer Y, Winters K. Washington, DC, American Psychiatric Publishing, 2011, pp 113–142

Fishman M: Placement criteria and strategies for adolescent treatment matching, in Principles of Addiction Medicine, 5th Edition. Edited by Ries R, Fiellin D. Philadelphia, PA, Lippincott Williams & Wilkins, 2014, pp 1627–1646

Fishman M, Winstanley EL, Curran E, et al: Treatment of opioid dependence in adolescents and young adults with extended release naltrexone: preliminary case-series and feasibility. Addiction 105(9):1669–1676, 2010 20626723

Fishman M, Curran E, Shah S, et al: Treatment outcomes with relapse prevention medications for opioid dependence in youth. Poster presented at the College on Problems of Drug Dependence Annual Meeting. Boca Raton, FL, June 22, 2011

Gastfriend DR (ed): Addiction Treatment Matching: Research Foundations of the American Society of Addiction Medicine (ASAM) Patient Placement Criteria. Binghamton, NY, Haworth Medical Press, 2003

Gastfriend DR, McLellan AT: Treatment matching: theoretic basis and practical implications. Med Clin North Am 81(4):945–966, 1997 9222262

Geller B, Cooper TB, Sun K, et al: Double-blind and placebo-controlled study of lithium for adolescent bipolar disorders with secondary substance dependency. J Am Acad Child Adolesc Psychiatry 37(2):171–178, 1998 9473913

Gray KM, Carpenter MJ, Baker NL, et al: A double-blind randomized controlled trial of N-acetylcysteine in cannabis-dependent adolescents. Am J Psychiatry 169(8):805–812, 2012 22706327

Hawkins JD, Catalano RF, Miller JY: Risk and protective factors for alcohol and other drug problems in adolescence and early adulthood: implications for substance abuse prevention. Psychol Bull 112(1):64–105, 1992 1529040

Kaminer Y, Winters KC: Proposed DSM-5 substance use disorders for adolescents: if you build it, will they come? Am J Addict 21(3):280–281, author reply 282, 2012 22494232

Kaminer Y, Goldberg P, Connor DF: Psychotropic medications and substances of abuse interactions in youth. Subst Abus 31(1):53–57, 2010 20391270

Kuepper R, van Os J, Lieb R, et al: Continued cannabis use and risk of incidence and persistence of psychotic symptoms: 10 year follow-up cohort study. BMJ 342:d738, 2011 21363868

Lee JD, Grossman E, DiRocco D, et al: Extended-release naltrexone for treatment of alcohol dependence in primary care. J Subst Abuse Treat 39(1):14–21, 2010 20363090

Leibenluft E: Severe mood dysregulation, irritability, and the diagnostic boundaries of bipolar disorder in youths. Am J Psychiatry 168(2):129–142, 2011 21123313

Marsch LA, Bickel WK, Badger GJ, et al: Comparison of pharmacological treatments for opioid-dependent adolescents: a randomized controlled trial. Arch Gen Psychiatry 62(10):1157–1164, 2005 16203961

Matson SC, Hobson G, Abdel-Rasoul M, et al: A retrospective study of retention of opioid-dependent adolescents and young adults in an outpatient buprenorphine/naloxone clinic. J Addict Med 8(3):176–182, 2014 24695018

MeeLee D, Shulman G, Fishman M, et al: The ASAM Criteria: Treatment Criteria for Addictive, Substance-Related, and Co-occurring Conditions. Philadelphia, PA, Lippincott Williams & Wilkins, 2013

Meyer RE: Psychopathology and Addictive Disorders. New York, Guilford, 1986

Pecoraro A, Fishman M, Ma M, et al: Pharmacologically assisted treatment of opioid-dependent youth. Paediatr Drugs 15(6):449–458, 2013 23912754

Pugatch M, Knight JR, McGuiness P, et al: A group therapy program for opioid dependent adolescents and their parents. Subst Abus 35(4):435–441, 2014 25174347

Riggs PD: Stimulant medication for ADHD not associated with subsequent substance use disorders. Evid Based Med 19(2):78, 2014

Riggs PD, Leon SL, Mikulich SK, Pottle LC, et al: An open trial of bupropion for ADHD in adolescents with substance use disorders and conduct disorder. J Am Acad Child Adolesc Psychiatry 37(12):1271–1278, 1998 9847499

Riggs PD, Hall SK, Mikulich-Gilbertson SK, et al: A randomized controlled trial of pemoline for attention-deficit/hyperactivity disorder in substance-abusing adolescents. J Am Acad Child Adolesc Psychiatry 43(4):420–429, 2004 15187802

Riggs PD, Mikulich-Gilbertson SK, Davies RD, et al: A randomized controlled trial of fluoxetine and cognitive behavioral therapy in adolescents with major depression, behavior problems, and substance use disorders. Arch Pediatr Adolesc Med 161(11):1026–1034, 2007 17984403

Riggs PD, Winhusen T, Davies RD, et al: Randomized controlled trial of osmotic-release methylphenidate with cognitive-behavioral therapy in adolescents with attention-deficit/hyperactivity disorder and substance use disorders. J Am Acad Child Adolesc Psychiatry 50(9):903–914, 2011 21871372

Roy AK, Lopes V, Klein RG: Disruptive mood dysregulation disorder: a new diagnostic approach to chronic irritability in youth. Am J Psychiatry 171(9):918–924, 2014 25178749

Sterling S, Weisner C, Hinman A, et al: Access to treatment for adolescents with substance use and co-occurring disorders: challenges and opportunities. J Am Acad Child Adolesc Psychiatry 49(7):637–646, quiz 725–726, 2010 20610133

Stevens L, Dennis M, Fishman M: Using the new GAIN patient placement summary to support individual treatment planning, placement and program evaluation. Workshop at the Joint Meeting on Adolescent Treatment Effectiveness, Baltimore, MD, March 2006

Subramaniam G, Stitzer M, Clemmey P, et al: Baseline depressive symptoms predict poor substance use outcome following adolescent residential treatment. J Am Acad Child Adolesc Psychiatry 46(8):1062–1069, 2007 17667484

Subramaniam G, Warden D, Minhajuddin A, et al: Predictors of abstinence: National Institute of Drug Abuse multisite buprenorphine/naloxone treatment trial in opioid dependent youth. J Am Acad Child Adolesc Psychiatry 50(11):1120–1128, 2011 22024000

Tamm L, Trello-Rishel K, Riggs P, et al: Predictors of treatment response in adolescents with comorbid substance use disorder and attention-deficit/hyperactivity disorder. J Subst Abuse Treat 44(2):224–230, 2013 22889694

Thurstone C, Riggs PD, Salomonsen-Sautel S, et al: Randomized, controlled trial of atomoxetine for attention-deficit/hyperactivity disorder in adolescents with substance use disorder. J Am Acad Child Adolesc Psychiatry 49(6):573–582, 2010 20494267

Volpicelli JR, Pettinati HM, McLellan AT, et al: Combining Medication and Psychosocial Treatments for Addictions: The BRENDA Approach. New York, Guilford, 2001

Warden D, Subramaniam GA, Carmody T, et al: Predictors of attrition with buprenorphine/naloxone treatment in opioid dependent youth. Addict Behav 37(9):1046–1053, 2012 22626890

Woody GE, Poole SA, Subramaniam G, et al: Extended vs short-term buprenorphine-naloxone for treatment of opioid-addicted youth: a randomized trial. JAMA 300(17):2003–2011, 2008 18984887

CHAPTER 3

Screening, Assessment, and Treatment Options for Youths With a Substance Use Disorder

Yifrah Kaminer, M.D., M.B.A.
Ken C. Winters, Ph.D.
John Kelly, Ph.D.

When a clinician is faced with an adolescent who is suspected of having or known to have a substance use problem, it is important to integrate the assessment process with treatment decisions. The initial phase involves efficient identification of substance use and related problems, psychiatric comorbidity, and psychosocial maladjustment (Tarter 1990). The clinician can achieve this objective through the use of screening instruments as a brief first step for assessment of drug use before moving, once it becomes clear that the adolescent may meet criteria for substance use disorder (SUD), to the second step of comprehensive assessment of problem severity. The end result of this assessment is a diagnostic summary that identifies the adolescent's treatment needs (Winters et al. 2008). Finally, the clinician develops an integrative treatment plan to target multidimensional areas of dysfunction, which include psychiatric comorbidity (Winters and Kaminer 2008) as well as potential problems in the school, family, peer, and legal domains. Reports on performance of pediatricians who customarily see youth for periodic checkups and address their medical needs have not been encouraging regarding the physicians' attention to substance use and risk behaviors. Fewer than half of the pediatricians surveyed reported screening adolescents for use of tobacco, alcohol, and other drugs, and fewer than a quarter acknowledged feeling comfortable conducting a comprehensive assessment and offering or making referral for treatment (Halpern-Felsher et al. 2000; Price et al. 2007). The reasons for these troubling figures include the following: insufficient time, lack of training to manage positive screens, need to triage competing medical problems, lack of treatment resources, and unfamiliarity with screening tools (Van Hook et al. 2007).

Clinicians who work with youth should receive formal training in the assessment of substance use and use disorders and should master at least one screening tool and one comprehensive assessment instrument. On the basis of our own clinical and teaching experience, the quantity and quality of training devoted to the screening and assessment of youth substance use, abuse, and dependence in medical schools and psychiatric residency/fellowship training are often insufficient. Little, if any, training is given on how to screen and assess for substance involvement and related problems and on what tools are available to assist with this process. Therefore, the objectives of this chapter are, first, to introduce several established screeners and comprehensive assessments that can be used in any physician's office; second, to address brief interventions for adolescent SUD; and, third, to summarize other major approaches typically used when intensive, longer-term treatment is warranted.

Assessment Domains

Drug Involvement

One major content domain for assessment is the teenager's drug involvement. Relevant variables are age at onset of first and regular drug use; lifetime and recent (e.g., past year) frequency of use and quantity of specific drugs; drug-related consequences and problems, including DSM-5 (American Psychiatric Association 2013) symptoms of an SUD; and reasons for drug use (e.g., psychological benefits).

DSM-5 offers both continuity and changes to the DSM system. As in DSM-IV (American Psychiatric Association 1994), none of the criteria in DSM-5 directly refer to onset, quantity, and frequency variables. A major difference in DSM-5, however, is that there is no longer the distinction between abuse and dependence. In DSM-5, a single SUD for various substance classes is proposed, using a set of 11 symptoms for all substances. Ten of these symptoms were in the DSM-IV abuse and dependence group of symptoms; the eleventh symptom, persistent craving, is new in DSM-5. Individuals are assigned a diagnosis based on how many symptoms on that list the individual meets: no disorder (0–1), mild (2–3), moderate (4–5), or severe (6 or more). The pros and cons of the proposed DSM-5 criteria for adolescents have been discussed in the literature (Kaminer and Winters 2012; Winters et al. 2011). Positives include the combined criterion set to diagnose a single SUD and the elimination of the DSM-IV "legal problems" symptom, which tends to be less relevant for younger teenagers. Nonetheless, several existing criteria—tolerance, withdrawal, hazardous use, and craving—have questionable validity when applied to adolescent drug users.

Biopsychosocial Factors

Another major area for assessment involves the various individual, environmental, and biological factors that impact the onset, development, and maintenance of drug use behaviors. These factors work together to increase (risk factors) or decrease (protective factors) an individual's drug involvement (Clark and Winters 2002). Prevention programs target these factors in their program curriculum, and intervention and treatment programs can personalize treatment by focusing on those factors that are particularly relevant to the client's recovery (Shoham and Insel 2011). The following is a list of core biopsychosocial factors: family history of substance use and SUDs; deviant behavior; peer behavior; self-control; legal problems; psychological and emotional functioning; community population density and level of crime; social connectedness to caring adults and institutions; parenting practices; coping skills; school connectedness; and involvement in conventional activities.

Biological Markers

Drug urinalysis is an important component of the assessment of any substance use and the treatment plan for SUD. The validity of self-report of drug use is challenging because youths in the community, school, and justice system–related settings may either deny use or underreport the amounts, frequency, and latency of drug used (Buchan et al. 2002). It has been suggested that underreporting may be due to social desirability and legal and other perceived consequences. In contrast to self-report only, drug testing provides objective information regarding drug use to those who screen for substance use or treat adolescents with SUD. In addition to chemically screening samples of patient fluids or tissue (e.g., saliva, hair, skin) for drugs of abuse (or their metabolites), clinicians may gain information about the adolescent's status by testing other biological markers that correspond to drug and alcohol use. A *biomarker* is any material or substance used as an indicator of a biologic state. Biomarkers may range from those that directly detect the substance and/or its metabolites to biomarkers that signal end organ damage from chronic substance use. Biomarkers can be useful in adolescent clinical populations by contributing to screening and diagnostic efforts and identifying relapse, continued use, and occult use of substances in patients already identified as having SUDs. Biomarkers, in conjunction with clinical suspicion and rating scales, aid in the screening and diagnosis of substance use disorders (Arias et al. 2011). In addition to their use by clinicians, biomarker tests can be used in the home setting by parents and are available over the counter. For further review of the ethical, legal, and practical considerations of drug testing for youth in school, home, and clinical settings as well as concordance between self-collateral report and drug testing, please refer to a comprehensive review (e.g., Arias et al. 2011).

Screening and Comprehensive Assessment

In this section, we provide an overview of psychometrically sound instruments and measures used for screening and comprehensively assessing a teenager suspected of having a drug problem. The screening process briefly assesses whether or not a person may have a drug problem; a "positive" screen leads to a comprehensive assessment in which detailed information is gathered to assist in determining a diagnosis and planning treatment. All of the tools noted below were developed specifically for youths and are well researched in terms of psychometric properties.

Screening Instruments

There are three types of screening tools based on drug focus: alcohol only, all drugs (including alcohol), and nonalcoholic drugs.

Alcohol Screens

The 24-item Adolescent Drinking Inventory (ADI; Harrell and Wirtz 1989) examines adolescent problem drinking by measuring psychological symptoms, physical symptoms, social symptoms, and loss of control. Scoring of the ADI provides a single score with cutoffs and two research subscale scores (self-medicating drinking and rebellious drinking). The 23-item Rutgers Alcohol Problem Index (RAPI; Martens et al. 2007; White and Labouvie 1989) addresses alcohol use problems in multiple areas of functioning: family life, social relations, psychological adjustment, delinquency, physical problems, and neuropsychological adjustment. The third tool in this group is the Alcohol Screening Protocol for Youth (National Institute on Alcohol Abuse and Alcoholism 2011). This empirically derived tool was based on a collaborative effort by the National Institute on Alcohol Abuse and Alcoholism, the American Academy of Pediatrics, clinical researchers, and health practitioners. The tool consists of only two questions. One focuses on whether or not the youth has friends who drink alcohol, and the other is about personal drinking frequency.

Drug Screens

The 14-item Adolescent Alcohol and Drug Involvement Scale (AADIS; Moberg 2003) measures drug abuse problem severity. The CRAFFT (Kelly et al. 2004; Knight et al. 2002, 2003) is a specialized six-item screen designed to be administered verbally during a primary care interview to address both alcohol and drug use. Its name is a mnemonic device to assist physicians in incorporating six questions during their primary care exams; the trigger words are car, relax, alone, forget, family or friends, and trouble. The GAIN–Short Screener (GAIN-SS; Dennis et al. 2006) is a 3- to 5-minute screener used to quickly identify those who would likely have a disorder based on the full companion instrument, the Global Appraisal of Individual Needs (GAIN; Dennis 1999). The 40-item Personal Experience Screening Questionnaire (PESQ; Winters 1992) consists of a problem severity scale, as well as items on drug use history, psychosocial problems, and response distortion tendencies ("faking good" and "faking bad"). The 81-item Adolescent Substance Abuse Subtle Screening Inventory-2 (SASSI-A2; Miller 2002) yields scores for several scales, including Face Valid Alcohol, Face Valid Other Drug, Obvious Attributes, Subtle Attributes, and Defensiveness.

Nonalcoholic Drug Screens

One screening tool that can be used to examine adolescents' use of nonalcoholic drugs is the Drug Abuse Screening Test for Adolescents (DAST-A; Martino et al. 2000). This tool was adapted from Skinner's (1982) adult tool, the Drug Abuse Screening Test.

Comprehensive Assessment Instruments

Numerous diagnostic interviews, problem-focused interviews, and multiscale questionnaires have been developed for assessing youths suspected of having substance use problems.

Diagnostic Interviews

The majority of the diagnostic interviews in the adolescent field are structured. This format directs the interviewer to read verbatim a series of questions in a decision-tree format, and the answers to these questions are restricted to a few predefined alternatives. The respondent is assigned the responsibility of interpreting the question and deciding on a reply.

There are two well-researched psychiatric diagnostic interviews that address SUDs and other psychiatric disorders. The Diagnostic Interview for Children and Adolescents–Revised (DICA-R; Reich et al. 1992) is a structured interview that is used widely among researchers and clinicians. An instrument that has undergone several adaptations is the Diagnostic Interview Schedule for Children (DISC; Costello et al. 1985; Shaffer et al. 1993). Its DSM-IV version is the DISC-IV (Shaffer et al. 1996, 2000). Separate forms of the interview exist for the child and the parent.

Other diagnostic interviews focus primarily on diagnostic criteria for SUDs. The Adolescent Diagnostic Interview (ADI; Winters and Henly 1993) assesses DSM-IV diagnostic symptoms associated with SUDs, as well as psychosocial stressors, level of functioning, and several adolescent psychiatric disorders. The Customary Drinking and Drug Use Record (CDDR; Brown et al. 1998) measures alcohol and other drug use consumption, DSM-IV substance dependence symptoms (including a detailed assessment of withdrawal symptoms), and several types of consequences of drug involvement. There are both lifetime and prior 2 years versions of the CDDR. The third instrument in this subgroup is the GAIN (Dennis 1999). The GAIN has eight core sections: background, substance use, physical health, risk behaviors and disease prevention, mental and emotional health, environment and living situation, legal, and vocational.

Problem-Focused Interviews

Comprehensive problem-focused interviews measure several problem areas associated with adolescent drug involvement but do not provide a specific diagnostic assessment of SUDs. These interviews assess drug use history and related consequences, as well as several functioning difficulties often experienced by adolescents who abuse drugs.

The Teen Addiction Severity Index (T-ASI; Kaminer et al. 1991) consists of seven content areas: chemical use, school status, employment-support status, family relationships, legal status, peer-social relationships, and psychiatric status. A medical status section was not included because it was deemed to be less relevant to adolescent drug abusers. Adolescent and interviewer severity ratings are elicited on a five-point scale for each content area. Kaminer et al. (1998) also developed a health service utilization tool that compliments the T-ASI, the Teen Treatment Services Review (T-TSR). This interview examines the type and number of services that the youths received during the treatment episode. The Comprehensive Addiction Severity Index for Adolescents (CASI-A; Meyers et al. 1995) measures education, substance use, use of free time, leisure activities, peer relationships, family (including family history and intrafamilial abuse), psychiatric status, and legal history. At the end of several major topics, space is provided for the assessor's comments, severity ratings, and quality ratings of the respondent's answers.

Multiscale Questionnaires

Other comprehensive instruments are self-administered, multiscale questionnaires. Although these instruments vary considerably in terms of administration length (some as short as 20 minutes), they share several characteristics: scales are provided for both drug use problem severity and psychosocial risk factors; strategies are included for detecting response distortion tendencies; norms are provided; and the option of computer administration and scoring is available. Four examples of instruments in this category are the Adolescent Self-Assessment Profile–II (ASAP-II; Wanberg 1998), Hilson Adolescent Profile (HAP; Inwald et al. 1986), Juvenile Automated Substance Abuse Evaluation (JASAE; Ellis 1987), and Personal Experience Inventory (PEI; Winters and Henly 1994).

Assessment Recommendations

Clinicians who work with youth should receive formal training in either medical school or residency in the assessment of substance use and use disorders and should master at least one screen and one comprehensive assessment instrument. The measures described in this section are all suitable not only for initial evaluation but also for periodic reevaluations to measure outcomes of treatment. In choosing which assessment tools to use, clinicians should consider length of administration time, resources in the clinic for training (i.e., professional workforce, funding for time allocated for evaluation, potential reimbursement), and periodic administration to measure multidimensional outcomes. Parameters of quality assurance for the curriculum training material and competence in administration and interpretation after training should be established. Finally, adolescents with SUD may be better served if current programs enable trainees to be more involved with their evaluation and treatment.

Treatment Options

Brief Interventions

Since the mid-1990s, significant progress has been made in the development of evidence-based practice treatment protocols for youths with SUD (Williams and Chang 2000). The focus of more recent interventions has been on several therapeutic approaches and modalities, including cognitive-behavioral therapy (CBT), motivational interviewing (MI), family- and community-based therapies, 12-step/fellowship meetings, contingency management, and integrated interventions (Becker and Curry 2008; Dennis et al. 2004). Most interventions have been provided in outpatient settings, where the vast majority of youths are treated. Despite prominent differences in theory, design, and methodology, studies employing various treatment modalities in youths with SUD have reported remarkably similar outcomes (Waldron and Turner 2008). About 60% of adolescents continued to vacillate in and out of recovery 3 months after discharge from treatment programs (Dennis et al. 2004; Kaminer et al. 2002; Winters et al. 2000). These findings point to the increased need to understand the specific differences between mechanisms of behavior change of therapeutic approaches that carry diverse names and that are distinguished by different ideologies, hypotheses, and technologies (Waldron and Turner 2008).

Most evidence-based treatments are also theory based; however, tests of the mechanisms of action suggested by the theories on which the interventions are based often do not yield positive results (Morgenstern and Longabaugh 2000; Morgenstern and McKay 2007). Some theorists have argued that positive treatment effects are due primarily to what are referred to as "nonspecific" therapeutic factors, such as an empathic and caring therapist, and the structure and support provided by regularly scheduled treatment sessions over a prolonged period of time. Magill (2009) concluded that what is known about treatment process to date is what researchers have chosen to measure. Therefore, it is unclear how unique and exclusive treatment processes are to specific interventions. Evidence points to a common process of change.

Within the addiction field, the search for critical conditions that are necessary and sufficient to induce change has led to the identification of six critical elements, recalled using the acronym FRAMES (Miller and Sanchez 1994): 1) feedback regarding personal risk or impairment, 2) emphasis on personal responsibility for change, 3) clear advice to change, 4) a menu of alternative change options, 5) therapist empathy, and 6) facilitation of participant optimism about the potential to change and self-efficacy. Therapeutic interventions containing some or all of these elements have been effective in initiating change and reducing alcohol use. Baseline and posttreatment assessments conducted by empathic and caring staff contain some or all of the components or active ingredients of FRAMES. Consequently, these interactions might be effective in initiating change and reducing substance use, although a priori they were not intended to be therapeutic.

Cognitive-Behavioral Therapy

The majority of CBT approaches integrate strategies derived from classical conditioning, operant perspectives, and social learning. Such interventions typically involve identifying contextual factors, such as settings, situations, or states, that may serve as potential "triggers" for substance abuse or relapse (Marlatt and Gordon 1985; Witkiewitz and Marlatt 2004). Operant perspectives view substance abuse as a behavior that follows an antecedent (i.e., a trigger) and that may lead to negative consequences. This sequence is the focus of exploration in functional analysis conducted with the patient to identify triggers for substance use behavior. The social learning model incorporates the influence of environmental events on the acquisition of behavior but also recognizes the role of cognitive processes in determining behavior (Bandura 1977, 1986).

CBT approaches view substance use and related problems as learned behaviors that are initiated and maintained in the context of environmental factors. CBT hypothesizes that those who do not make progress in treatment or who relapse either lack or are deficient in the coping skills necessary to deal with life stressors and high-risk situations. Therefore, improvement in these skills will increase self-efficacy or confidence in the ability to refrain from drug use (Waldron and Kaminer 2004). Self-efficacy appears to be a partial mediator of treatment outcome. In a large multicenter study on the treatment of adults with cannabis use disorders, increase in self-efficacy from pretreatment to posttreatment was a more powerful predictor of decrease in drug use than was change in coping skills (Litt et al. 2003). In addition, early abstinence appears to be important, to the extent that it increases self-efficacy (Litt et al. 2008). Nevertheless, contrary to expectations, the CBT treatment group did not experience greater coping skills acquisition than did an MI comparison group. Similarly, in an adolescent treatment study, self-efficacy was found to be directly correlated with treatment outcome, even when controlling for drug-positive urine in treatment and regardless of therapeutic approach (Burleson and Kaminer 2005). In other words, regardless of the "theory-driven" CBT, it did not produce higher levels of self-efficacy compared with interpersonal treatment.

Few studies have focused on the hypothesized mechanisms of change underlying CBT in youths. Most notably, coping factors have been identified as significant predictors of treatment outcome (Myers et al. 1993).

CBT sessions characteristically include modeling, behavior rehearsal, feedback, and homework assignments. It is important to take into account the adolescent's age and developmental level. Moreover, many youths may not have had sufficient opportunity to acquire certain social and coping skills normally developed during adolescence because of their heavy drug use, and therefore components may need to be incorporated to address basic skill deficits.

The most influential psychosocial intervention study conducted with youth was the Cannabis Youth Treatment (CYT) study, a randomized noncontrolled field experiment in which five interventions, in various combinations, were compared across four implementation sites (Dennis et al. 2004). The study was designed to address the differential efficacy of the treatments implemented and the effect of treatment dose on outcome. Two group CBT interventions were offered. Both began with two individual motivational enhancement therapy (MET) sessions, which were followed by either three CBT sessions (MET/CBT-5; Sampl and Kadden 2001) or 10 CBT sessions (MET/CBT-12; Webb et al. 2002). A third intervention represented a family-based add-on intervention involving MET/CBT-12 plus a 6-week family psychoeducational intervention (Hamilton et al. 2001). In addition, a 12-session individual Adolescent Community Reinforcement Approach (Godley et al. 2001) and a 12-week multidimensional family therapy (MDFT) condition (Liddle 2002) were included. The five treatment models were evaluated in two arms, in a community-based program and an academic medical center. Although not all five models were implemented within treatment sites, the replication of the MET/CBT-5 intervention across all four sites made it possible to study site differences and conduct quasi-experimental comparisons of the interventions across study arms.

Overall, a total of 600 adolescents ages 13–18 were randomly assigned to one of three interventions. With follow-up rates of 98% at 3 months and 94% at 12 months, Dennis et al. (2004) reported that all five interventions produced significant reductions in cannabis use and negative consequences of use from pretreatment to the 3-month follow-up, and these reductions were sustained through the 12-month follow-up. In addition, changes in marijuana use were accompanied by reductions in behavioral problems, family problems, school problems, school absences, argumentativeness, violence, and illegal activity. In terms of cost-effectiveness ratio, MDFT was found to be higher than other interventions (French et al. 2002).

Consistent empirical support has been found for group CBT for substance-abusing adolescents (Burleson et al. 2006; Dennis et al. 2004). These findings stand in contrast to the iatrogenic "deviant" peer-group effects reported for group interventions (Dishion et al. 1999, 2001). In neither the CYT study group interventions mentioned earlier in this section nor in the Waldron et al. (2001) and Kaminer et al. (2002) interventions in outpatient settings, which included a significant percentage of adolescents with conduct disorders, did therapists experience any severe or unmanageable problems related to conducting group therapy (e.g., need to eject subjects, need to discontinue a session, physical abuse). It appears that diverse referral sources allow for a mix of adolescents who are manageable in a group setting once a clearly communicated and signed behavioral contract for ground rules is introduced. Experienced therapists should be able to address inappropriate behavior and to troubleshoot other issues, particularly when using a manual-driven treatment (Apodaca and Longabaugh 2009).

Brief Motivational Interventions

The theoretical basis of brief motivational intervention (BMI) is grounded in client-centered therapy, particular therapists' "accurate empathy" (Rogers 1957), social learning theory (Bandura 1977), CBT (Marlatt and Gordon 1985), and the transtheoretical paradigm of change (Prochaska et al. 1992). This theoretical basis, in turn, resulted in the shift from viewing motivation as a "trait" to a "state" (Maisto et al. 1999). BMIs utilize a harm reduction approach that is tailored to the needs of the individual. BMI appeals to clinicians because of its short course (i.e., from one to five sessions), the increased rapport with patients, and the improved commitment of the patient to change. The manual for the use of MET with alcoholic adult patients was reported in Project MATCH (1997), whereas the CYT study provided the MET manual for youth (Sampl and Kadden 2001).

The transtheoretical model describes five stages of change through which people progress in the process of modifying problem behaviors; these stages are precontemplation, contemplation, determination, action, and maintenance. The MET approach addresses where the client currently is in the cycle of change and assists him or her to move through the stages toward action and maintenance. Miller and Rollnick (2002) developed MI, emphasizing that the term *motivational interviewing* pertains both to a style of relating to others and a set of techniques to facilitate that process. They described five main strategies that are used in applying this approach: 1) expressing empathy, 2) developing discrepancy, 3) avoiding argumentation, 4) rolling with resistance, and 5) supporting self-efficacy. It is important for a clinician to respond to a client's needs in a way perceived as helpful yet to keep the responsibility for change on the client. MI decreases the likelihood of being drawn into a power struggle and arguing with the resistant (i.e., precontemplator) or ambivalent (i.e., contemplator) client about the need to change. More specifically, employing an empathic style is demonstrated by reflective listening techniques and a warm attitude. Developing discrepancy is achieved through inquiring about the patient's short- and long-term goals and exploring how the addictive behavior affects the process of achieving these goals. Avoiding argumentation and rolling with resistance are achieved by avoiding debates about beliefs, perceptions, or behaviors; acknowledging the differences between individuals' positions; and being able to accept and tolerate other opinions and to change without becoming defensive.

Although increased motivation or readiness to change does not appear to be the mechanism or mediator of behavior change (Borsari et al. 2009), several studies of youths emphasize the importance of readiness to change in predicting treatment outcomes. Godley et al. (2007) reported that motivated adolescents were three times more likely than nonmotivated youths to remain abstinent during aftercare and to show improved engagement. Higher motivation to abstain predicted fewer days of marijuana use in adolescents (King et al. 2009). Chung and Maisto (2009) reported that there was a reciprocal association between motivation to change and substance use. Furthermore, a majority of adolescents reported that substance abuse treatment helped to increase their readiness to change substance use behavior. MI was suggested to increase *change talk*, a construct describing more assertive statements about the wish to limit or stop using drugs, which was associated with better outcomes in adults (Moyers et al. 2007) and youths (Baer et al. 2008); however, the mechanisms that foster change talk in youths have not yet been identified. Chung and Maisto (2009) suggest investigating social network characteristics that might affect motivation to change.

BMIs for youth have been useful (Monti et al. 2001; Tevyaw and Monti 2004). In a study in which people ages 16–20 years were randomized to a single session of MI designed to reduce illicit drug use or to a nonintervention control group, McCambridge and Strang (2004) reported a significant decrease in cannabis use among the MI subjects at 12-week follow-up compared with subjects in the control group. Several earlier studies successfully employed BMI following a negative event, such as alcohol-related trauma and referral to the emergency room. These interventions capitalized on a "teachable moment"; that is, the salience of an alcohol-related event may increase sense of vulnerability and make an adolescent more receptive to intervention (Spirito et al. 2004).

BMI can be a very attractive treatment option for adolescents. "It is not necessary for adolescents to admit to or acknowledge having substance use problems in order to benefit from BMI, because BMI can be applied to individuals within a range of readiness to change" (Tevyaw and Monti 2004, p. 65). BMI alone may not be sufficient for adolescents with high-severity SUD or with psychiatric comorbidity. However, front-loading BMI onto adolescent treatments such as CBT, as successfully reported in the CYT study (Dennis et al. 2004), might affect proximal outcomes by improving engagement and by providing feedback to increase readiness for change.

Family Therapy

Adolescent substance abuse treatments that involve family members and seek to change or influence an adolescent's environment have demonstrated considerable efficacy in several randomized clinical trials (Dennis et al. 2004; Rigter et al. 2005; Vaughn and Howard 2008). A shared assumption among approaches is that adolescents are part of multiple systems, which are critical to incorporate as change agents or to address during treatment (Dakof et al. 2011). Family therapy includes several forms of manualized interventions for adolescent substance abuse, including multisystemic therapy (MST), the Adolescent Community Reinforcement Approach (A-CRA), MDFT, and brief strategic family therapy (BSFT).

Multisystemic Therapy

MST is an intensive (up to 60 hours) home-based intervention for families that addresses multiple systems, including schools, peer groups, parenting skills, communication skills, family relations, and other cognitive-behavioral change (Henggeler et al. 1998). The approach incorporates structural and strategic family therapy and CBT (Henggeler and Borduin 1995). A pivotal strategy is incorporating an ecological approach by providing the intervention in the adolescent's home and community. Such an approach removes one of the most important barriers to treatment—that is, bringing the teen and his or her family to the clinic. Henggeler et al. (2006) reported the findings from a randomized controlled study that compared outcomes for substance-abusing juvenile offenders assigned to family court with usual services (FC), drug court with usual services (DC), drug court with MST (DC/MST), or drug court with MST and contingency management (DC/MST/CM). In regard to substance use outcome, DC/MST and DC/MST/CM did not produce a better outcome than DC alone. Similar findings were found for rearrest rates and out-of-home placement. These outcomes suggest the need for cost-effective analyses to determine whether addition of MST services to drug courts is justified.

With the goal of assessing the impact of MST on behavioral and psychosocial outcomes for youths and families, Littell et al. (2005) identified 35 MST outcome studies, of which 8 met inclusion criteria for their review. They concluded that available evidence does not support the hypothesis that MST is consistently more effective than usual services or other interventions for youths with social, emotional, or behavioral problems. The authors asserted that MST has no evidence of harmful effects compared with alternative services, that the approach has several advantages over other approaches in that it is a comprehensive intervention based on current knowledge of youth and family problems, and that MST is well documented and studied.

Adolescent Community Reinforcement Approach

A-CRA has been widely implemented in over 50 treatment agencies in 20 states in the United States. The intervention was originally developed as an approach to treat adults with alcohol use disorder (Azrin et al. 1982). It was adapted for adolescents, manualized, and evaluated as part of the CYT study (Godley et al. 2001). A-CRA also has been evaluated in randomized clinical trials of assertive continuing care (Godley et al. 2007) and as an intervention with homeless adolescents (Slesnick et al. 2007).

The overall style of A-CRA is behavioral or cognitive-behavioral. Therapists are trained to identify each adolescent's and caregiver's individual reinforcers. Then the therapist helps the adolescent and family recognize the relationships between attaining reinforcers and reducing or stopping substance use. These reinforcers can be used as therapists discuss with adolescents and parents why it is important to attend sessions, learn and practice new skills, and sample periods of not using.

Another primary goal of A-CRA is to increase the adolescent's family, social, and educational/vocational reinforcers, so that the adolescent's environment will increasingly support recovery. Conversely, if an adolescent uses alcohol or other drugs, then a time-out from these reinforcers occurs (based on Hunt and Azrin 1973). To facilitate engagement and retention, the therapist uses warmth, makes understanding statements, and is nonjudgmental.

The A-CRA manual developed for the CYT study (Godley et al. 2001) outlines an outpatient program that targets youths ages 12–18 with DSM-IV diagnoses of cannabis, alcohol, and/or other SUDs. However, A-CRA also has been implemented in intensive outpatient and residential treatment settings. A-CRA includes guidelines for three types of sessions: adolescents alone, parents/caregivers alone, and adolescents and parents/caregivers together. Treatment begins with an overview of what the adolescent can expect, and emphasizes that the goal of therapy is to help the adolescent have a more satisfying life.

Subsequent sessions are very flexible, and the clinician draws from a toolbox of 17 treatment procedures to help adolescents improve their quality of life and decrease or eliminate alcohol and/or drug use. Some procedures, such as anger management and job-seeking skills, will be used only if needed by a particular adolescent. Two sessions are designed for caregivers alone and two more for caregivers and adolescents together to work on improving their relationship(s). These four sessions with caregivers are considered the minimum number; more can be added if needed. Role-playing/behavioral rehearsal is a critical component of the skills training components (e.g., drug refusal, problem solving). Every session ends with a mutually agreed upon homework assignment to either practice skills learned during sessions or engage in a new prosocial activity after potential barriers to completing the assignment are discussed and addressed through problem solving. To reinforce completion of homework, which helps ensure generalization of skills learned in sessions to the adolescent's natural environment, each session begins with a review of the homework assignment.

Multidimensional Family Therapy

MDFT combines drug counseling with multiple systems assessment and intervention, both inside and outside the family. This manualized approach is developmentally and ecologically oriented and is delivered in 16–25 sessions over 4–6 months in the home or office.

The model is used widely as an effective science-based treatment for adolescent SUDs and delinquency (e.g., Liddle et al. 2008, 2009; Wal-

dron and Turner 2008). MDFT is theory driven, combining aspects of
several theoretical frameworks (i.e., family systems theory, developmental psychology, and the risk and protective model of adolescent substance abuse). It incorporates key elements of adolescent drug
treatment, including comprehensive assessment, an integrated treatment approach, family involvement, developmentally appropriate interventions, specialized engagement and retention protocols, attention
to qualifications of staff and their ongoing training, gender and cultural
competence, and a focus on a broad range of outcomes (Liddle et al.
2006).

MDFT is both a tailored and flexible treatment delivery system and,
depending on the needs of the youth and family, can be conducted from
one to three times per week over the course of 3–6 months, both in the
home and in the clinic. Therapists work simultaneously in four interde-
pendent treatment domains—the adolescent, parent, family, and community—each of which is addressed in three stages: 1) building a
foundation for change, 2) facilitating individual and family change, and
3) solidifying changes. At various points throughout treatment, the
therapist meets alone with the adolescent, alone with the parent(s), or
conjointly with the adolescent and parent(s), depending on the treatment domain and specific problem being addressed.

The MDFT treatment team typically includes a therapist assistant
who, in a highly coordinated collaboration with the therapist, works
with the family in the context of important institutions that influence
their lives. For example, the therapist assistant might help the parents
find a more appropriate school placement for their teen, obtain needed
economic assistance such as food stamps and Medicaid, or procure
mental health or substance abuse treatment services for themselves, the
teen, or other children in the family.

MDFT and A-CRA are similar in several ways, even though some of
the underlying theories, therapeutic guidelines, and methods differ. Although A-CRA, MDFT, and other efficacious treatments for adolescent
substance abuse have distinct therapeutic formats and methods that differentiate them, Dennis et al. (2004) suggested that carefully designed
and implemented interventions will result in generally favorable outcomes regardless of specific therapeutic model, techniques, or methods.

Brief Strategic Family Therapy

BSFT was developed and refined for Hispanic families with youths who
have behavior problems by Szapocznik et al. (2002). BSFT is structured
so that the entire family meets once weekly for 8–12 weeks and includes

specialized engagement strategies. The effectiveness of BSFT was reported by Santisteban et al. (2003), who randomly assigned youths to BSFT or group therapy and assessed youths posttreatment. Although youths in both conditions showed significant reductions in substance use, those assigned to BSFT showed significantly more improvement in drug use, conduct problems, delinquency fostered by peer group, and family functioning than did those in group therapy. The differential improvement in family functioning among youths in BSFT is significant in that this is the proposed mediator of change for the intervention.

Using a social ecological formulation (Bronfenbrenner 1979) to guide treatment intervention, Slesnick and Prestopnik (2005) compared ecologically based family therapy conducted in the home (EBFT) with treatment as usual (TAU) through the local shelter for primary drug-abusing runaway adolescents. Overall, youths receiving EBFT showed a greater reduction in overall substance use compared with those assigned to TAU. Gender and ethnicity did not differentially influence outcome. However, an interaction was found between abuse history, time, and modality. Among youths who reported physical and sexual abuse, those assigned to EBFT reported fewer problem consequences and reported a reduction in the number of different drugs used over time compared with those receiving TAU. Both EBFT and TAU groups showed significant improvements over time on measures of psychological and family functioning.

According to Slesnick et al. (2008), few studies have compared family therapies with one another, and no evidence is available to suggest that one type of family therapy is superior to another, because all share the underlying conceptual framework that individual problems are best understood and addressed at the level of family interaction. In sum, outcome research has provided support for the positive impact of family therapy on reducing alcohol and drug use, increasing engagement and retention in treatment, reducing internalizing and externalizing problems, improving family interaction, and increasing the adolescent's involvement in school.

Twelve-Step Mutual-Help Programs and Youth

Professional treatment approaches targeting adolescent SUDs in the United States often incorporate the 12-step philosophy and practices of community mutual-help organizations (MHOs) such as Alcoholics Anonymous (AA) and Narcotics Anonymous (NA) (Drug Strategies 2003; Roman and Blum 1999). In addition, most treatment programs encourage attendance and refer youths to community AA and NA groups following treatment to help prevent relapse and support recovery (Knudsen et al. 2008).

In theory, community MHOs such as AA and NA possess certain elements that make them attractive as adjuncts to formal care. Meetings are available in most communities several times a day, notably at times of high relapse risk, such as evenings and weekends, when professional care is often unavailable. Between meetings, sponsors (MHO mentors) and other fellowship members often make themselves available on demand (e.g., by telephone) 7 days a week at any time. Because a major precursor to adolescent relapse is association with pretreatment substance-using friends, the socially oriented abstinence-focused structure of AA and NA could serve as a useful antidote by providing access to a new, recovery-specific social network that reduces exposure to social situations in which alcohol and drugs might be present. Also of note is the fact that AA and NA groups can be attended free of charge (or with voluntary contributions) for as long as an individual desires.

Developmentally related differences between adolescents and adults suggest, however, that 12-step fellowships may not be an ideal fit for youths. For instance, compared with adults, adolescents on average possess less addiction severity and related sequelae and lower substance-related problem recognition and motivation for abstinence (e.g., Stewart and Brown 1995; Tims et al. 2002). They are also substantially younger than the majority of AA and NA members (e.g., Alcoholics Anonymous 2012). Furthermore, some youths may feel less comfortable with the degree of spiritual or religious emphasis in AA and NA. Conceivably, such differences might signify a poor fit with 12-step fellowships' unwavering emphasis on abstinence and spiritual growth.

Following a call for greater research on AA by the Institute of Medicine (1990), evidence accumulated during the past 25 years regarding the benefits of adult 12-step MHO participation (e.g., Kelly and Yeterian 2011) has led influential organizations such as the American Psychiatric Association and the Department of Veterans Affairs to include standard referral to these groups in their clinical practice guidelines (American Psychiatric Association 1995; Veterans Health Administration 2001). However, a lingering question for providers of adolescent SUD treatment is to what extent clinical resources (if any) should be devoted to facilitating posttreatment 12-step MHO participation.

Compared with adults, less is known about the empirical relationships between AA or NA participation and recovery or benefits among young people, but the quantity and quality of the evidence has increased (Kelly and Myers 2007; Sussman 2010). Several prospective empirical studies of increasing scientific rigor have emerged during the past 15 years of examining AA or NA participation and its relation to adolescent substance use outcomes following treatment. These studies have shown that adolescents who participate in AA or NA post-treatment have much lower relapse rates (Chi et al. 2009; Kennedy and Minami 1993), have more abstinent days (Kelly et al. 2008), and are more likely to be completely abstinent (Hsieh et al. 1998; Kelly et al. 2000). A prospective 8-year follow-up study of adolescents treated initially for SUD at the average age of 16 found that for every 12-step meeting youths attended over the 8-year period, they gained an additional 2 days of abstinence, over and above the effects of other factors associated with good outcome. Also, it was found that attending one meeting per week was associated with significant benefit, whereas attending two to three meetings per week was associated with complete abstinence. Other studies have found that youths who become more actively involved in MHOs (e.g., obtain and use a sponsor, participate verbally during meetings) have better outcomes posttreatment (Kelly et al. 2002, 2008) and experience benefit over and above the recovery benefits derived from AA or NA attendance alone (Dow and Kelly 2012; Kelly and Urbanoski 2012).

Some evidence suggests that the characteristics of certain 12-step groups may moderate the likelihood of participation and derived benefits. Kelly et al. (2005) examined the relationship between the age composition of 12-step groups and adolescents' frequency of attendance, degree of involvement, and substance use outcomes. The greater the age similarity between adolescent study participants and other 12-step attendees, the more likely youths were to rate 12-step attendance as being important to recovery, to attend 12-step meetings more frequently, and to have better treatment outcomes. This age-matching effect appeared to diminish over time, however, such that adolescents who continued to attend mostly teenage meetings derived progressively less benefit. This early, but diminishing, age-matching effect was replicated in a young adult sample (Labbe et al. 2013). Findings from these studies suggest that age similarity may be helpful for engaging youths in 12-step MHOs and that it is associated with more abstinence early in posttreatment but that adolescents may need gradual access to a broader range of meetings with more of an age mix, including older individuals with longer-term sobriety and life experience.

The empirical focus on MHO effects in adults has moved beyond asking whether they are effective to asking how they work (Kelly et al. 2009). Less work has been conducted in this regard using adolescent samples (Chi et al. 2009; Kelly et al. 2000, 2002, 2014). Findings suggest that although young MHO participants and adult MHO participants benefit from 12-step MHOs to similar degrees, the ways in which the two groups benefit differ. Studies have found that youths may benefit from the continual remotivating aspects of 12-step meetings (i.e., exposure to successful recovery role models, support for abstinence/recovery lifestyles, continual reminders of past negative consequences associated with active use). Whereas adults appear to benefit mostly from the social network changes associated with 12-step participation, adolescents and young adults do not appear to benefit in this way, perhaps because they find it more difficult to make new social contacts at meetings because fewer people are their own age (Kelly et al. 2014).

Contingency Management

An approach that has not been explored extensively in youths with SUD is the CM reinforcement that provides rewards for drug-free urinalysis. It has been hypothesized that drug abstinence can be improved by providing tangible incentives that are contingent on providing objective evidence of abstinence.

Petry (2000) delineated a strategy for CM that involves rearranging the substance user's environment so that 1) drug use and abstinence are readily detected, 2) drug abstinence is positively reinforced, 3) drug use results in an immediate loss of reinforcement, and 4) the density of reinforcement derived from nondrug sources is increased to compete with the reinforcing effects of drugs. Higgins et al. (1995) stressed the following core strengths of CM: 1) conceptual clarity, 2) empiricism and operationalism, 3) compatibility with pharmacotherapies, 4) clinical breadth, and 5) demonstrable efficacy.

An abstinence reinforcement system used in combination with an intensive behavioral treatment program has produced positive short-term outcomes in adult cannabis abusers for up to 35% of participants during treatment (Budney et al. 2000, 2006; Kadden et al. 2007). However, maintenance of treatment gains when the reinforcement was no longer available after treatment completion was poor.

The few CM studies targeting abstinence in youths with SUD have mostly involved noncontrolled, nonrandomized, very small samples that have generated acceptable feasibility and demonstrated preliminary promising efficacy of CM among adolescents in reducing use of mainly cannabis and tobacco (Kamon et al. 2005; Stanger and Budney 2010; Tevyaw et al. 2007). A randomized controlled study of CM plus

MST compared with MST only in juvenile drug courts did not show significant improvement for the addition of CM (Henggeler et al. 2006).

Some success has been reported for the use of an abstinence-contingent reward system. Kamon et al. (2005) showed the feasibility of a voucher-based, contingent reward system integrated with individual-based CBT for marijuana use and related disorders for 19 youths and their parents. Subsequently, Stanger et al. (2009) conducted a randomized trial involving 69 adolescents and their parents; both conditions received individualized MET and CBT, but only one condition also received family therapy. Stanger and Budney (2010) concluded that despite compelling evidence regarding the efficacy and the wide acceptability and applicability of these procedures in adults, only limited evidence supports employing CM procedures with adolescents. Therefore, continued research on CM procedures with youth, which includes a component examining what might differentiate the mechanism of change in adolescent CM intervention compared with adults, could be useful. This limited evidence might be associated with brain maturity level and developmental delayed-discounting phenomenon (Kaminer et al. 2014).

Adaptive Treatment and Aftercare

In general, it is sensible to refer to patients as either good, partial, or poor responders to treatment. The term *relapse prevention* has traditionally applied only to those who have achieved sobriety or abstinence. Patients who have not improved will be unlikely to respond to more of the same treatment. Therefore, clinicians should change and adapt patients' treatment by implementing an alternative sequential treatment plan similar to the pharmacological algorithm commonly used for psychiatric disorders in youth (e.g., depression, attention-deficit/hyperactivity disorder).

Historically, *aftercare* (known also as continued care) referred to maintenance interventions (e.g., group counseling, fellowship meetings) following a successful course of an index biopsychosocial treatment for SUD. Step-down care (i.e., referral to successively lower-intensity treatment episodes) is the most common form of aftercare (MacKay 2009). The step-down model, however, has not proven to be a common course for adolescents. A more typical course is for adolescents to either discontinue their acute care episode prematurely or experience relapse relatively soon after discharge without being involved in aftercare. The American Society of Addiction Medicine (2001) thus defined *continuing care* as flexible services that provide patients with SUD the type of treatment needed at any given time. This definition of continuing care implies that for many and perhaps most patients, SUD is ongoing and may recur in the same manner as other chronic diseases. Although this definition is well recognized in practice, even the best-intended referrals are more likely to result in failure to show without assertive interaction by a clinician (Godley et al. 2007).

Addiction treatment researchers have reported positive outcomes of aftercare or continuing care in randomized controlled trials involving adolescents with SUD. Godley et al. (2007) reported on an assertive continuing care protocol. This manualized approach (Godley et al. 2006) includes a combination of community visits (home, school, and other locations), case management, and A-CRA (Godley et al. 2001).

Because the vast majority of adolescents receive their index care episode in outpatient treatment, studies are needed to extend the understanding of aftercare or continuing care following outpatient treatment. Kaminer et al. (2008) conducted an aftercare study with adolescents who were randomly assigned after completion of treatment to one of the following: a five-session face-to-face booster course of CBT, a brief telephone intervention, or no active aftercare. At the end of the 3-month aftercare phase, the likelihood of relapse, days of alcohol use, and days of heavy alcohol use were significantly greater for adolescents with no active aftercare than for those in the active aftercare conditions. This study provides experimental support that during the aftercare phase, active aftercare prevents relapse. Post-aftercare outcomes are still needed to assess long-term effectiveness of active aftercare.

Future strategies for aftercare should incorporate use of communication technologies embraced by youths in contemporary society. Most youths today, including those receiving SUD treatment, have mobile phones. The brief telephone protocol of Kaminer and Napolitano (2010) is a flexible protocol that can be paired with assertive patient-locating procedures. A short message service texting version of the protocol could also be tested, because many adolescents increasingly prefer this mode of communication over voice. In one survey of treated youths, over 90% reported having Myspace.com profiles (Kaminer and Godley 2010), underscoring just how ubiquitous Web-based social networking has become among adolescents. Future research on adaptive treatment for adolescents should be mated to tracking technologies that are clearly embraced by youths to increase the chances of long-term retention, monitoring, support, and, when necessary, reintervention. Finally, the gap between clinical care and science persists in clinical care of youth. To promote delivery of evidence-based effective care, a meta-systematic approach should be adopted (Kazak et al. 2010).

Summary and Future Directions

Engaging and retaining adolescents in any kind of SUD treatment is a challenge. Low problem recognition and low motivation can make it difficult to obtain detailed information during an assessment and to achieve meaningful behavior change. Fortunately, clinicians have standardized screening and assessment tools, and a range of well-researched treatment approaches are available. Future research directions should focus on understanding the mechanisms of change of different interventions at various critical points of treatment, improving short- and long-term outcomes, and maintaining treatment gains in aftercare programs. Focus on adaptive treatments for poor responders and rapid relapsers is imperative. Finally, examining the transportability of interventions into other treatment modalities, such as phone (Kaminer and Napolitano 2010) or Internet interventions, as well as into other community settings, is desirable.

KEY POINTS

- Screening, comprehensive assessment, triage, and referral to treatment is the recommended sequence.

- The use of a validated and developmentally informed instrument is key to effective assessments.

- Youths with substance use disorders (SUDS) should be referred for specialty treatment.

- There is no obvious difference in the effectiveness of various single-modality interventions in treating SUD. Therefore, comprehensive interventions and the inclusion of drug urinalysis are preferable.

- Continuity of care, including posttreatment interventions, is pivotal in preventing or delaying relapse.

References

Alcoholics Anonymous: Alcoholics Anonymous 2011 Membership Survey. New York, Alcoholics Anonymous World Services, 2012

American Psychiatric Association: Diagnostic and Statistical Manual of Mental Disorders, 4th Edition. Washington, DC, American Psychiatric Association, 1994

American Psychiatric Association: Practice guideline for psychiatric evaluation of adults. Am J Psychiatry 152(11 suppl):63–80, 1995 9565542

American Psychiatric Association: Diagnostic and Statistical Manual of Mental Disorders, 5th Edition. Arlington, VA, American Psychiatric Association, 2013

American Society of Addiction Medicine: Patient Placement Criteria for the Treatment of Substance-Related Disorders, 2nd Edition. Chevy Chase, MD, American Society of Addiction Medicine, 2001

Apodaca TR, Longabaugh R: Mechanisms of change in motivational interviewing: a review and preliminary evaluation of the evidence. Addiction 104(5):705–715, 2009 19413785

Arias JE, Arias AJ, Kaminer Y: Biomarkers testing for substance use in adolescents, in Clinical Manual of Adolescent Substance Abuse Treatment. Edited by Kaminer Y, Winters KC. Washington, DC, American Psychiatric Publishing, 2011 pp 83–112

Azrin NH, Sisson RW, Meyers R, et al: Alcoholism treatment by disulfiram and community reinforcement therapy. J Behav Ther Exp Psychiatry 13(2):105–112, 1982 7130406

Baer JS, Beadnell B, Garrett SB, et al: Adolescent change language within a brief motivational intervention and substance use outcomes. Psychol Addict Behav 22(4):570–575, 2008 19071983

Bandura A: Social Learning Theory. Englewood Cliffs, NJ, Prentice Hall, 1977

Bandura A: Social Foundations of Thought and Action: A Social Cognitive Theory. Englewood Cliffs, NJ, Prentice Hall, 1986

Becker SJ, Curry JF: Outpatient interventions for adolescent substance abuse: a quality of evidence review. J Consult Clin Psychol 76(4):531–543, 2008 18665683

Borsari B, Murphy JG, Carey KB: Readiness to change in brief motivational interventions: a requisite condition for drinking reductions? Addict Behav 34(2):232–235, 2009 18990500

Bronfenbrenner U: The Ecology of Human Development. Cambridge, MA, Harvard University Press, 1979

Brown SA, Myers MG, Lippke L, et al: Psychometric evaluation of the Customary Drinking and Drug Use Record (CDDR): a measure of adolescent alcohol and drug involvement. J Stud Alcohol 59(4):427–438, 1998 9647425

Buchan BJ, Dennis M, Tims FM, et al: Cannabis use: consistency and validity of self-report, on-site urine testing and laboratory testing. Addiction 97(suppl 1):98–108, 2002 12460132

Budney AJ, Higgins ST, Radonovich KJ, et al: Adding voucher-based incentives to coping skills and motivational enhancement improves outcomes during treatment for marijuana dependence. J Consult Clin Psychol 68(6):1051–1061, 2000 11142539

Budney AJ, Moore BA, Rocha HL, et al: Clinical trial of abstinence-based vouchers and cognitive-behavioral therapy for cannabis dependence. J Consult Clin Psychol 74(2):307–316, 2006 16649875

Burleson J, Kaminer Y: Self-efficacy as a predictor of treatment outcome in adolescent substance use disorders. Addict Behav 20(9):1751–1764, 2005 16095844

Burleson JA, Kaminer Y, Dennis ML: Absence of iatrogenic or contagion effects in adolescent group therapy: findings from the Cannabis Youth Treatment (CYT) study. Am J Addict 15 (suppl 1):4–15, 2006 17182415

Chi FW, Kaskutas LA, Sterling S, et al: Twelve-Step affiliation and 3-year substance use outcomes among adolescents: social support and religious service attendance as potential mediators. Addiction 104(6):927–939, 2009 19344442

Chung T, Maisto SA: "What I got from treatment": predictors of treatment content received and association of treatment content with 6-month outcomes in adolescents. J Subst Abuse Treat 37(2):171–181, 2009 19339134

Clark DB, Winters KC: Measuring risks and outcomes in substance use disorders prevention research. J Consult Clin Psychol 70(6):1207–1223, 2002 12472298

Costello EJ, Edelbrock CS, Costello AJ: Validity of the NIMH Diagnostic Interview Schedule for Children: a comparison between psychiatric and pediatric referrals. J Abnorm Child Psychol 13(4):579–595, 1985 4078188

Dakof GA, Godley SH, Smith JE: The adolescent community reinforcement approach and multidimensional family therapy: addressing relapse during treatment, in Clinical Manual of Adolescent Substance Abuse Treatment. Edited by Kaminer Y, Winters KC. Washington, DC, American Psychiatric Publishing, 2011, pp 239–268

Dennis ML: Global Appraisal of Individual Needs (GAIN): Administration Guide for the GAIN and Related Measures. Normal, IL, Chestnut Health Systems, 1999

Dennis M, Godley SH, Diamond G, et al: The Cannabis Youth Treatment (CYT) study: main findings from two randomized trials. J Subst Abuse Treat 27(3):197–213, 2004 15501373

Dennis ML, Chan YF, Funk RR: Development and validation of the GAIN Short Screener (GSS) for internalizing, externalizing and substance use disorders and crime/violence problems among adolescents and adults. Am J Addict 15 (suppl 1):80–91, 2006 17182423

Dishion TJ, McCord J, Poulin F: When interventions harm: peer groups and problem behavior. Am Psychol 54(9):755–764, 1999 10510665

Dishion TJ, Poulin F, Burraston B: Peer group dynamics associated with iatrogenic effects in group interventions with high-risk young adolescents. New Dir Child Adolesc Dev 91(91):79–92, 2001 11280015

Dow SJ, Kelly JF: Listening to youth: adolescents' self-reported reasons for alcohol and drug use as a unique predictor of treatment response and outcome (abstract). Alcohol Clin Exp Res 36 (suppl s1):158A, 2012

Drug Strategies: Treating Teens: A Guide to Adolescent Programs. Washington, DC, Drug Strategies, 2003

Ellis BR: Juvenile Automated Substance Abuse Evaluation (JASAE). Clarkston, MI, ADE Incorporated, 1987

French MT, Roebuck MC, Dennis ML, et al: The economic cost of outpatient marijuana treatment for adolescents: findings from a multi-site field experiment. Addiction 97 (suppl 1):84–97, 2002 12460131

Godley MD, Godley SH, Dennis ML, et al: The effect of assertive continuing care on continuing care linkage, adherence and abstinence following residential treatment for adolescents with substance use disorders. Addiction 102(1):81–93, 2007 17207126

Godley SH, Meyers RS, Smith JE: The Adolescent Community Reinforcement Approach For Adolescent Cannabis Users (Cannabis Youth Treatment Series [CYT], Vol 4). Rockville, MD, Center for Substance Abuse Treatment, 2001

Godley SH, Godley MD, Karvinen T, et al: The Assertive Continuing Care Protocol: A Clinician's Manual for Working With Adolescents After Residential Treatment of Alcohol and Other Substance Use Disorders, 2nd Edition. Bloomington, IL, Lighthouse Institute, 2006

Halpern-Felsher BL, Ozer EM, Millstein SG, et al: Preventive services in a health maintenance organization: how well do pediatricians screen and educate adolescent patients? Arch Pediatr Adolesc Med 154(2):173–179, 2000 10665605

Hamilton NL, Brantley LB, Tims FM: Family Support Network for Adolescent Cannabis Users. (Cannabis Youth Treatment Series [CYT], Vol 4). Rockville, MD, Center for Substance Abuse Treatament, 2001

Harrell A, Wirtz PM: Screening for adolescent problem drinking: validation of a multidimensional instrument for case identification. Psychol Assess 1(1):61–63, 1989

Henggeler SW, Borduin CM: Multisystemic treatment of serious juvenile offenders and their families, in Home-Based Services for Troubled Children. Edited by Schwartz IM, AuClaire P. Lincoln, University of Nebraska Press, 1995, pp 113–130

Henggeler SW, Schoenwald SK, Borduin CM: Multisystemic Treatment of Antisocial Behavior in Children And Adolescents. New York, Guilford, 1998

Henggeler SW, Halliday-Boykins CA, Cunningham PB, et al: Juvenile drug court: enhancing outcomes by integrating evidence-based treatments. J Consult Clin Psychol 74(1):42–54, 2006 16551142

Higgins ST, Budney AJ, Bickel WK: Outpatient behavioral treatment for cocaine dependence: 1-year outcome. Exp Clin Psychopharmacol 3(2):205–212, 1995

Hsieh S, Hoffmann NG, Hollister CD: The relationship between pre-, during-, post-treatment factors, and adolescent substance abuse behaviors. Addict Behav 23(4):477–488, 1998 9698976

Hunt GM, Azrin NH: A community-reinforcement approach to alcoholism. Behav Res Ther 11(1):91–104, 1973 4781962

Institute of Medicine: Broadening the Base of Treatment for Alcohol Problems. Washington, DC, National Academies Press, 1990

Inwald RE, Brobst MA, Morissey RF: Identifying and predicting adolescent behavioral problems by using a new profile. Juvenile Justice Digest 14:1–9, 1986

Kadden RM, Litt MD, Kabela-Cormier E, et al: Abstinence rates following behavioral treatments for marijuana dependence. Addict Behav 32(6):1220–1236, 2007 16996224

Kaminer Y, Godley M: From assessment reactivity to aftercare for adolescent substance abuse: are we there yet? Child Adolesc Psychiatr Clin N Am 19(3):577–590, 2010 20682222

Kaminer Y, Napolitano C: Brief Telephone Continuing Care Therapy for Adolescents. Center City, MN, Hazelden, 2010

Kaminer Y, Winters KC: Proposed DSM-5 substance use disorders for adolescents: if you build it, will they come? Am J Addict 21(3):280–281, 2012 22494232

Kaminer Y, Bukstein O, Tarter RE: The Teen-Addiction Severity Index: rationale and reliability. Int J Addict 26(2):219–226, 1991 1889921

Kaminer Y, Blitz C, Burleson JA, et al: The Teen Treatment Services Review (T-TSR). J Subst Abuse Treat 15(4):291–300, 1998 9650137

Kaminer Y, Burleson J, Goldberger R: Cognitive-behavioral coping skills and psychoeducation therapies for adolescent substance abuse. J Nerv Ment Dis 190(11):737–745, 2002 12436013

Kaminer Y, Burleson JA, Burke RH: Efficacy of outpatient aftercare for adolescents with alcohol use disorders: a randomized controlled study. J Am Acad Child Adolesc Psychiatry 47(12):1405–1412, 2008 18978635

Kaminer Y, Burleson J, Burke R, et al: The efficacy of contingency management for adolescent cannabis use disorder: a controlled study. Subst Abuse J 35(4):391–398 2014

Kamon J, Budney A, Stanger C: A contingency management intervention for adolescent marijuana abuse and conduct problems. J Am Acad Child Adolesc Psychiatry 44(6):513–521, 2005 15908833

Kazak AE, Hoagwood K, Weisz JR, et al: A meta-systems approach to evidence-based practice for children and adolescents. Am Psychol 65(2):85–97, 2010 20141264

Kelly JF, Myers MG: Adolescents' participation in Alcoholics Anonymous and Narcotics Anonymous: review, implications and future directions. J Psychoactive Drugs 39(3):259–269, 2007 18159779

Kelly JF, Urbanoski K: Youth recovery contexts: the incremental effects of 12-step attendance and involvement on adolescent outpatient outcomes. Alcohol Clin Exp Res 36(7):1219–1229, 2012 22509904

Kelly JF, Yeterian JD: The role of mutual-help groups in extending the framework of treatment. Alcohol Res Health 33(4):350–355, 2011 23580019

Kelly JF, Myers MG, Brown SA: A multivariate process model of adolescent 12-step attendance and substance use outcome following inpatient treatment. Psychol Addict Behav 14(4):376–389, 2000 11130156

Kelly JF, Myers MG, Brown SA: Do adolescents affiliate with 12-step groups? A multivriate process model of effects. J Stud Alcohol 63(3):293–304, 2002 12086130

Kelly JF, Myers MG, Brown SA: The effects of age composition of 12-step groups on adolescent 12-step participation and substance use outcome. J Child Adolesc Subst Abuse 15(1):63–72, 2005 18080000

Kelly JF, Brown SA, Abrantes A, et al: Social recovery model: an 8-year investigation of adolescent 12-step group involvement following inpatient treatment. Alcohol Clin Exp Res 32(8):1468–1478, 2008 18557829

Kelly JF, Magill M, Stout RL: How do people recover from alcohol dependence? A systematic review of the research on mechanisms of behavior change in Alcoholics Anonymous. Addict Res Theory 17(3):236–259, 2009

Kelly JF, Stout RL, Greene MC, et al: Young adults, social networks, and addiction recovery: post treatment changes in social ties and their role as a mediator of 12-step participation. PLoS One 9(6):e100121, 2014 24945357

Kelly TM, Donovan JE, Chung T, et al: Alcohol use disorders among emergency department-treated older adolescents: a new brief screen (RUFT-Cut) using the AUDIT, CAGE, CRAFFT, and RAPS-QF. Alcohol Clin Exp Res 28(5):746–753, 2004 15166649

Kennedy BP, Minami M: The Beech Hill Hospital/Outward Bound Adolescent Chemical Dependency Treatment Program. J Subst Abuse Treat 10(4):395–406, 1993 8411298

King KM, Chung T, Maisto SA: Adolescents' thoughts about abstinence curb the return of marijuana use during and after treatment. J Consult Clin Psychol 77(3):554–565, 2009 19485595

Knight JR, Sherritt L, Shrier LA, et al: Validity of the CRAFFT substance abuse screening test among adolescent clinic patients. Arch Pediatr Adolesc Med 156(6):607–614, 2002 12038895

Knight J, Sherritt L, Harris SK, et al: Validity of brief alcohol screening tests among adolescents: a comparison of the AUDIT, POSIT, CAGE and CRAFFT. Alcohol Clin Exp Res 27(1):67–73, 2003 12544008

Knudsen HK, Ducharme LJ, Roman PM, et al: Service Delivery and Use of Evidence-Based Treatment Practices in Adolescent Substance Abuse Treatment Settings: Project Report, June 2008. Lexington, University of Kentucky, and Athens, University of Georgia, 2008

Labbe AK, Greene C, Bergman BG, et al: The importance of age composition of 12-step meetings as a moderating factor in the relation between young adults' 12-step participation and abstinence. Drug Alcohol Depend 133(2):541–547, 2013 23938074

Liddle HA: Multidimensional Family Therapy Treatment for Adolescent Cannabis Users (Cannabis Youth Treatment Series [CYT], Vol 5). Rockville, MD, Center for Substance Abuse Treatment, 2002

Liddle HA, Rowe CL, Gonzalez A, et al: Changing provider practices, program environment, and improving outcomes by transporting multidimensional family therapy to an adolescent drug treatment setting. Am J Addict 15 (suppl 1):102–112, 2006 17182425

Liddle HA, Dakof GA, Turner RM, et al: Treating adolescent drug abuse: a randomized trial comparing multidimensional family therapy and cognitive behavior therapy. Addiction 103(10):1660–1670, 2008 18705691

Liddle HA, Rowe CL, Dakof GA, et al: Multidimensional family therapy for young adolescent substance abuse: twelve-month outcomes of a randomized controlled trial. J Consult Clin Psychol 77(1):12–25, 2009 19170450

Litt MD, Kadden RM, Cooney NL, et al: Coping skills and treatment outcomes in cognitive-behavioral and interactional group therapy for alcoholism. J Consult Clin Psychol 71(1):118–128, 2003 12602432

Litt MD, Kadden RM, Kabela-Cormier E, et al: Coping skills training and contingency management treatments for marijuana dependence: exploring mechanisms of behavior change. Addiction 103(4):638–648, 2008 18339108

Littell JH, Popa M, Forsythe B: Multisystemic therapy for social, emotional, and behavioral problems in youth aged 10–17. Cochrane Database Syst Rev (4):CD004797, 2005 16235382

MacKay JR: Treating Substance Use Disorders With Adaptive Continuing Care. Washington, DC, American Psychological Association, 2009

Magill M: Treatment mechanisms: shifting evaluation priorities in alcoholism research. Brown Univ Dig Addict Theory Appl: DATA 28(9):8, 2009

Maisto SA, Conigliaro J, McNeil M, et al: Factor structure of the SOCRATES in a sample of primary care patients. Addict Behav 24(6):879–892, 1999 10628520

Marlatt GA, Gordon JR: Relapse Prevention: Maintenance Strategies in the Treatment of Addictive Behaviors. New York, Guilford, 1985

Martens MP, Neighbors C, Dams-O'Connor K, et al: The factor structure of a dichotomously scored Rutgers Alcohol Problem Index. J Stud Alcohol Drugs 68(4):597–606, 2007 17568966

Martino S, Grilo CM, Fehon DC: Development of the Drug Abuse Screening Test for Adolescents (DAST-A). Addict Behav 25(1):57–70, 2000 10708319

McCambridge J, Strang J: The efficacy of single-session motivational interviewing in reducing drug consumption and perceptions of drug-related risk and harm among young people: results from a multi-site cluster randomized trial. Addiction 99(1):39–52, 2004 14678061

Meyers K, McLellan AT, Jaeger JL, et al: The development of the Comprehensive Addiction Severity Index for Adolescents (CASI-A): an interview for assessing multiple problems of adolescents. J Subst Abuse Treat 12(3):181–193, 1995 7474026

Miller G: Adolescent Substance Abuse Subtle Screening Inventory-2. Springville, IN, SASSI Institute, 2002

Miller WR, Rollnick S: Motivational Interviewing: Preparing People for Change, 2nd Edition. New York, Guilford, 2002

Miller WR, Sanchez VC: Motivating young adults for treatment and lifestyle change, in Alcohol Use and Misuse by Young Adults. Edited by Howard GS, Nathan PE. Notre Dame, IN, University of Notre Dame Press, 1994, pp 55–81

Moberg DP: Screening for Alcohol and Other Drug Problems Using the Adolescent Alcohol and Drug Involvement Scale (AADIS). Madison, Center for Health Policy and Program Evaluation, University of Wisconsin–Madison, 2003

Monti PM, Colby SM, O'Leary TA: Adolescents, Alcohol, and Substance Abuse: Reaching Teens Through Brief Interventions. New York, Guilford, 2001

Morgenstern J, Longabaugh R: Cognitive-behavioral treatment for alcohol dependence: a review of evidence for its hypothesized mechanisms of action. Addiction 95(10):1475–1490, 2000 11070524

Morgenstern J, McKay JR: Rethinking the paradigms that inform behavioral treatment research for substance use disorders. Addiction 102(9):1377–1389, 2007 17610541

Moyers TB, Martin T, Christopher PJ, et al: Client language as a mediator of motivational interviewing efficacy: where is the evidence? Alcohol Clin Exp Res 31(10 suppl):40s–47s, 2007 17880345

Myers MG, Brown SA, Mott MA: Coping as a predictor of adolescent substance abuse treatment outcome. J Subst Abuse 5(1):15–29, 1993 8329878

National Institute on Alcohol Abuse and Alcoholism: Alcohol Screening and Brief Intervention for Youth: A Practitioner's Guide. Rockville, MD, National Institute on Alcohol Abuse and Alcoholism, 2011

Petry NM: A comprehensive guide to the application of contingency management procedures in clinical settings. Drug Alcohol Depend 58(1–2):9–25, 2000 10669051

Price JH, Jordan TR, Dake JA: Pediatricians' use of the 5 A's and nicotine replacement therapy with adolescent smokers. J Community Health 32(2):85–101, 2007 17571523

Prochaska JO, DiClemente CC, Norcross JC: In search of how people change: applications to addictive behaviors. Am Psychol 47(9):1102–1114, 1992 1329589

Project MATCH: Matching Alcoholism Treatments to Client Heterogeneity: Project MATCH posttreatment drinking outcomes. J Stud Alcohol 58(1):7–29, 1997 8979210

Reich W, Shayla JJ, Taibelson C: The Diagnostic Interview for Children and Adolescents–Revised (DICA-R). St. Louis, MO, Washington University, 1992

Rigter H, Van Gageldonk A, Ketelaars T: Treatment and Other Interventions Targeting Drug Use and Addiction: State of the Art 2004. Utrecht, The Netherlands, National Drug Monitor, 2005

Rogers CR: The necessary and sufficient conditions of therapeutic personality change. J Consult Psychol 21(2):95–103, 1957 13416422

Roman PM, Blum TC: National Treatment Center Study (Summary 3). Athens, University of Georgia, 1999

Sampl S, Kadden R: Motivational Enhancement Therapy and Cognitive Behavioral Therapy for Adolescent Cannabis Users: 5 Sessions (Cannabis Youth Treatment Series [CYT], Vol 1). Rockville, MD, Center for Substance Abuse Treatment, 2001

Santisteban DA, Coatsworth JD, Perez-Vidal A, et al: Efficacy of brief strategic family therapy in modifying Hispanic adolescent behavior problems and substance use. J Fam Psychol 17(1):121–133, 2003 12666468

Shaffer D, Schwab-Stone M, Fisher P, et al: Revised version of the Diagnostic Interview Schedule for Children (DISC-R), I: preparation, field testing, interrater reliability, and acceptability. J Am Acad Child Adolesc Psychiatry 32(3):643–650, 1993

Shaffer D, Fisher P, Dulcan M: The NIMH Diagnostic Interview Schedule for Children Version 2.3 (DISC-2.3): description, acceptability, prevalence rates, and performance in the MECA Study. Methods for the Epidemiology of Child and Adolescent Mental Disorders Study. J Am Acad Child Adolesc Psychiatry 35(7):865–877, 1996 8768346

Shaffer D, Fisher P, Lucas CP, et al: NIMH Diagnostic Interview Schedule for Children Version IV (NIMH DISC-IV): description, differences from previous versions, and reliability of some common diagnoses. J Am Acad Child Adolesc Psychiatry 39(1):28–38, 2000 10638065

Shoham V, Insel TR: Rebooting for whom? Portfolios, technology, and personalized intervention. Perspect Psychol Sci 6(5):478–482, 2011

Skinner H: Development and Validation of a Lifetime Alcohol Consumption Assessment Procedure. Substudy No. 1248. Toronto, ON, Canada, Addict Research Foundation, 1982

Slesnick N, Prestopnik JL: Perceptions of the family environment and youth behaviors: alcohol-abusing runaway adolescents and their primary caretakers. Fam J Alex Va 12(3):243–253, 2005 18776946

Slesnick N, Prestopnik JL, Meyers RJ, et al: Treatment outcome for street-living, homeless youth. Addict Behav 32(6):1237–1251, 2007 16989957

Slesnick N, Kaminer Y, Kelly J: Most common psychosocial interventions for adolescent substance use disorders, in Adolescent Substance Abuse: Psychiatric Comorbidities and High-Risk Behaviors. Edited by Kaminer Y, Bukstein O. New York, Routledge, 2008, pp 111–134

Spirito A, Monti PM, Barnett NP, et al: A randomized clinical trial of a brief motivational intervention for alcohol-positive adolescents treated in an emergency department. J Pediatr 145(3):396–402, 2004 15343198

Stanger C, Budney AJ: Contingency management approaches for adolescent substance use disorders. Child Adolesc Psychiatr Clin N Am 19(3):547–562, 2010 20682220

Stanger C, Budney AJ, Kamon JL, et al: A randomized trial of contingency management for adolescent marijuana abuse and dependence. Drug Alcohol Depend 105(3):240–247, 2009 19717250

Stewart DG, Brown SA: Withdrawal and dependency symptoms among adolescent alcohol and drug abusers. Addiction 90(5):627–635, 1995 7795499

Sussman S: A review of Alcoholics Anonymous/Narcotics Anonymous programs for teens. Eval Health Prof 33(1):26–55, 2010 20164105

Szapocznik J, Hervis OE, Schwartz S: Brief Strategic Family Therapy for Adolescent Drug Abuse. Rockville, MD, National Institute on Drug Abuse, 2002

Tarter RE: Evaluation and treatment of adolescent substance abuse: a decision tree method. Am J Drug Alcohol Abuse 16(1–2):1–46, 1990 2330931

Tevyaw TO, Monti PM: Motivational enhancement and other brief interventions for adolescent substance abuse: foundations, applications and evaluations. Addiction 99 (suppl 2):63–75, 2004 15488106

Tevyaw TO, Gwaltney CJ, Tidey JW, et al: Contingency management for adolescent smokers: an exploratory study. J Child Adolesc Subst Abuse 16(4):23–44, 2007

Tims FM, Dennis ML, Hamilton N, et al: Characteristics and problems of 600 adolescent cannabis abusers in outpatient treatment. Addiction 97 (suppl 1):46–57, 2002 12460128

Van Hook S, Harris SK, Brooks T, et al: The "Six T's": barriers to screening teens for substance abuse in primary care. J Adolesc Health 40(5):456–461, 2007 17448404

Vaughn MG, Howard MO: Adolescent substance abuse treatment, in Readings in Evidence-Based Social Work: Syntheses of the Intervention Knowledge Base. Edited by Vaughn MG, Howard M, Thyer BA. Thousand Oaks, CA, Sage, 2008, pp 171–187

Veterans Health Administration: Management of Substance Use Disorders in the Primary and Specialty Care. Washington, DC, Office of Quality and Performance and the Veterans Affairs and Department of Defense Development Work Group, 2001

Waldron HB, Kaminer Y: On the learning curve: the emerging evidence supporting cognitive-behavioral therapies for adolescent substance abuse. Addiction 99 (suppl 2):93–105, 2004 15488108

Waldron HB, Turner CW: Evidence-based psychosocial treatments for adolescent substance abuse. J Clin Child Adolesc Psychol 37(1):238–261, 2008 18444060

Waldron HB, Slesnick N, Brody JL, et al: Treatment outcomes for adolescent substance abuse at 4- and 7-month assessment. J Consult Clin Psychol 69(5):802–813, 2001 11680557

Wanberg K: User's Guide to the Adolescent Self-Assessment Profile–II (ASAP-II). Arvada, CO, Center for Addictions Research and Evaluation, 1998

Webb C, Scudder M, Kaminer Y, et al: Motivational Enhancement Therapy and Cognitive Behavioral Therapy for Adolescent Cannabis Users: 7 Sessions (Cannabis Youth Treatment Series [CYT], Vol 1). Rockville, MD, Center for Substance Abuse Treatment, 2002

White HR, Labouvie EW: Towards the assessment of adolescent problem drinking. J Stud Alcohol 50(1):30–37, 1989 2927120

Williams RJ, Chang SY: A comprehensive and comparative review of adolescent substance abuse treatment outcome. Clinical Psychology: Science and Practice 7(2):138–166, 2000

Winters KC: Development of an adolescent alcohol and other drug abuse screening scale: Personal Experience Screening Questionnaire. Addict Behav 17(5):479–490, 1992 1332434

Winters KC, Henly GA: Adolescent Diagnostic Interview Schedule and Manual. Los Angeles, CA, Western Psychological Services, 1993

Winters KC, Henly GA: Personal Experience Inventory and Manual. Los Angeles, CA, Western Psychological Services, 1994

Winters KC, Kaminer Y: Screening and assessing adolescent substance use disorders in clinical populations. J Am Acad Child Adolesc Psychiatry 47(7):740–744, 2008 18574399

Winters KC, Stinchfield RD, Opland E, et al: The effectiveness of the Minnesota Model approach in the treatment of adolescent drug abusers. Addiction 95(4):601–612, 2000 10829335

Winters KC, Stinchfield R, Bukstein OG: Assessing adolescent substance use and abuse, in Adolescent Substance Abuse: Psychiatric Comorbidity and High-Risk Behaviors. Edited by Kaminer Y, Bukstein OG. New York, Routledge, 2008, pp 53–86

Winters KC, Martin CS, Chung T: Substance use disorders in DSM-V when applied to adolescents. Addiction 106(5):882–884, 2011 21477236

Witkiewitz K, Marlatt GA: Relapse prevention for alcohol and drug problems: that was Zen, this is Tao. Am Psychol 59(4):224–235, 2004 15149263

CHAPTER 4

Conduct Disorder and Delinquency and Substance Use Disorders

Oscar G. Bukstein, M.D., M.P.H.

Drug and alcohol use are ubiquitous among adolescents in the United States. Johnston et al. (2013) reported that 35.8% of high school students reported any illicit drug use and 48.4% reported any alcohol use. Among high school seniors, these figures increased to 50.4% and 68.2%, respectively. Fortunately, problem or pathological use is much more circumscribed, with findings from a nationally representative sample of U.S. youth indicating that the lifetime prevalence of an alcohol use disorder is approximately 8% and of illicit drug use disorders is 2%–3% (Merikangas et al. 2010). Those adolescents with substance use disorders (SUDs) also have a high prevalence of other psychiatric disorders, especially conduct disorder (CD) (Armstrong and Costello 2002). Although CD represents a discrete diagnosis, subsumed under the concept are aggression, problem behavior, deviant social behavior, and delinquency. Although each of these labels differs in its context, they all connote social deviance. For the purposes of simplicity, I use the term *conduct disorder* when discussing the general aspects of social deviance as well as the specific DSM-5 (American Psychiatric Association 2013) entity. I also specifically discuss aggression and delinquency and the relationship of these conditions with substance use and SUDs, including the prevalence of this comorbidity, the role of CD in the development of

SUDs, and finally how CD is relevant in the assessment and treatment of SUDs.

Epidemiology

Conduct disorder, as defined in DSM-5, is "a repetitive and persistent pattern of behavior in which the basic rights of others or major age-appropriate societal norms or rules are violated" (American Psychiatric Association 2013, p. 469). CD is characterized by aggressive, deceptive, and/or destructive behavior that usually begins in childhood or adolescence. CD symptoms are among the most common presented problems for psychiatric referral among children and adolescents in the United States (Loeber et al. 2000). Youths diagnosed with CD report higher levels of distress and impairment in almost all domains of functioning compared with youths with other psychiatric disorders (Lambert et al. 2001). Conduct problems during childhood or adolescence are associated with significantly increased risk of other mental disorders, legal problems, and premature mortality (Loeber et al. 2000).

Substance use is a common comorbid condition among youths with disruptive and oppositional defiant disorders. The estimated lifetime prevalence of CD in the United States is 9.5% (12.0% among males and 7.1% among females), and the median age at onset is 11.6 years (Nock et al. 2006). Lifetime prevalence of oppositional defiant disorder is estimated to be 10.2% (males, 11.2%; females, 9.2%). Of individuals with lifetime oppositional defiant disorder, 92.4% meet criteria for at least one other lifetime DSM-IV (American Psychiatric Association 1994) disorder, including SUD in 47.2% (Nock et al. 2007). A literature review of community studies of adolescent substance use, abuse, or dependence found that comorbidity with disruptive behavior disorders is high. The median prevalence of substance-related disorders was 46% among those with disruptive behavior disorders but was only 7%–8% among those without disruptive behavior disorders; the odds ratios had a median of 4, indicating a fourfold increase of risk for disruptive behavior disorder in substance-using or substance-abusing youths (Armstrong and Costello 2002). Not surprisingly, 38% of youths receiving SUD treatment have been found to have CD (Castel et al. 2006).

A majority of the diagnosable youths in the juvenile system also have a co-occurring SUD (Teplin et al. 2002). CD is the most common diagnosis among juvenile offenders, but other mental health disorders are also prevalent in these adolescents; in fact, 60% of males in juvenile detention have diagnoses other than CD (Teplin et al. 2002). McClelland et al. (2004) found a high prevalence rate of multiple SUDs among juvenile detainees in Cook County, Illinois. Nearly half the detainees had one or more SUDs, with 21% having two or more. Of those detainees with an SUD, nearly half had multiple SUDs, the most prevalent involving alcohol and cannabis use disorders.

Etiology

CD has been identified in many research studies as a precursor to SUDs (e.g., Armstrong and Costello 2002; Fergusson et al. 2007). Several investigators report evidence that behavior problems and aggression at a younger age predict later adolescent illicit substance use (Mason et al. 2007), escalations in use over time (Hussong et al. 1998), and later diagnoses of substance abuse and dependence (Chassin et al. 1999).

The age at onset of CD is often a harbinger of severity. Children with CD who had an earlier onset of substance use are more likely to abuse multiple substances in comparison with children without CD (Lynskey and Fergusson 1995). A New Zealand population study of nearly 1,000 children found that conduct problems at age 8 predicted alcohol and illicit drug use at age 15 (Lynskey and Fergusson 1995). Similarly, Hopfer et al. (2013), in a longitudinal study of community subjects, found that CD was associated with elevated risk for initiation of all substances, with comparatively greater risk of initiating illicit substance use at age 15 years. By age 18, the adjusted hazard ratios remained significant except for alcohol. At age 21, the adjusted hazard ratios were significant only for cocaine, amphetamines, inhalants, and club drugs. McCarty et al. (2012) found that any alcohol use at ages 12–14 predicted parent-reported, but not self-reported, CD symptoms the following year, over and above prior CD symptoms.

Although attention-deficit/hyperactivity disorder (ADHD) is common among adolescents with SUDs, the association between conduct and attentional problems explains the later relationship between attentional problems and SUDs (Fergusson et al. 2007). The presence of ADHD may worsen the severity of the SUD (Molina and Pelham 2003).

Numerous risk factors are associated with CD, including prenatal factors such as in utero exposure to alcohol and tobacco use (Baer et al. 2003), poor parental monitoring (Dishion and Kavanagh 2003), ineffective discipline (Frick et al. 1992), parent-child conflict (Burt et al. 2003), and parent substance abuse (Frick et al. 1992). The overlap in the risk factors that have been identified for both CD and SUDs is consistent with the notion of common pathways in the development of both disorders and may serve to explain the high correlation of CD and SUDs.

Although many studies have found that early-onset CD predicts later substance use, additional research indicates that early onset of substance use is predictive of symptoms of CD and later criminality. Synthesis of this research suggests that the relationship between the two disorders is reciprocal (for review, see Loeber et al. 2000). This seeming reciprocity may be in part peer related, because adolescents with elevated use patterns in early adolescence may have been more likely to associate with deviant peers over time (Kiesner et al. 2010), and these associations, not substance use, may have been the proximal risk factor exacerbating or precipitating the development of CD symptoms (Dishion et al. 2010). Rather than one disorder predicting the other, the two disorders share common etiology that manifests differently, possibly depending on environmental contexts.

Research indicates that both CD and SUDs are highly heritable and that the same genes play a role in this heritability (Dick 2007). Other research indicates that 11%–35% of association between CD and alcohol dependence can be accounted for by genetic factors (Slutske et al. 1998). A number of researchers have proposed that the high genetic covariation between CD and SUDs may be explained by a single latent factor referred to as behavioral disinhibition (Iacono et al. 2008).

Another similarity between CD and SUDs is dysfunction of reward centers. A hypofunctioning reward system may result in a propensity toward risk taking and reckless behavior, potentially reflecting insensitivity to reward and an inability to delay gratification, resulting in poor decision making (Gatzke-Kopp et al. 2009).

The use of alcohol and drugs may be part of a pattern of antisocial and rule-breaking behavior common to CD. In many respects, substance use is another deviant behavior and could be included with other symptoms of CD, although the opportunity to use presents in late childhood or early adolescence. Substance use may trap adolescents into more persistent patterns of antisocial behavior (Hussong et al. 2004).

The relationship between deviant social behavior and SUDs continues into adulthood. National surveys of adult populations have consistently demonstrated that persons with adult antisocial personality disorder, which requires adolescent CD as a precursor, have high rates of SUD as well as more severe SUD (Loeber et al. 2002). Adolescents with CD who use substances are also at increased risk of developing antisocial personality disorder (Loeber et al. 2002).

Aggression

Early aggression has clearly been associated with later substance use (Rappaport and Thomas 2004). Aggression is a common risk factor for CD and SUDs; it is a behavior pattern that is a primary characteristic of childhood-onset CD, and a high level of aggression in childhood serves as a risk factor for substance use and other negative outcomes during adolescence and adulthood (Lynskey and Fergusson 1995). Symptoms associated with CD in childhood, especially aggression, have consistently been associated with substance-using behaviors later in adolescence (Armstrong and Costello 2002). Childhood anger problems, which are a common precursor to aggression, were predictive of subsequent substance use by adolescents (and by adults) (Swaim et al. 1989). Several longitudinal studies reported that preadolescent levels of aggression are predictive of boys' subsequent adolescent use of alcohol, marijuana, and other drugs and of delinquent activity (Lochman and Wayland 1994).

A reciprocal relationship exists between aggression and substance use or SUDs: aggression predicts substance use, and substance use predicts aggression (Rappaport and Thomas 2004). The relationship between aggression and substance use appears to be influenced by the presence of associated symptoms of depression and impulsivity as well as by a family history of alcoholism and drug abuse and involvement with peers or gangs using drugs (Lipsey and Derzon 1998). The physiological effects of intoxication in conjunction with situational provocation could also facilitate risk that adolescents will engage in aggressive and antisocial behavior (Felson and Staff 2010). White et al. (2002) reported that adolescents who reported committing offenses against persons were more often under the influence of alcohol or drugs than were those who committed general theft. Aggressive acts were more often related to self-reported acute alcohol use than to marijuana use. Those adolescents who reported committing illegal acts under the influence were more likely to report committing offenses with other people and being arrested more often than those who did not. Offenses committed under the influence were more prevalent among heavier alcohol and drug users, more serious offenders, more impulsive youths, and youths with more deviant peers. The relationship between marijuana and violence or aggression may be due to selection effects, because these behaviors tend to co-occur in certain individuals, not because one behavior causes the other; in other words, both are influenced by shared risk factors and/or an underlying tendency toward deviance (Wei et al.

2004). Similarly, drinkers are much more likely than nondrinkers to commit violence *while sober*, suggesting that a considerable portion of the relationship between prevalence of drinking and violence is spurious (Felson et al. 2008). In many respects, persistent aggression is not only a symptom of CD but also a marker for a more severe clinical picture of CD.

Another CD symptom, bullying, has received increased attention. Studies have found that boys who reported being bullies at age 8 were more likely than nonbullies or victims to report illicit drug use or a greater magnitude of drug use at age 18 (Niemelä et al. 2011). Kaltiala-Heino et al. (2000) concluded that bullies were 4.8 times more likely to engage in frequent excessive drinking and 8.2 times more likely to use other substances than were those not engaged in bullying.

Delinquency

A number of studies have shown that youths with substance abuse or mental health disorders consistently have higher offending rates than those without disorders (Loeber and Farrington 2000) and that early substance use predicts subsequent criminal behavior in adolescents (Loeber and Farrington 2000). Researchers have also reported that the presence of co-occurring disorders increases the chances of criminal involvement in emerging adulthood (Loeber and Farrington 2000) and that both the presence and number of comorbid disorders within a sample of substance-abusing and delinquent adolescents predicts subsequent negative outcomes, including arrest (Loeber and Farrington 2000).

The comorbidity of SUDs and externalizing disorders such as CD appears to be particularly problematic for a range of outcomes, including high school dropout, dysfunctional family relationships, and general delinquency (Chassin et al. 2004). Involvement with drugs or alcohol increases the likelihood of continued and serious contact with the juvenile justice system. Higher levels of involvement with substance use increase the rate of offending, the severity of the committed offense, and the duration of antisocial behavior (Sealock et al. 1997). The younger a person is at onset of substance use, the more likely it is that he or she will become a severe and chronic offender (e.g., Loeber et al. 2000). Consistent involvement of youth with the juvenile justice system may be associated with the likelihood of increased emotional and mental problems (Robertson et al. 2004).

Using data from a longitudinal study of serious adolescent offenders, Chassin et al. (2009) and Mulvey et al. (2010) evaluated the association of mental health problems with three distinct outcomes (rearrest, self-reported antisocial activity, and diminished gainful activity) and tested whether having a mental health problem contributed any unique explanatory power regarding these outcomes over and above other criminogenic risk factors. They also examined whether mental health problems moderated the relationship between risk factors and outcomes. The presence of an SUD showed consistent associations with the outcomes. Youths with an SUD were more likely to continue offending over the 7 years and were less likely to spend time working or in school than were those with no substance use issues. In addition, having an SUD magnified the impact of other risk factors related to continued offending. Having an SUD made things significantly worse. Greater substance use is highly correlated with increased offending at each time point. Researchers who follow adolescent offenders over time find that substance use at one age is one of the most consistent indicators of continued serious offending at a later age (D'Amico et al. 2008).

Criminal behavior and substance use follow parallel courses over time, suggesting a reciprocal relationship between the two behaviors (Sullivan and Hamilton 2007). Some of the same factors that put an individual at risk for involvement in criminality, especially CD, also place the adolescent at risk for problems with substance use (Iacono et al. 2008). Parental SUDs, poor parenting, conflictual family environments, and constitutional factors such as sensation seeking and behavioral disinhibition place an adolescent at higher risk of using drugs and alcohol and/or engaging in illegal acts (Hawkins et al. 1992).

In the United States, drug violations account for 11.6% of all juvenile arrests, and juvenile arrests account for 12.4% of all arrests for drug violations (Puzzanchera 2013). Not all youths who are adjudicated delinquent have CD. Although drug offenses are highly correlated with other offenses (Mulvey et al. 2010), associating the behavior of those youths following a specialty offending career with only drug- and/or alcohol-related offenses and subsequent violations of probation or other status offenses confuses the crime-SUD relationship. The elimination of repeated arrests as part of the DSM abuse criteria in DSM-5 was, in part, based on this confusion (American Psychiatric Association 2013).

A specific issue related to juvenile justice and SUDs is drug dealing. Large numbers of youths with juvenile justice system involvement have a history of illicit drug selling (Floyd et al. 2010). In one study, drug dealing among white youths was associated with use of marijuana, hallucinogens, and cocaine; prescription drug misuse; availability of cocaine; and socioeconomic status. In contrast, drug dealing among black youths was associated with marijuana use and availability of crack and marijuana (Floyd et al. 2010). Friedman et al. (2003) found that young black men involved in drug trade who used illegal drugs only used marijuana. Factors other than individual substance use (e.g., contextual factors) are likely driving involvement in drug trade among black youths. The extant literature suggests that social and economic factors play a significant role in the involvement of black youths in the drug economy (Floyd et al. 2010).

Racial disparities were also demonstrated in a study of arrests (Kakade et al. 2012). African American adolescents were less likely than whites to have engaged in drug use or drug selling, but they were more likely to have been arrested; they were 2.5 times as likely as whites to have been arrested multiple times and 1.6 times as likely to have been arrested once. This disparity could not be explained by differences in the two groups' rates of drug-related and other illegal behaviors.

Assessment

Given the importance of CD and particularly aggression in marking more severe cases of SUD in terms of prognosis and treatment response, the clinician should capture a patient's history of deviant social behaviors, including aggressive behaviors and delinquency. CD symptoms and behaviors, including aggression, are also risk factors for the onset of substance use and the development of SUDs and therefore are a staple of any clinical evaluation of children and adolescents, whether in mental health or primary care settings. In a mental health setting, inquiry into CD risk factors, because they are shared with those of SUDs, is useful to determine overall risk status. Questions about drug dealing and delinquency related to substance use are also important.

Prevention

Among the principles for effective prevention programs proposed by the National Institute on Drug Abuse (2003) and relevant to CD are that prevention programs should enhance protective factors and reverse or reduce risk factors and that programs should do so as early as possible and persistently, as needed. For indicated prevention programs targeting salient risk factors, early-onset CD, aggression, and other deviant social behaviors are often the determining characteristics and the proximal targets for the program outcome (Committee on the Prevention of

Mental Disorders and Substance Abuse Among Children, Youth, and Young Adults 2009).

Treatment of Youths With Conduct Problems and SUDs

Evidence supports that comorbid CD and SUDs negatively impact treatment outcomes for both disorders (Grella et al. 2001). Typically, the selection of treatment interventions for adolescents with SUDs and CD aggression and/or delinquency requires the same general considerations made for all adolescents with SUDs. Consistent with a broader view of treatment that targets other salient domains of adolescent functioning, a comprehensive treatment plan for an adolescent who has CD and/or aggression with or without delinquent behavior would include increasing prosocial behaviors through the adolescent's involvement with a prosocial peer group. Improvement in adolescent problem solving and impulse control may be among the individual targets, whereas family functioning and parent-adolescent communication are among the family-oriented treatment targets.

Cuellar et al. (2004) examined the association of mental health and substance abuse treatment with reductions in detention rates for juveniles in the Colorado child welfare system. They found that individuals who received treatment had lower probabilities of being detained for any offense. A meta-analysis of the effects of outpatient treatment on substance use outcomes for adolescents with SUDs showed no differences in effectiveness related to the severity of delinquency (Tanner-Smith et al. 2013). However, Tripodi and Bender (2011), who conducted a systematic review on the effectiveness of treatment of alcohol and marijuana use in juvenile offenders and compared the results with previous meta-analyses of community studies (Bender et al. 2011; Tripodi et al. 2010), concluded that effect sizes are smaller among juvenile offender samples than among community samples. Substance-abusing juvenile offenders may therefore be more difficult to treat for both offending and substance use behavior. Van der Put et al. (2014) reported that substance-using offenders, especially those with substance use problems (SUPs, substance use causing psychosocial problems), had more risk factors and fewer protective factors than abstaining youths (i.e., those who had not used drugs or alcohol in the preceding 6 months) in the domains of school, use of free time, relationships, family, attitude, aggression, and skills. The associations between most of the risk and/or protective factors and recidivism were stronger in the abstaining group than in the SUP group. Substance use uniquely predicted recidivism, suggesting that general interventions for juvenile offenders addressing risk and protective factors with the aim of reducing recidivism may be less effective for offenders with SUPs and that SUPs should be addressed specifically in treatment. This finding is consistent with findings of Henggeler et al. (1999, 2006), who reported that the well-documented capacity of multisystemic therapy (MST) to reduce rearrest rates (Henggeler et al. 1999) did not emerge in substance-abusing juvenile offenders. These findings suggest that changing offending behavior may be more difficult with increasing levels of SUPs. Overall, substance abuse treatment appears to have a small to moderate effect on alcohol and marijuana use reduction for juvenile offenders (Tripodi and Bender 2011). An increased risk for the development of antisocial personality disorder remains even after intensive treatment for SUDs (Myers et al. 1998).

Many of the evidence-based interventions shown to be effective for reducing substance use have also targeted CD symptoms and behaviors. Because many of the risk and protective factors are the same for both SUD and CD, particularly since CD is often a precursor to SUDs, effective treatment approaches should target a broad set of deviant social behaviors.

Multidimensional Family Therapy

In comparison with a control group receiving peer-group therapy, multidimensional family therapy participants experienced a faster decrease in reported involvement with delinquent peers from intake to treatment termination, a difference associated with a medium effect size (Cohen's $d=0.67$) (Liddle et al. 2009). Although this variable continued to improve across the 6- and 12-month follow-ups, the difference between groups was not significant. Self-reports of disruptive behaviors in school decreased from intake to treatment termination among participants in both conditions, but multidimensional family therapy participants reported fewer school disruptions than peer-group therapy participants across the treatment period. Participants' self-reports of academic and school conduct problems decreased from intake to treatment termination across both treatment conditions.

Brief Strategic Family Therapy

Adolescents who participated in brief strategic family therapy showed a significantly greater reduction in conduct problems than adolescents in the comparison condition, who received a participatory-learning group intervention (Santisteban et al. 2003). The adolescents in the brief strategic family therapy group also showed a significantly greater reduction in socialized aggression than adolescents in the comparison condition.

Functional Family Therapy

From baseline to the 4-month follow-up assessment, adolescents who received functional family therapy (FFT) for adolescent alcohol and drug abuse had lower scores on the Delinquent Behavior subscale of the Youth Self-Report than did adolescents who received psychoeducational group therapy, a result that continued through the 4- to 19-month follow-up assessments (French et al. 2000). From the 4- to 19-month follow-up assessments, there was no significant difference in Delinquent Behavior subscale scores between teens who received FFT for adolescent alcohol and drug abuse and those who received joint FFT for adolescent alcohol and drug abuse plus cognitive-behavioral treatment individual therapy.

Family Behavior Therapy

Among youths who used substances, the mean number of problems reported on the Quay Problem Behavior Checklist decreased from 22.5 to 14.3 for those in family behavior therapy but remained essentially unchanged for those in supportive therapy (Azrin et al. 2001). Multiple measures of conduct problems showed significant pretreatment to posttreatment improvements in youths diagnosed with CD. Posttreatment improvement was maintained at 6-month follow-up. Improvements observed in adolescents receiving family behavior therapy were similar to those observed for clients receiving individual cognitive therapy.

Multisystemic Therapy

In a study comparing youths receiving treatment as usual with youths receiving MST, the latter were arrested about half as often in the posttreatment period. Recidivism rates were 42% for the youths engaged in MST compared with 62% for youths receiving usual services (Henggeler et al. 1992, 1993). In a second study, MST was more effective than individual therapy in preventing rearrests for violent offenses during the follow-up period (Henggeler et al. 1992, 1993). At the end of 4 years of follow-up, the rate of criminal recidivism (rearrest) for the MST completers (22%) was less than one-third the overall rate for individual therapy completers (71%). At 13.7 years after treatment, MST participants (then age 29 years) showed significantly lower rates of criminal recidivism (50%) than comparable youths, who had received treatment as usual (81%). MST participants had on average 73 fewer days of incarceration than youths receiving usual services. More than two-thirds (68%) of youths in the usual services group were incarcerated after treatment, compared with only 20% of the MST group. Almost 14 years after treatment, MST youths had been sentenced to less than half as many days of incarceration as the comparison youths.

Multidimensional Treatment Foster Care

Multidimensional treatment foster care (MTFC) is a behavioral treatment alternative to residential placement for youths who have problems with chronic antisocial behavior, emotional disturbance, and delinquency, rather than specifically substance use or SUDs. In a study by Chamberlain and Smith (2003), although nearly all of the MTFC participants showed high levels of substance use, they neither received specific substance use treatment (e.g., substance use counseling) nor attended substance use support groups (e.g., Alcoholics Anonymous). Despite lack of a specific focus on substance use treatment, a significant effect was found for substance use from the MTFC intervention. At 12-month follow-up, no statistically significant differences between groups were found for reported alcohol, tobacco, or marijuana use; however, MTFC participants did have a significant decrease in their reported use of other drugs relative to the comparison group. At 18-month follow-up, MTFC participants had a significant decrease in reported tobacco use, marijuana use, and other drug use relative to the comparison group, who had received residential placement. No statistically significant difference between groups was observed for alcohol use at the 18-month assessment.

Treatment of Delinquent Adolescents

Serious Offenders

Chassin et al. (2009) examined drug treatment–related reductions in alcohol and marijuana use, cigarette smoking, and commission of non-drug offenses among male adolescents who had been adjudicated of a serious (almost exclusively a felony) offense. Results indicated that the treatment for drug use that these adolescents experienced had significant effects on substance use, which could not be explained solely by incarceration in controlled environments. Progress in reducing cigarette smoking and criminal offending was found only for treatments that included family involvement. However, low rates of family involvement in treatment reflect the types of services that are actually received by serious juvenile offenders, especially in more secure institutional settings than in community settings (Mulvey et al. 2007).

Motivational Interviewing

Feldstein and Ginsburg (2006) suggest four reasons to support the adaptation of motivational interviewing (MI) to the juvenile justice setting. First, the research indicates robust support for MI's efficacy in helping adolescents reduce their use of marijuana, which is the most predominant substance used within the juvenile justice population. Second, during a brief MI session administered upon entry into emergency rooms, MI has demonstrated efficacy in reducing other substance use, as well as in increasing feelings of self-efficacy. This finding provides support for using MI during the teachable moment of entry into the juvenile justice system. Third, MI has shown promise as an intervention with adult offender populations, indicating its probable efficacy with a comparable, although younger, population. Fourth, MI appears to be an appropriate developmental match for adolescents, overlapping well with adolescents' cognitive and emotional abilities and limitations. Although several reports of MI use in delinquent populations did not find differences between the MI and control groups, evaluation of the Connecticut Motivational Interviewing and Strength-Based Case Management (MI/SBCM) Initiatives (Justice Research Center 2012) found that recidivism rates for youths involved in the MI/SBCM Initiatives were significantly lower than those for youths supervised under the previous model. The MI/SBCM approach resulted in recidivism reductions for both males and females, with stronger effects observed with males.

Contingency Management

Stanger and Budney (2010) reported high expectations for the use of contingency management as an adjunct to other treatment modalities for treating adolescents with SUDs. Henggeler et al. (2006) used contingency management in juvenile drug court (JDC); individuals were randomly assigned either to a condition in which therapists were trained to deliver contingency management in combination with family engagement strategies or to continue their usual services. The study found that drug court was more effective than family court services in decreasing rates of adolescent substance use and criminal behavior. These reductions may have been due to the substantially increased surveillance of youths associated with drug court. The "relative reductions in antisocial behavior did not translate to corresponding decreases in rearrest or incarceration" (Henggeler et al. 2006, p. 42), thus no significant effect was found for contingency management for these distal outcomes.

Iatrogenic Effects of Group Therapies With Deviant Youths

Although group modalities (e.g., cognitive-behavioral therapy) are part of many of the evidence-based interventions for adolescents with SUDs as well as those with SUDs plus CD and/or delinquent behavior, the work of Dishion et al. (1999) has suggested that group work for youth may be iatrogenic—that is, youths might increase deviant behaviors because of peer contagion or deviancy training. Subsequent research has questioned aspects of the deviancy training hypothesis (Mager et al. 2005), pointing to inadequate support for peer contagion affecting those in treatment. A comprehensive meta-analytic review of the literature proposed that previous results on deviancy training may be attributed to inadequate treatment or to deviant youths put together for other than treatment purposes (Weiss et al. 2005), a result found in other studies (Shapiro et al. 2010). Although it is possible that good treatment interventions and structure would compensate for any propensity for peer contagion and deviancy training, clinicians should be vigilant and monitor for such adverse behaviors. For some youths with CD/delinquent behavior, group settings may not be indicated, and individual or family interventions would be a safer alternative.

Drug Courts

Because a considerable percentage of youths are in the juvenile justice system as a result of drug offenses, the number of JDCs is expanding, with 447 JDCs as of June 30, 2013 (National Institute of Justice 2014). Compared with the already substantial literature on adult drug courts and their effectiveness in reducing recidivism (U.S. General Accounting Office 2005), support for the effectiveness of JDCs is limited (Fradella et al. 2009). Several evaluations report that JDC youths fare better than non-JDC youths on measures of recidivism during and after the program (Anspach and Ferguson 2005), whereas other reports show no advantage of JDCs over usual interventions. One study compared JDC with standard probation; the two groups of youths did not significantly differ at any of the follow-up time intervals on alcohol and/or other drug offenses, although JDC youths had statistically significantly fewer delinquency and/or criminal offenses than probationers at all follow-up points, with the difference between the groups increasing with longer follow-up periods (Hickert et al. 2011).

General Considerations in Treating Youths With SUDs and Conduct Disorder and/or Delinquent Behavior

The literature suggests several lessons regarding intervention for adolescents having SUDs and CD and/or delinquent behavior. Owing to the increase in multiple comorbidities in addition to the persistence and severity of CD and offending behaviors, these youths are a severely impaired group with many liabilities that attenuate treatment response. Although attending to risk and protective factors as a general principle of treatment should continue, specifically addressing substance use behavior with evidence-based interventions is essential for this population. Several recent innovations (i.e., MI, contingency management, drug courts) address the common occurrence of poor motivation seen in youths with CD and/or delinquent behavior (Chassin 2008; Tripodi and Bender 2011).

Finally, the need for external structure and the possibility of peer contagion and/or deviance training in adolescent group settings prompt increased consideration of family-based interventions rather than group interventions. If group interventions are used, facilitators should closely monitor youths for undue negative peer influence.

Summary and Future Directions

Adolescents with SUD and CD and/or engaged in delinquent behavior are among the most difficult patients to treat because of multiple psychiatric comorbidities, poor environmental background, and poor parental and other environmental supports. An adolescent with CD and engaged in delinquent behavior and persistent aggressive behavior should be highly suspect of having an SUD unless an assessment proves otherwise. Interventions should address substance use behaviors in addition to related environmental contexts as well as risk and protective factors. Future research and development of prevention and treatment programs should consider expansion of community-based paradigms—particularly alternative venues such as school-based and after-school programming, various "doses" of intervention, the use of booster sessions and other aftercare options, and the influence of identification and treatment of other comorbid psychopathology on SUD and CD/delinquency outcomes.

KEY POINTS

- Early and persistent conduct (behavior) problems and aggression are prominent risk factors for the development of substance use disorders.

- The presence of substance use disorder predicts the likelihood of continued and serious contact with the juvenile justice system.

- Many of the evidence-based interventions shown to be effective for reducing substance use have also targeted and improved conduct disorder symptoms and behaviors. Positive effects on cigarette smoking and criminal offending are increased for treatments that include family involvement.

- Drug treatment reduces alcohol and marijuana use, cigarette smoking, and nondrug offending among male adolescents adjudicated of a serious (almost exclusively a felony) offense.

- Drug courts for juveniles adjudicated of drug- or alcohol-related offenses appear to improve substance use outcomes when compared with family courts, and these outcomes are enhanced with the use of evidence-based interventions.

References

American Psychiatric Association: Diagnostic and Statistical Manual of Mental Disorders, 4th Edition. Washington, DC, American Psychiatric Association, 1994

American Psychiatric Association: Diagnostic and Statistical Manual of Mental Disorders, 5th Edition. Arlington, VA, American Psychiatric Association, 2013

Anspach D, Ferguson A: Part II: Outcome Evaluation of Maine's Statewide Juvenile Drug Treatment Court Program. Portland, University of Southern Maine, 2005

Armstrong TD, Costello EJ: Community studies on adolescent substance use, abuse, or dependence and psychiatric comorbidity. J Consult Clin Psychol 70(6):1224–1239, 2002 12472299

Azrin NH, Donohue B, Teichner GA, et al: A controlled evaluation and description of individual-cognitive problem solving and family behavior therapies in dually diagnosed conduct-disordered and substance-dependent youth. J Child Adolesc Subst Abuse 11(1):1–44, 2001

Baer JS, Sampson PD, Barr HM, et al: A 21-year longitudinal analysis of the effects of prenatal alcohol exposure on young adult drinking. Arch Gen Psychiatry 60(4):377–385, 2003 12695315

Bender K, Tripodi SJ, Sarteschi C, et al: A meta-analysis of interventions to reduce adolescent cannabis use. Res Soc Work Pract 21(2):153–164, 2011

Burt SA, Krueger RF, McGue M, et al: Parent-child conflict and the comorbidity among childhood externalizing disorders. Arch Gen Psychiatry 60(5):505–513, 2003 12742872

Castel S, Rush B, Urbanoski K, et al: Overlap of clusters of psychiatric symptoms among clients of a comprehensive addiction treatment service. Psychol Addict Behav 20(1):28–35, 2006 16536662

Chamberlain P, Smith DK: Antisocial behavior in children and adolescents: the Oregon Multidimensional Treatment Foster Care Model, in Evidence-Based Psychotherapies for Children and Adolescents. Edited by Kazdin AE, Weisz JR. New York, Guilford, 2003, pp 282–300

Chassin L: Juvenile justice and substance use. Future Child18(2):165–183, 2008 21338002

Chassin L, Pitts SC, Delucia SC Todd M: A longitudinal study of children of alcoholics: Predicting young adult substance use disorders, anxiety and depression. J Abnorm Psychol 108(1):106–119, 1999 10066997

Chassin L, Flora DB, King KM: Trajectories of alcohol and drug use and dependence from adolescence to adulthood: the effects of familial alcoholism and personality. J Abnorm Psychol 113(4):483–498, 2004 15535782

Chassin L, Knight G, Vargas-Chanes D, et al: Substance use treatment outcomes in a sample of male serious juvenile offenders. J Subst Abuse Treat 36(2):183–194, 2009 18657942

Committee on the Prevention of Mental Disorders and Substance Abuse Among Children, Youth, and Young Adults: Research Advances and Promising Interventions: Preventing Mental, Emotional, and Behavioral Disorders Among Young People: Progress and Possibilities, Edited by O'Connell ME, Boat T, Warner KE. Washington, DC, National Academies Press, 2009

Cuellar AE, Markowitz S, Libby AM: Mental health and substance abuse treatment and juvenile crime. J Ment Health Policy Econ 7:59–68, 2004 15208466

D'Amico EJ, Edelen MO, Miles JNV, et al: The longitudinal association between substance use and delinquency among high-risk youth. Drug Alcohol Depend 93(1–2):85–92, 2008 17977669

Dick DM: Identification of genes influencing a spectrum of externalizing psychopathology. Curr Dir Psychol Sci 16(6):331–335, 2007

Dishion TJ, Kavanagh K: Intervening in Adolescent Problem Behavior: A Family Centered Approach. New York, Guilford, 2003

Dishion TJ, McCord J, Poulin F: When interventions harm: peer groups and problem behavior. Am Psychol 54(9):755–764, 1999 10510665

Dishion TJ, Véronneau MH, Myers MW: Cascading peer dynamics underlying the progression from problem behavior to violence in early to late adolescence. Dev Psychopathol 22(3):603–619, 2010 20576182

Feldstein SW, Ginsburg JID: Motivational interviewing with dually diagnosed adolescents in juvenile justice settings. Brief Treatment and Crisis Intervention 6(3):218–233, 2006

Felson RB, Staff J: The effects of alcohol intoxication on violent versus other offending. Crim Justice Behav 37(12):1343–1360, 2010

Felson RB, Teasdale B, Burchfield KB: The influence of being under the influence: alcohol effects on adolescent violence. J Res Crime Delinq 45(2):119–141, 2008

Fergusson DM, Horwood LJ, Ridder EM: Conduct and attentional problems in childhood and adolescence and later substance use, abuse and dependence: results of a 25-year longitudinal study. Drug Alcohol Depend 88 (suppl 1):S14–S26, 2007 17292565

Floyd LJ, Alexandre PK, Hedden SL, et al: Adolescent drug dealing and race/ethnicity: a population-based study of the differential impact of substance use on involvement in drug trade. Am J Drug Alcohol Abuse 36(2):87–91, 2010 20337503

Fradella H, Fischer R, Hagan Kleinpeter C, et al: Latino youth in the juvenile drug court of Orange County, California. J Ethn Crim Justice 7(4):271–292, 2009

French MT, McGeary KA, Chitwood DD, et al: Chronic drug use and crime. Subst Abus 21(2):95–109, 2000 12466650

Frick PJ, Lahey BB, Loeber R, et al: Familial risk factors to oppositional defiant disorder and conduct disorder: parental psychopathology and maternal parenting. J Consult Clin Psychol 60(1):49–55, 1992 1556285

Friedman AS, Terras A, Glassman K: The differential disinhibition effect of marijuana use on violent behavior: a comparison of this effect on a conventional, non-delinquent group versus a delinquent or deviant group. J Addict Dis 22(3):63–78, 2003 14621345

Gatzke-Kopp LM, Beauchaine TP, Shannon KE, et al: Neurological correlates of reward responding in adolescents with and without externalizing behavior disorders. J Abnorm Psychol 118(1):203–213, 2009 19222326

Grella CE, Hser YI, Joshi V, et al: Drug treatment outcomes for adolescents with comorbid mental and substance use disorders. J Nerv Ment Dis 189(6):384–392, 2001 11434639

Hawkins JD, Catalano RF, Miller JY: Risk and protective factors for alcohol and other drug problems in adolescence and early adulthood: implications for substance abuse prevention. Psychol Bull 112(1):64–105, 1992 1529040

Henggeler SW, Melton GB, Smith LA: Family preservation using multisystemic therapy: an effective alternative to incarcerating serious juvenile offenders. J Consult Clin Psychol 60(6):953–961, 1992 1460157

Henggeler SW, Melton GB, Smith LA, et al: Family preservation using multisystemic treatment: long-term follow-up to a clinical trial with serious juvenile offenders. J Child Fam Stud 2(4):283–293, 1993

Henggeler SW, Pickrel SG, Brondino MJ: Multisystemic treatment of substance abusing and dependent delinquents: outcomes, treatment fidelity, and transportability. Ment Health Serv Res 1(3):171–184, 1999 11258740

Henggeler SW, Halliday-Boykins CA, Cunningham PB, et al: Juvenile drug court: enhancing outcomes by integrating evidence-based treatments. J Consult Clin Psychol 74(1):42–54, 2006 16551142

Hickert A, Becker E, Próspero M, et al: Impact of juvenile drug courts on drug use and criminal behavior. Journal of Juvenile Justice 1:1, 2011. Available at: http://www.journalofjuvjustice.org/jojj0101/article05.htm. Accessed July 30, 2014.

Hopfer C, Salomonsen-Sautel S, Mikulich-Gilbertson S, et al: Conduct disorder and initiation of substance use: A prospective longitudinal study. J Am Acad Child Adolesc Psychiatry 52(5):511–518, 2013 23622852

Hussong AM, Curran PJ, Chassin L: Pathways of risk for accelerated heavy alcohol use among adolescent children of alcoholic parents. J Abnorm Child Psychol 26(6):453–466, 1998 9915652

Hussong AM, Curran PJ, Moffitt TE, et al: Substance abuse hinders desistance in young adults' antisocial behavior. Dev Psychopathol 16(4):1029–1046, 2004 15704826

Iacono WG, Malone SM, McGue M: Behavioral disinhibition and the development of early-onset addiction: common and specific influences. Annu Rev Clin Psychol 4:325–348, 2008 18370620

Johnston LD, O'Malley PM, Miech RA, et al: 2013 Overview: Key Findings on Adolescent Drug Use. Monitoring the Future: National Results on Drug Use, 1975–2013. Ann Arbor, University of Michigan Institute for Social Research, 2013. Available at: http://www.monitoringthefuture.org//pubs/monographs/mtf-overview2013.pdf. Accessed May 25, 2014.

Justice Research Center: Evaluation of the Connecticut Motivational Interviewing and Strength-Based Case Management Initiatives, 2007-10: Final Outcome Evaluation Report. 2012. Available at: http://www.jud.ct.gov/cssd/research/juvprob/Eval_CT_MI_SBCM_Initiative.pdf. Accessed July 2014.

Kakade M, Duarte CS, Liu X, et al: Adolescent substance use and other illegal behaviors and racial disparities in criminal justice system involvement: findings from a U.S. national survey. Am J Public Health 102(7):1307–1310, 2012 22594721

Kaltiala-Heino R, Rimpelä M, Rantanen P, et al: Bullying at school—an indicator of adolescents at risk for mental disorders. J Adolesc 23(6):661–674, 2000 11161331

Kiesner J, Poulin F, Dishion TJ: Adolescent substance use with friends: moderating and mediating effects of parental monitoring and peer activity contexts. Merrill Palmer Q (Wayne State Univ Press) 56(4):529–556, 2010 21165170

Lambert EW, Wahler RG, Andrade AR, et al: Looking for the disorder in conduct disorder. J Abnorm Psychol 110(1):110–123, 2001 11265675

Liddle HA, Rowe CL, Dakof GA, et al: Multidimensional family therapy for young adolescent substance abuse: twelve-month outcomes of a randomized controlled trial. J Consult Clin Psychol 77(1):12–25, 2009 19170450

Lipsey MW, Derzon JH: Predictors of violent or serious delinquency in adolescence and early adulthood: a synthesis of longitudinal research, in Serious and Violent Juvenile Offenders. Edited by Loeber R, Farrington DP. Thousand Oaks, CA, Sage, 1998, pp 86–105

Lochman JE, Wayland KK: Aggression, social acceptance, and race as predictors of negative adolescent outcomes. J Am Acad Child Adolesc Psychiatry 33(7):1026–1035, 1994 7961341

Loeber R, Farrington DP: Young children who commit crime: epidemiology, developmental origins, risk factors, early interventions, and policy implications. Dev Psychopathol 12(4):737–762, 2000 11202042

Loeber R, Burke JD, Lahey BB, et al: Oppositional defiant and conduct disorder: a review of the past 10 years, part I. J Am Acad Child Adolesc Psychiatry 39(12):1468–1484, 2000 11128323

Loeber R, Burke JD, Lahey BB: What are adolescent antecedents to antisocial personality disorder? Crim Behav Ment Health 12(1):24–36, 2002 12357255

Lynskey MT, Fergusson DM: Childhood conduct problems, attention deficit behaviors, and adolescent alcohol, tobacco, and illicit drug use. J Abnorm Child Psychol 23(3):281–302, 1995 7642838

Mager W, Milich R, Harris MJ, et al: Intervention groups for adolescents with conduct problems: is aggregation harmful or helpful? J Abnorm Child Psychol 33(3):349–362, 2005 15957562

Mason WA, Hitchings JE, McMahon RJ, et al: A test of three alternative hypotheses regarding the effects of early delinquency on adolescent psychosocial functioning and substance involvement. J Abnorm Child Psychol 35(5):831–843, 2007 17534712

McCarty CA, Wymbs BT, King KM, et al: Developmental consistency in associations between depressive symptoms and alcohol use in early adolescence. J Stud Alcohol Drugs 73(3):444–453, 2012 22456249

McClelland GM, Elkington KS, Teplin LA Abram KM: Multiple substance use disorders in juvenile detainees. J Am Acad Child Adolesc Psychiatry 43(10):1215–1224, 2004 15381888

Merikangas KR, He JP, Burstein M, et al: Lifetime prevalence of mental disorders in U.S. adolescents: results from the National Comorbidity Survey Replication—Adolescent Supplement (NCS-A). J Am Acad Child Adolesc Psychiatry 49(10):980–989, 2010 20855043

Molina BS, Pelham WE Jr: Childhood predictors of adolescent substance use in a longitudinal study of children with ADHD. J Abnorm Psychol 112(3):497–507, 2003 12943028

Mulvey EP, Schubert CA, Chung HL: Service use after court involvement in a sample of serious adolescent offenders. Child Youth Serv Rev 29(4):518–544, 2007 19907667

Mulvey EP, Schubert CA, Chassin L: Substance Use and Delinquent Behavior Among Serious Adolescent Offenders. Washington, DC, Office of Juvenile Justice and Delinquency Prevention, 2010

Myers MG, Stewart DG, Brown SA: Progression from conduct disorder to antisocial personality disorder following treatment for adolescent substance abuse. Am J Psychiatry 155(4):479–485, 1998 9545992

National Institute of Justice: Drug Courts, 2014. Available at: http://www.nij.gov/topics/courts/drug-courts/Pages/welcome.aspx. Accessed July 30, 2014.

National Institute on Drug Abuse: Preventing Drug Use Among Children and Adolescents: A Research-Based Guide for Parents, Educators, and Community Leaders, 2nd Edition. Rockville, MD, National Institute on Drug Abuse/National Institutes of Health, 2003

Niemelä S, Brunstein-Klomek A, Sillanmäki L, et al: Childhood bullying behaviors at age eight and substance use at age 18 among males: a nationwide prospective study. Addict Behav 36(3):256–260, 2011 21146319

Nock MK, Kazdin AE, Hiripi E, et al: Prevalence, subtypes, and correlates of DSM-IV conduct disorder in the National Comorbidity Survey Replication. Psychol Med 36(5):699–710, 2006 16438742

Nock MK, Kazdin AE, Hiripi E, et al: Lifetime prevalence, correlates, and persistence of oppositional defiant disorder: results from the National Comorbidity Survey Replication. J Child Psychol Psychiatry 48(7):703–713, 2007 17593151

Puzzanchera C: Juvenile arrests 2011, in Juvenile Offenders and Victims: National Report Series, Office of Juvenile Justice and Delinquency Prevention, December 2013. Available at: http://www.ojjdp.gov/pubs/244476.pdf. Accessed August 4, 2014.

Rappaport N, Thomas C: Recent research findings on aggressive and violent behavior in youth: implications for clinical assessment and intervention. J Adolesc Health 35(4):260–277, 2004 15450540

Robertson AA, Dill L, Husain J, Undesser C: Prevalence of mental illness and substance abuse disorders among incarcerated juvenile offenders in Mississippi. Child Psychiatry Hum Dev 35(1)55–74, 2004 15626325

Santisteban DA, Coatsworth JD, Perez-Vidal A, et al: Efficacy of brief strategic family therapy in modifying Hispanic adolescent behavior problems and substance use. J Fam Psychol 17(1):121–133, 2003 12666468

Sealock MD, Gottfredson DC, Gallagher CA: Drug treatment for juvenile offenders: some good and bad news. J Res Crime Delinq 34(2):210–236, 1997

Shapiro CJ, Smith BH, Malone PS, et al: Natural experiment in deviant peer exposure and youth recidivism. J Clin Child Adolesc Psychol 39(2):242–251, 2010 20390815

Slutske WS, Heath AC, Dinwiddie SH: Common genetic risk factors for conduct disorder and alcohol dependence. J Abnorm Psychol 107(3):363–374, 1998 9715572

Stanger C, Budney AJ: Contingency management approaches for adolescent substance use disorders. Child Adolesc Psychiatr Clin N Am 19(3):547–562, 2010 20682220

Sullivan CJ, Hamilton ZK: Exploring careers in deviance: a joint trajectory analysis of criminal behavior and substance use in an offender population. Deviant Behav 28(6):497–523, 2007

Swaim RC, Oetting ER, Edwards RW, et al: Links from emotional distress to adolescent drug use: a path model. J Consult Clin Psychol 57(2):227–231, 1989 2708609

Tanner-Smith EE, Wilson SJ, Lipsey MW: The comparative effectiveness of outpatient treatment for adolescent substance abuse: a meta-analysis. J Subst Abuse Treat 44(2):145–158, 2013 22763198

Teplin LA, Abram KM, McClelland GM, et al: Psychiatric disorders in youth in juvenile detention. Arch Gen Psychiatry 59(12):1133–1143, 2002 12470130

Tripodi SJ, Bender K: Substance abuse treatment for juvenile offenders: a review of quasi-experimental and experimental research. J Crim Justice 39(3):246–252, 2011

Tripodi SJ, Bender K, Litschge C, et al: Interventions for reducing adolescent alcohol abuse: a meta-analytic review. Arch Pediatr Adolesc Med 164(1):85–91, 2010 20048247

U.S. General Accounting Office: Adult Drug Courts: Evidence Indicates Recidivism Reductions and Mixed Results for Other Outcomes. Washington, DC, U.S. General Accounting Office, 2005

Van der Put CE, Creemers HE, Hoeve M: Differences between juvenile offenders with and without substance use problems in the prevalence and impact of risk and protective factors for criminal recidivism. Drug Alcohol Depend 134:267–274, 2014 24238911

Wei E, Loeber R, White HR: Teasing apart the developmental associations between alcohol and marijuana use and violence. J Contemp Crim Justice 20(2):166–183, 2004

Weiss B, Caron A, Ball S, et al: Iatrogenic effects of group treatment for antisocial youths. J Consult Clin Psychol 73(6):1036–1044, 2005 16392977

White HR, Tice PC, Loeber R, et al: Illegal acts committed by adolescents under the influence of alcohol and drugs. J Res Crime Delinq 39(2):131–152, 2002

CHAPTER 5

Attention-Deficit/Hyperactivity Disorder and Substance Use Disorders

Timothy E. Wilens, M.D.
Courtney A. Zulauf, B.A.

Substance use disorders (SUDs) begin in adolescence or early adulthood and affect up to 30% of U.S. adults. It is estimated that 9% of adolescents manifest a drug use disorder, and 6% meet criteria for an alcohol use disorder (Merikangas et al. 2010). Increased severity of SUD, decreased efforts to seek treatment, and prolonged duration of SUD in adulthood are all predicted by childhood-onset SUD (Johnson et al. 2000). Early-onset SUD is associated with elevated rates of academic failure, suicidal behaviors, and other dangerous behaviors (Brook et al. 1996). Increasingly, the connection between early-onset SUD and attention-deficit/hyperactivity disorder (ADHD) is emerging as an area of intense study and concern.

ADHD is one of the most prevalent neurobehavioral disorders in children and adolescents. ADHD has an onset in early childhood and affects 6%–9% of children and adolescents (Merikangas et al. 2011). Moreover, in approximately 50% of individuals with ADHD, the disorder persists into adulthood (Wilens and Spencer 2010), such that 4%–5% of adults worldwide are affected by the disorder.

This research was supported by grant K24 DA016264, awarded to T.E. Wilens, M.D.

Given the apparent risks associated with having an SUD, as well as the high rate of ADHD in adolescents, the overlap between the two disorders is relevant to research as well as clinical practice in developmental pediatrics, psychology, and psychiatry, with implications for diagnosis.

Features and Diagnosis of ADHD

The essential features encompassing the diagnosis of ADHD from DSM-5 (American Psychiatric Association 2013) are listed in Box 5–1. ADHD begins in childhood and has a requirement that several symptoms be present before age 12 years. This criterion conveys the importance of a substantial clinical presentation during childhood. Furthermore, manifestations of the disorder must be present in more than one setting (e.g., at school, in interpersonal relationships). A critical clinical feature of ADHD is that it has a *persistent* pattern of inattention and/or hyperactivity-impulsivity that interferes with functioning or development. *Hyperactivity* manifests as excessive motor activity when it is not appropriate, such as excessive fidgeting, tapping, talking, or internal restlessness. *Inattention* refers to wandering off task, lacking persistence, having difficulty sustaining focus, and being disorganized, and is not due to defiance or lack of ability. *Impulsivity* refers to hasty actions that occur in the moment without forethought of consequences and/or that have potential for undue harm to the individual.

Box 5–1.   DSM-5 Criteria for Attention-Deficit/Hyperactivity Disorder

---

A. A persistent pattern of inattention and/or hyperactivity-impulsivity that interferes with functioning or development, as characterized by (1) and/or (2):

1. **Inattention:** Six (or more) of the following symptoms have persisted for at least 6 months to a degree that is inconsistent with developmental level and that negatively impacts directly on social and academic/occupational activities:

    Note: The symptoms are not solely a manifestation of oppositional behavior, defiance, hostility, or failure to understand tasks or instructions. For older adolescents and adults (age 17 and older), at least five symptoms are required.

    a. Often fails to give close attention to details or makes careless mistakes in schoolwork, at work, or during other activities (e.g., overlooks or misses details, work is inaccurate).

    b. Often has difficulty sustaining attention in tasks or play activities (e.g., has difficulty remaining focused during lectures, conversations, or lengthy reading).

    c. Often does not seem to listen when spoken to directly (e.g., mind seems elsewhere, even in the absence of any obvious distraction).

    d. Often does not follow through on instructions and fails to finish schoolwork, chores, or duties in the workplace (e.g., starts tasks but quickly loses focus and is easily sidetracked).

    e. Often has difficulty organizing tasks and activities (e.g., difficulty managing sequential tasks; difficulty keeping materials and belongings in order; messy, disorganized work; has poor time management; fails to meet deadlines).

    f. Often avoids, dislikes, or is reluctant to engage in tasks that require sustained mental effort (e.g., schoolwork or homework; for older adolescents and adults, preparing reports, completing forms, reviewing lengthy papers).

    g. Often loses things necessary for tasks or activities (e.g., school materials, pencils, books, tools, wallets, keys, paperwork, eyeglasses, mobile telephones).

    h. Is often easily distracted by extraneous stimuli (for older adolescents and adults, may include unrelated thoughts).

    i. Is often forgetful in daily activities (e.g., doing chores, running errands; for older adolescents and adults, returning calls, paying bills, keeping appointments).

2. **Hyperactivity and impulsivity:** Six (or more) of the following symptoms have persisted for at least 6 months to a degree that is inconsistent with developmental level and that negatively impacts directly on social and academic/occupational activities:

    Note: The symptoms are not solely a manifestation of oppositional behavior, defiance, hostility, or a failure to understand tasks or instructions. For older adolescents and adults (age 17 and older), at least five symptoms are required.

    a. Often fidgets with or taps hands or feet or squirms in seat.

    b. Often leaves seat in situations when remaining seated is expected (e.g., leaves his or her place in the classroom, in the office or other workplace, or in other situations that require remaining in place).

    c. Often runs about or climbs in situations where it is inappropriate. (**Note:** In adolescents or adults, may be limited to feeling restless.)

    d. Often unable to play or engage in leisure activities quietly.

    e. Is often "on the go," acting as if "driven by a motor" (e.g., is unable to be or uncomfortable being still for extended time, as in restaurants, meetings; may be experienced by others as being restless or difficult to keep up with).

    f. Often talks excessively.

    g. Often blurts out an answer before a question has been completed (e.g., completes people's sentences; cannot wait for turn in conversation).

    h. Often has difficulty waiting his or her turn (e.g., while waiting in line).

    i. Often interrupts or intrudes on others (e.g., butts into conversations, games, or activities; may start using other people's things without asking or receiving permission; for adolescents and adults, may intrude into or take over what others are doing).

B. Several inattentive or hyperactive-impulsive symptoms were present prior to age 12 years.

C. Several inattentive or hyperactive-impulsive symptoms are present in two or more settings (e.g., at home, school, or work; with friends or relatives; in other activities).

D. There is clear evidence that the symptoms interfere with, or reduce the quality of, social, academic, or occupational functioning.

E. The symptoms do not occur exclusively during the course of schizophrenia or another psychotic disorder and are not better explained by another mental disorder (e.g., mood disorder, anxiety disorder, dissociative disorder, personality disorder, substance intoxication or withdrawal).

Specify whether:

314.01 (F90.2) Combined presentation: If both Criterion A1 (inattention) and Criterion A2 (hyperactivity-impulsivity) are met for the past 6 months.

314.00 (F90.0) Predominantly inattentive presentation: If Criterion A1 (inattention) is met but Criterion A2 (hyperactivity-impulsivity) is not met for the past 6 months.

314.01 (F90.1) Predominantly hyperactive/impulsive presentation: If Criterion A2 (hyperactivity-impulsivity) is met and Criterion A1 (inattention) is not met for the past 6 months.

Specify if:

In partial remission: When full criteria were previously met, fewer than the full criteria have been met for the past 6 months, and the symptoms still result in impairment in social, academic, or occupational functioning.

Specify current severity:

Mild: Few, if any, symptoms in excess of those required to make the diagnosis are present, and symptoms result in no more than minor impairments in social or occupational functioning.

Moderate: Symptoms or functional impairment between "mild" and "severe" are present.

Severe: Many symptoms in excess of those required to make the diagnosis, or several symptoms that are particularly severe, are present, or the symptoms result in marked impairment in social or occupational functioning.

Several noteworthy changes to the diagnostic criteria for ADHD in DSM-5 are particularly relevant when discussing comorbid SUDs. The age at onset requirement has been modified from onset of symptoms before age 7 years to onset before age 12 years. Also, subtypes have been replaced with presentation specifiers that align directly to prior subtypes. Last, a comorbid diagnosis with autism spectrum disorder is now allowed.

Etiology and Clinical Course of ADHD

ADHD is most often identified during the elementary school years, but identification may be delayed in individuals with higher IQ or inattentive subtype without concurrent disruptive comorbidity. In most individuals, symptoms of hyperactivity become less obvious in adolescence and adulthood, but difficulties with inattention and impulsivity typically persist and are associated with dysfunction. In adults, inattention, restlessness, and impulsivity may remain problematic even when hyperactivity diminishes. Long-term controlled follow-up studies have demonstrated the persistence of ADHD, with childhood cases continuing into adolescence for approximately three-quarters of cases and into adulthood for half of cases (Wilens and Spencer 2010).

Compared with their peers without ADHD, adolescents with ADHD have more disturbances in social relations and underachieve academically despite adequate intellectual abilities (Biederman et al. 2010). ADHD is also frequently associated with co-occurring learning and psychiatric problems across the life span (Wilens and Spencer 2010, 2011). Of no surprise, SUDs are among the most problematic disorders that co-occur with ADHD (Wilens et al. 2011b).

Relationship of ADHD With SUD

A growing literature has demonstrated that children with ADHD are at an elevated risk for developing an SUD compared with their non-ADHD counterparts (Chang et al. 2012; Charach et al. 2011; Groenman et al. 2013) (Figure 5–1). In a meta-analytic review, Charach et al. (2011) noted a substantially higher likelihood of cigarette smoking (2.4-fold increase) and SUD (1.5-fold increase) in youths with ADHD compared with those without ADHD. Groenman et al. (2013) reported in a 4-year follow-up that youths with ADHD were at a heightened risk for developing an SUD or nicotine dependence, independent of conduct disorder. Furthermore, Chang et al. (2012) followed 1,480 pairs of twins from childhood to adolescence and found that the hyperactive/impulsive symptoms of ADHD predicted early-onset tobacco use and that those children with persistent hyperactivity/impulsivity were at a pronounced risk for early onset of both tobacco and alcohol use.

Adolescents with ADHD, compared with peers without ADHD, not only have an increased risk for SUD but also seem to generally have an earlier onset and more chronic path (Wilens et al. 1997). For instance, in a case-control study, Kousha et al. (2011) found that adolescents with ADHD had a younger age at onset for SUD, a shorter period between the first use of a substance and developing a fulminant SUD, greater functional impairment, and more severe use of substances.

A large body of literature has also reported that adolescents and adults with SUD have higher rates of ADHD than those without SUD (for review, see Frodl 2010 and van Emmerik-van Oortmerssen et al. 2012). Studies incorporating structured psychiatric diagnostic interviews assessing ADHD and other disorders in substance-abusing groups have indicated that from one-quarter of adults to one-half of adolescents with SUD have ADHD (Frodl 2010; van Emmerik-van Oortmerssen et al. 2012). For instance, in a meta-analysis, 29 studies assessing rates of ADHD with SUD were examined across all age groups, and 23% of individuals with SUD were reported to manifest ADHD (van Emmerik-van Oortmerssen et al. 2012). Recently, the International ADHD in Substance Use Disorders Prevalence study reported data on 3,558 treatment-seeking subjects with SUD from 10 countries and found that 41% of subjects screened positive for ADHD (van de Glind et al. 2013). Furthermore, data from a large multisite study of mainly cannabis-abusing youths indicated that ADHD is the second most common psychiatric comorbidity, with 40%–50% of both girls and boys manifesting full criteria for ADHD (Dennis et al. 2004). Data ascertained from adult groups with SUD also show earlier onset and more severe SUD associated with ADHD (Carroll and Rounsaville 1993).

Despite the relatively high risk for ADHD among SUD groups, ADHD appears to be underidentified in the setting of addiction treatment. For example, work in an addiction treatment center indicated that although 3% of youths were identified in the records as having ADHD, systematic assessment of patients for ADHD identified a rate of 44% (McAweeney et al. 2010). Although the precise reasons for this variance are unclear, the underreporting of rates may be the result of differences in substance of abuse, variations in diagnostic assessment, lack of knowledge that ADHD is a major comorbidity with SUD, and/or the

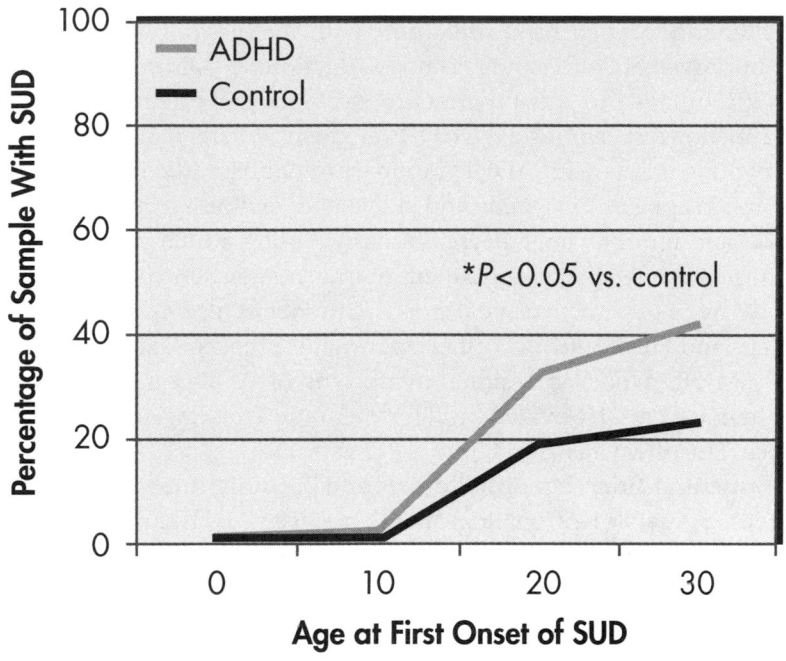

FIGURE 5–1.   Onset of substance use disorder (SUD) in never-treated adults with attention-deficit/hyperactivity disorder (ADHD).

ADHD was ascertained retrospectively. Control group consists of individuals without ADHD.

Source.   Adapted from Wilens et al. 1997.

lack of identification of ADHD previously in treatment-seeking patients with SUD.

Possible Explanations for Relationship Between ADHD and SUD

Although an increasing body of literature shows an intriguing link between ADHD and SUD, the nature of the relationship remains unclear. One possible explanation is that a subgroup of individuals with ADHD may be self-medicating—that is, their substance use helps them to relieve painful affects or to experience or control emotions (Khantzian 1997). One study suggested that the developmental progression from ADHD to conduct disorder and eventual SUD may be related to demoralization and failure (Mannuzza et al. 1989). Other evidence of self-medication includes data indicating a preference for drugs over alcohol in both adolescents (Hartsough and Lambert 1987) and adults (Biederman et al. 1995) with ADHD. Of interest, the use of nicotinic agents (Jacobsen et al. 2005) and the use of nicotinic agents for ADHD (Wilens and Decker 2007) have resulted in adolescents and adults both with and without ADHD indicating improved attention and executive functioning—although Wilens et al. (2011b) failed to show that neuropsychologically defined executive dysfunction drives SUD in ADHD. Previously, Wilens et al. (2007) found that young adults with ADHD reported initiating and continuing their self-medicating with nicotine and substances of abuse to attenuate their mood and improve their sleep. Similarly, young adults who use marijuana report often that it calms their internal restlessness (possibly due to the decay of hyperactive symptoms) (Kaminer et al. 2008; Wilens 2006; Wilens and Fusillo 2007). Further data suggest that college-age students with ADHD who had residual symptoms of ADHD independent of treatment were at elevated risk for cigarette smoking and substance abuse (Upadhyaya et al. 2005).

Structural brain abnormalities found in individuals with ADHD suggest a possible neurobiological link between ADHD and SUD. These abnormalities have included smaller volumes in the frontal cortex, cerebellum, and subcortical structures (Wilens and Spencer 2010). Functional imaging studies have demonstrated that individuals with both ADHD and SUD may have deficits in anterior cingulate activation and in the frontosubcortical systems. Another possibility is that variances in the differential development of the frontal/executive/inhibitory and the limbic/reward systems in ADHD (and conduct disorder) may account for the increased risk for SUD (Casey and Jones 2010). In addition, dopamine systems and striatal involvement are similar for the two disorders (Frodl 2010). A recent study comparing striatal dopamine transporter density in treatment-naive adolescents with ADHD or with ADHD and SUD and in healthy control subjects found that adolescents with ADHD and SUD had lower striatal density compared with those without SUD (Silva et al. 2014); the authors speculate that substance use may be responsible for the lower striatal density, a possibility that may support the self-medication theory in adolescents with ADHD. However, findings from a large and well-constructed multisite study of 1,593 adolescents indicate that there may, in fact, be completely different neurocircuitry involved in both disorders (Whelan et al. 2012).

Moreover, the extant literature has shown that siblings, parents, and offspring of individuals with SUD share the etiologies of ADHD and SUD as well as several genes (Faraone and Biederman 2004). Furthermore, gestational exposure to nicotine or alcohol has been linked consistently to an elevated risk for ADHD in offspring (Schmitz et al. 2006). Hence, family and genetic contributions (Faraone and Biederman 2004) and exposure to parental SUD (Yule et al. 2013) may be other possible explanations linking SUD and ADHD.

Role of Comorbidity

The possible role of comorbid disorders is an important consideration when assessing the link between ADHD and SUD in adolescents and young adults. Most frequently, co-occurring conduct disorder or bipolar disorder has been shown to be associated with a heightened risk for SUD among subjects with ADHD (Wilens et al. 2011b). A few studies have gone so far as to suggest that the link between SUD and ADHD disappears after controlling for comorbid conduct disorder (Lee et al. 2011). However, because of limitations in referral and selection biases, which may have introduced higher than normal levels of conduct disorder, results from these studies need to be approached with great caution. In fact, several population-based studies using dimensional approaches to selection have demonstrated a significant independent link between ADHD and SUD (Burke et al. 2007). For example, in a community-based sample of 968 adolescents, Szobot et al. (2007) found that after controlling for conduct disorder, adolescents with ADHD continued to present a significantly higher risk for SUD compared with peers without ADHD. Moreover, in a case-controlled follow-up study of ADHD, Wilens et al. (2011b) showed that although baseline conduct disorder beget a much higher risk for SUD at 10-year follow-up (a 2.47-fold increase), ADHD continued to be a risk for SUD even in the absence of concurrent conduct disorder (a 1.6-fold increase). Clearly, although ADHD alone places an individual at increased risk for SUD, comorbid conduct disorder or bipolar disorder places an individual at heightened risk for the development of SUD.

Relationship Between Psychopharmacology Treatment for ADHD and Later SUD

Pharmacotherapy remains a fundamental treatment for ADHD. Despite concerns that early stimulant treatment may increase the rates of later SUD, data do not appear to support this possibility. Humphreys et al. (2013) conducted a large meta-analysis of 15 longitudinal studies. After the authors conducted separate random-effects analyses on various substance outcomes, the results suggested that treating ADHD with medications did not influence later substance use. Over 10 years ago, our group conducted the only other meta-analysis on this topic and found that stimulant treatment for ADHD significantly *reduced* later substance problems, particularly in adolescents relative to adults (Wilens et al. 2003).

Several studies not included in the review by Humphreys et al. (2013) are noteworthy. Overall, these studies either do not show an effect of medication treatment on SUD or do show that medication treatment improves SUD and related outcomes. One such study investigating a longer-term open trial of an extended-release form (osmotic-release oral system) of methylphenidate (OROS-MPH) showed that adolescents with ADHD treated with a stimulant were at lower risk than a matched group of untreated youths with ADHD for developing cigarette smoking (Hammerness et al. 2013) and SUD (Hammerness et al. 2012). In the largest study to date, Lichtenstein et al. (2012) reported on 25,656 young adults with ADHD who were followed for 5 years through the age when criminality and SUD would be likely to develop. Approximately half of the subjects were treated pharmacologically for their ADHD, and the authors reported significant reductions in criminality (41% for females and 32% for males); approximately 36% of crimes were drug related and a supposed proxy of SUD (Lichtenstein et al. 2012). Of interest, further analysis found that rates of criminality were lowest during periods when the patients were receiving medication for their ADHD. Another multisite study from Europe also showed diminished SUD in treated groups with ADHD (Konstenius et al. 2014). This 24-week follow-up study randomized 54 men, who were currently incarcerated and who had ADHD and amphetamine dependence, to receive either MPH or placebo in conjunction with weekly cognitive-behavioral therapy (CBT). Compared with the placebo group, the MPH-treated group experienced a reduction in ADHD symptoms, had a significantly higher proportion of drug-negative urine screens, and had a significantly higher treatment retention rate (Konstenius et al. 2014). Given the results from the very large Swedish registry study (Lichtenstein et al. 2012) and more recent prospective trials, it appears that although earlier findings were mixed, more recent findings have shown that medication treatment for ADHD substantially reduces the risk for SUD in general ADHD and high-risk ADHD groups.

Assessment and Interventions

Evaluation and treatment of comorbid ADHD and SUD should be part of a plan in which consideration is given to all aspects of the individual's life. Given that many individuals with comorbid ADHD and SUD are ages 16–26 years, an assessment and management strategy has been developed for this age group with SUD (Wilens et al. 2013), as summarized in Table 5–1. Briefly, a careful evaluation of the patient should be conducted, including psychiatric, addiction, social, cognitive, educational, medical, and family issues. A thorough history of substance use should be obtained, including past and current usage and treatments. Careful attention should be paid to the differential diagnosis(es), including medical and neurological conditions whose symptoms may overlap with ADHD or be a result of SUD (i.e., protracted withdrawal, intoxication, hyperactivity). Current psychosocial factors contributing to the clinical presentation need to be explored thoroughly. Similarly, a comprehensive assessment of educational abilities, achievement, performance, and dysfunction should be performed. Although no specific guidelines exist for evaluating the patient with active SUD, we consider at least 1 month of abstinence to be useful in accurately and reliably assessing a patient for ADHD symptoms. Data on this issue are limited; however, as part of a clinical trial in adults, Wilens et al. (2011a) found up to a 30% worsening of ADHD symptoms in the context of active alcohol use. Semistructured psychiatric interviews or validated rating scales of ADHD (Adler and Cohen 2004) are invaluable aids for the systematic diagnostic assessments of this group.

To meet the treatment needs of individuals with comorbid ADHD and SUD, both disorders should be taken into consideration. If possible, it is best to have some stabilization of the addiction prior to treating the ADHD, at least pharmacologically, given that the bulk of studies have not demonstrated positive outcomes for ADHD treatment in the context of active SUD. One intervention that may be useful for both ADHD and SUD is CBT that combines motivational interviewing with addiction and ADHD components. After stabilization of the addiction (stable low-level use or abstinence), medication may be introduced. Self-help groups offer a supportive treatment modality for many with SUD. In tandem with addiction treatment, SUD patients with ADHD require intervention(s) for the ADHD (and, if applicable, other additional comorbid psychiatric disorders). Education of the individual, family members, and other caregivers is a useful initial step to improve the recognition of the ADHD.

Role of Medication

Medication serves an important role in reducing the symptoms of ADHD and other concurrent psychiatric disorders. Effective agents for ADHD include stimulants, α-agonists, noradrenergic agents, and catecholaminergic antidepressants (Wilens and Spencer 2010).

TABLE 5–1. Components of treatment for co-occurring ADHD and SUD in adolescents and young adults

Comprehensive evaluation	Evaluation of mental health, addiction, social skills, cognition, education, medical and family issues
Substance use history	History of past and current usage and treatments
Diagnosis of ADHD	Clinical interview, structured interview, rating scales Review of childhood documents, discussion with significant other(s)
Decide level of care	If feasible, most effective to stabilize SUD first and/or use MI/CBT for comorbid condition; careful attention to treat ADHD medically
Psychotherapy	MI, CBT, skill-based training
Psychopharmacology	SUD: Anticraving agents, aversive agents, opioid replacement therapy, cigarette smoking cessation
	ADHD: Medications with low(er) abuse liability (nonstimulants, such as atomoxetine, bupropion, tricyclic antidepressants; extended-release stimulants, OROS methylphenidate, extended-release D-methylphenidate, extended-release D-amphetamine)
	Data suggest the use of nonstimulants as first-line agents (for core ADHD as well as often comorbid conditions, such as anxiety or mood disorders), followed by extended-release stimulant preparations.
	Immediate-release stimulants should be avoided because of the higher risk for misuse or diversion.
Parent work	Education, support, and directed coaching and problem solving
Recognize treatment issues	Stigma, access to care, denial of illness, insurance, adherence, unreasonable expectations, and uncomfortable side effects

Note. ADHD=attention-deficit/hyperactivity disorder; CBT=cognitive-behavioral therapy; MI=motivational interviewing; OROS=osmotic-release oral system; SUD=substance use disorder.

Although concerns have been raised that stimulants may worsen cigarette smoking in individuals with ADHD (Vansickel et al. 2011), prospective studies do not support that position (Hammerness et al. 2013; Winhusen et al. 2010). For instance, in a multisite, 11-week, placebo-controlled study of 255 smoking adults with ADHD treated with smoking cessation counseling and the nicotine patch, those also given OROS-MPH dosage up to 72 mg/day experienced improved ADHD but no effects on rates of cigarette smoking (Winhusen et al. 2010).

In general, although open studies are more encouraging, results from controlled trials with stimulants and/or bupropion suggest that ADHD pharmacotherapy used in adults with ADHD plus active SUD has meager effects on the ADHD or the substance use or cravings. Schubiner et al. (2002) reported the results of a prospective, double-blind, randomized trial of MPH in cocaine-abusing subjects with ADHD. Of the 48 subjects enrolled, 52% completed the 13-week trial. Although significant reductions in symptoms of ADHD were reported, no changes in cocaine use (based on self-report or urine toxicology screens) or cocaine craving were found in the MPH group. Similarly, in two well-conducted studies of MPH and/or bupropion in adults with cocaine addiction (±opioid replacement with methadone), Levin et al. (2006, 2007) found only small to no improvements in ADHD and SUD outcomes. Notably, in relation to MPH or bupropion administration, these investigators did not observe worsening of cocaine or other drug use. Consistent results were also shown from a multisite study of treatment of adolescents with ADHD and SUD (Riggs 2009). In this 16-week placebo-controlled study, 300 adolescents with mixed SUDs received placebo or OROS-MPH to 72 mg/day along with weekly individual CBT. Significant improvement compared with baseline occurred in both treatment arms; however, there was no significant improvement in ADHD (per investigator or parent) or SUD (per adolescent self-report) between treatment groups. Side effects were reminiscent of adolescent studies, and the medication was reported to be of low abuse liability (Winhusen et al. 2011).

Atomoxetine is a commonly studied drug because of its broad spectrum of activity in ADHD and its lack of abuse liability (Heil et al. 2002). In a 12-week multisite study in recently abstinent alcoholic individuals, Wilens et al. (2008b) found that compared with placebo, atomoxetine improved ADHD and recurrent episodes of heavy drinking but not relapse to heavy drinking. Similarly, in a small, 10-week, open-label study, atomoxetine treated ADHD symptoms and reduced the intensity, frequency, and length of cravings in recently abstinent adults with

SUD and comorbid ADHD (Adler et al. 2010). Atomoxetine administration in heavy drinkers relative to light drinkers or nondrinkers was associated with more side effects; however, neither serious adverse events nor evidence of impaired liver functioning emerged in the heavy drinkers in these relatively short-term trials (Adler et al. 2009). These promising data in abstinent alcoholic individuals need to be tempered against another placebo-controlled study of atomoxetine in *currently using* adolescents with SUD. Thurstone et al. (2010), in a 12-week study of 70 adolescents with ADHD and at least one active non-nicotine SUD, reported that no differences between ADHD scores or in use of substances between treatment groups emerged. Similar results were found by McRae-Clark et al. (2010) in 12-week, randomized controlled trial of atomoxetine or placebo in conjunction with motivational interviewing. Hence, when it comes to providing pharmacotherapy to current substance-abusing individuals with ADHD, the aggregate results indicate only minimal effects on ADHD and substance use (Levin et al. 2006, 2007; McRae-Clark et al. 2010; Riggs et al. 2011; Schubiner et al. 2002; Thurstone et al. 2010). However, providing treatment to groups of recently abstinent persons or groups at very high risk of SUD (e.g., incarcerated individuals) in a more "relapse-prevention" mode may protect against the onset of SUD (Konstenius et al. 2014; Wilens et al. 2008a).

Role of Psychotherapy

To date, no studies have directly examined in a controlled manner the possible beneficial role of psychotherapies for treating adolescents with ADHD and SUD (Zulauf et al. 2014). However, a growing body of literature demonstrates the success of CBT in reducing adults' ADHD symptoms (Emilsson et al. 2011; Philipsen et al. 2007; Safren et al. 2005) and SUD (Dennis et al. 2004). Furthermore, emerging data on adolescents with ADHD suggest that CBT may be effective as well. For instance, Antshel et al. (2012) examined a modified CBT intervention based on adult work (Safren et al. 2005) and observed improvements in core and associated symptoms across 82 adolescents who participated in the program. This study's results were similar to results from adult studies (Emilsson et al. 2011; Philipsen et al. 2007; Safren et al. 2005) that demonstrated the success of CBT in trials for reducing ADHD symptoms and SUD.

These findings that CBT is successful in treating either ADHD or SUD bring into question whether psychotherapies can contribute to treatment among adolescents and adults with both disorders (Zulauf et al. 2014). As mentioned in the subsection "Role of Medication," several randomized controlled trials of medication to treat subjects with ADHD and SUD have shown overall improvements in ADHD outcome across subjects, with no differences between groups (medication vs. placebo; Figure 5–2). Notably, all subjects in these studies received adjunct psychotherapies, either CBT or motivational interviewing, warranting the idea that the psychotherapy, and not the medication, explains the overall improvement in ADHD among substance abusers with ADHD (Zulauf et al. 2014). Owing to previous study designs, no concrete conclusions regarding the psychotherapies can be determined, and therefore further investigation into the role of psychotherapy alone in treating comorbid ADHD and SUD is needed (Riggs et al. 2011).

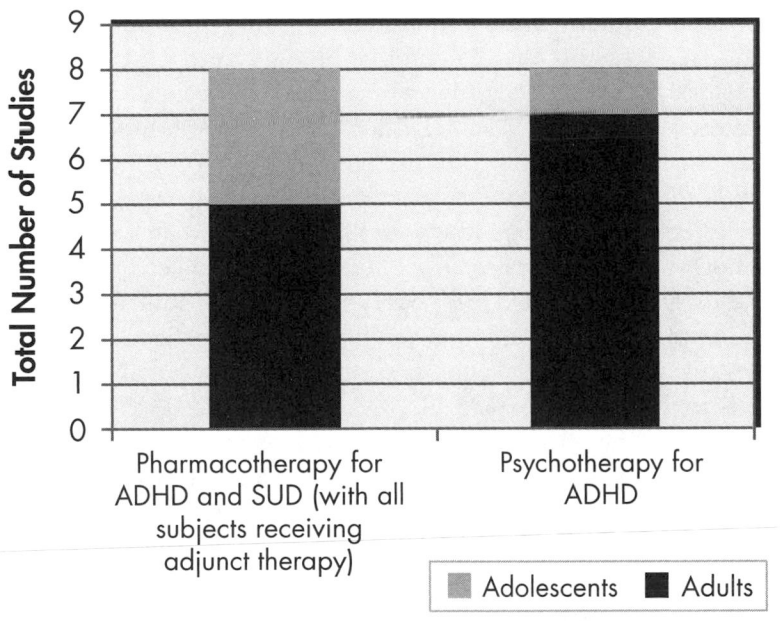

FIGURE 5–2.   Studies that have shown success in reducing symptoms of ADHD.

Trials of pharmacotherapy to treat subjects with ADHD and SUD have shown overall ADHD outcome improvements across subjects, with no differences between groups (medication vs. placebo). All of these studies used adjunct psychotherapies, warranting the conclusion that the psychotherapy, and not the medication, explains the overall improvement in ADHD. These findings suggest the need for investigation into the role of psychotherapy alone for comorbid ADHD and SUD. ADHD=attention-deficit/hyperactivity disorder; SUD=substance use disorder.
Source.   Data from Zulauf et al. 2014.

Diversion and Misuse of Stimulants

The wide use of medications to treat ADHD has led to growing concern regarding the misuse and diversion of stimulants (for review, see Wilens et al. 2008a), particularly among higher-risk groups such as those with SUD. The National Monitoring of Adolescent Prescription Stimulants Study surveyed 11,048 youths ages 10–18 years and found that 12% of those surveyed reported lifetime incoming/outgoing diversion of prescription stimulants (Cottler et al. 2013). Previous data suggested that approximately 5% of college students had misused stimulants (Teter et al. 2006). Table 5–2 reviews studies of misuse and diversion among college samples. The apparent increase in misuse and diversion may be due to the increased rate of prescribing stimulants for ADHD treatment; the medication is, therefore, more readily available.

There is evidence that those who misuse stimulants are more likely to have ADHD symptoms or neuropsychological problems that predate the misuse (Amelia et al. 2010). For example, in a secondary analysis of an Internet-based survey, young adults with higher Adult ADHD Self-Report Scale scores were significantly more likely to engage in nonmedical use of ADHD medications, whereas young adults with lower scores were less likely to engage in nonmedical use (i.e., use without a prescription or in a manner not prescribed) (Upadhyaya et al. 2010).

Research has indicated that peers are the leading source of diversion of prescription stimulants among adolescents and college students and that most young adults who misuse stimulants obtain them from friends, often for free (Arria et al. 2008; McCabe and Boyd 2005; Wilens et al. 2008a). One review conducted by Wilens et al. (2008a) found that among stimulant-receiving high school students with ADHD, 15% had given and 7% had sold their medications to other students. Similar results from a Web-based survey indicated that approximately 13.8% of lifetime prescribed users of controlled medications had traded, sold, given away, or loaned their medications (McCabe et al. 2011). Further analysis showed that being approached to divert medications, nonmedical use of prescription medications, externalizing behaviors, and being nonwhite were significantly associated with the diversion of controlled medications. Results from the Monitoring the Future study (McCabe and West 2013) showed that adolescents who used stimulants for nonmedical reasons (without a prescription) were at significantly greater risk for substance use behaviors than were peers who used stimulants only for medical reasons.

TABLE 5–2. Representative studies of misuse and diversion in college samples

Study authors	Ascertainment	Type of study	Age group	Misuse/diversion
Babcock and Byrne 2000	283 students at a public liberal arts college	Self-reported college survey via mail	Mean, 21 years	17% of sample reported having used MPH recreationally; 13% reported intranasal use
Low and Gendaszek 2002	Convenience sample of 150 undergraduates in a psychology class	Self-reported written survey	Mean, 20 years	36% reported illicit use of stimulants; use associated with use of cocaine and MDMA
Teter et al. 2003	Random sample of 2,250 undergraduates at large public university	Self-reported Web-based student life survey	Mean, 20.1±1.7 years	3% reported illicit MPH use (2% since junior high, 19% since high school, 79% since college)
Hall et al. 2005	381 undergraduate students	Student self-reported written survey via mail and in person	Mean, 19.4±1.7 years	17% of men and 11% of women reported illicit stimulant use for recreation and academics
McCabe and Boyd 2005; McCabe et al. 2006; Teter et al. 2005	Random sample of 9,161 undergraduates at large public university	Self-administered Web-based student life survey	Undergraduates	5.4% reported illicitly using stimulants; 68% reported obtaining drugs from peers; more binge drinking among illicit stimulant users Motivation: 58% concentration; 43% alertness; 43% get high; 14% other

TABLE 5–2. Representative studies of misuse and diversion in college samples *(continued)*

Study authors	Ascertainment	Type of study	Age group	Misuse/diversion
Upadhyaya et al. 2005	Convenience sample of 334 students from a state college	Self-reported survey conducted in class	Mean, 20.6 years	25% used medications to get high; 29% gave or sold medications
White et al. 2006	1,025 undergraduates	Web-based and paper surveys	17–24 years and older	16% reported misusing or abusing stimulants; 96% of them prefer MPH; 40% reported intranasal use
Teter et al. 2006	4,580 full-time college students	Self-administered Web-based survey	Mean, 20.0±2.0 years	8.3% reported lifetime illicit stimulant use; 5.9% past-year illicit use (76% Adderall, 25% Ritalin, 96% oral, 38% intranasal)
Arria et al. 2008	1,253 first-year college students	Cross-sectional study; structured interviews	17–19 years	18% misused stimulants; among those with ADHD, 26.7% overused their ADHD medication and 15.6% nonmedically used someone else's prescription stimulants
Rabiner et al. 2009	115 college students with a prescription for stimulants	Self-administered Web-based survey	Undergraduates	31% endorsed misuse of prescription medications; 8% reported intranasal use and 26% had diverted stimulants to peers

TABLE 5–2. Representative studies of misuse and diversion in college samples *(continued)*

Study authors	Ascertainment	Type of study	Age group	Misuse/diversion
Jardin et al. 2011	43 undergraduate students using prescription stimulants	Structured interviews and a battery of questionnaires	Mean, 20.7 years	Misusers significantly endorsed using greater number of illicit substances over past year
Sepúlveda et al. 2011	1,738 college students at a large Midwestern research university	Self-administered Web-based survey	Mean, 20.8 years	Of 55 students who reported use of prescribed stimulants for ADHD, 40% endorsed misuse; misusers were more likely to report additional substance use

Note. ADHD=attention-deficit/hyperactivity disorder; MDMA=methylenedioxymethamphetamine (Ecstasy); MPH=methylphenidate.
Source. Adapted from Zulauf et al. 2014.

Furthermore, stimulant misuse has generally been found to be related to other substances of abuse (McCabe et al. 2004), as well as to psychopathology such as depression (Poulin 2007), ADHD (Amelia et al. 2010; Upadhyaya et al. 2010), and conduct disorder (Wilens et al. 2006).

A growing database suggests that the formulation of the stimulant may impact the misuse of the medication. For instance, previous studies have shown extended-release MPH to be less popular relative to immediate-release MPH (Wilens et al. 2006). Hence, among older adolescents, college students, and individuals with SUD histories, it seems prudent to recommend the use of extended-release stimulants to help reduce misuse and diversion of this class of medication. Because of the seemingly high rates of misuse and diversion, clinicians need to educate parents and patients about the importance of safe storage and disposal of medications.

Summary and Future Directions

ADHD alone or particularly in combination with other psychiatric comorbidities is a risk factor for the development of cigarette smoking and SUD. ADHD is prevalent among adolescents and adults who have SUD. Individuals with ADHD and SUD have more complicated SUD, including earlier onsets, more complicated courses, and more difficulty with treatment. Early and sustained treatment of ADHD may reduce the ultimate risk for cigarette smoking and SUD. Treatment strategies for substance-abusing adolescents and adults with ADHD should focus on the addiction initially, if possible, and then the ADHD, with CBT as the preferred initial therapy. For those at high risk for using substances, pharmacotherapy for ADHD may help prevent relapses. The use of nonstimulants or the judicious use of extended-release stimulants is preferred when treating groups at high risk for diverting or misusing their medications. The growing trend of stimulant use by non-ADHD youths seeking cognitive enhancement ("smart pills") needs to be further studied, and the development of preventive strategies in academic institutes is warranted (Bagot and Kaminer 2014). Finally, future studies elucidating the biological and psychosocial mechanism(s) linking ADHD to cigarette smoking or SUD, as well as the protective effects of treatment on later addictive behaviors, are necessary.

KEY POINTS

- Individuals with attention-deficit/hyperactivity disorder (ADHD) are at elevated risk for cigarette smoking and substance use disorder (SUD) throughout their life span.

- All adolescent and adult patients with SUD should be screened for ADHD because of the high rates of comorbidity.

- Patients with SUD and ADHD should receive addiction treatment initially, followed by individual therapy or pharmacotherapy to treat ADHD.

- In groups that are at high risk for medication misuse, treatment with nonstimulants or carefully monitored extended-release stimulants is preferred.

References

Adler L, Cohen J: Diagnosis and evaluation of adults with ADHD. Psychiatr Clin North Am 27(2):187–201, 2004 15063992

Adler L, Wilens T, Zhang S, et al: Retrospective safety analysis of atomoxetine in adult ADHD patients with or without comorbid alcohol abuse and dependence. Am J Addict 18(5):393–401, 2009 19874159

Adler LA, Guida F, Irons S, et al: Open label pilot study of atomoxetine in adults with ADHD and substance use disorder. J Dual Diagn 6:196–207, 2010

Amelia AM, Garnier-Dykstra LM, Caldeira KM, et al: Persistent nonmedical use of prescription stimulants among college students: possible association with ADHD symptoms. J Atten Disord 15(5):347–356, 2010 20484709

American Psychiatric Association: Diagnostic and Statistical Manual of Mental Disorders, 5th Edition. Arlington, VA, American Psychiatric Association, 2013

Antshel KM, Faraone SV, Gordon M: Cognitive behavioral treatment outcomes in adolescent ADHD. J Atten Disord 18(6):483–495, 2012 22628140

Arria AM, Caldeira K, O'Grady KE, et al: Nonmedical use of prescription stimulants among college students: associations with attention-deficit-hyperactivity disorder and polydrug use. Pharmacotherapy 28(2):156–169, 2008 18225963

Babcock Q, Byrne T: Student perceptions of methylphenidate abuse at a public liberal arts college. J Am Coll Health 49(3):143–145, 2000 11125642

Bagot KS, Kaminer Y: Efficacy of stimulants for cognitive enhancement in non-attention deficit hyperactivity disorder youth: a systematic review. Addiction 109(4):547–557, 2014 24749160

Biederman J, Wilens T, Mick E, et al: Psychoactive substance use disorders in adults with attention deficit hyperactivity disorder (ADHD): effects of ADHD and psychiatric comorbidity. Am J Psychiatry 152(11):1652–1658, 1995 7485630

Biederman J, Petty CR, Monuteaux MC, et al: Adult psychiatric outcomes of girls with attention deficit hyperactivity disorder: 11-year follow-up in a longitudinal case-control study. Am J Psychiatry 167(4):409–417, 2010 20080984

Brook JS, Whiteman M, Finch SJ, et al: Young adult drug use and delinquency: childhood antecedents and adolescent mediators. J Am Acad Child Adolesc Psychiatry 35(12):1584–1592, 1996 8973064

Burke JD, Loeber R, White HR, et al: Inattention as a key predictor of tobacco use in adolescence. J Abnorm Psychol 116(2):249–259, 2007 17516758

Carroll KM, Rounsaville BJ: History and significance of childhood attention deficit disorder in treatment-seeking cocaine abusers. Compr Psychiatry 34(2):75–82, 1993 8485984

Casey BJ, Jones RM: Neurobiology of the adolescent brain and behavior: implications for substance use disorders. J Am Acad Child Adolesc Psychiatry 49(12):1189–1201, quiz 1285, 2010 21093769

Chang Z, Lichtenstein P, Larsson H: The effects of childhood ADHD symptoms on early onset substance use: a Swedish twin study. J Abnorm Child Psychol 40(3):425–435, 2012 21947618

Charach A, Yeung E, Climans T, et al: Childhood attention-deficit/hyperactivity disorder and future substance use disorders: comparative meta-analyses. J Am Acad Child Adolesc Psychiatry 50(1):9–21, 2011 21156266

Cottler LB, Striley CW, Lasopa SO: Assessing prescription stimulant use, misuse, and diversion among youth 10–18 years of age. Curr Opin Psychiatry 26(5):511–519, 2013 23896947

Dennis M, Godley SH, Diamond G, et al: The Cannabis Youth Treatment (CYT) study: main findings from two randomized trials. J Subst Abuse Treat 27(3):197–213, 2004 15501373

Emilsson B, Gudjonsson G, Sigurdsson JF, et al: Cognitive behaviour therapy in medication-treated adults with ADHD and persistent symptoms: a randomized controlled trial. BMC Psychiatry 11:116, 2011 21787431

Faraone SV, Biederman J: Neurobiology of attention deficit hyperactivity disorder, in Neurobiology of Mental Illness, 2nd Edition. Edited by Charney DS, Nestler EJ. New York, Oxford University Press, 2004, pp 979–999

Frodl T: Comorbidity of ADHD and substance use disorder (SUD): a neuroimaging perspective. J Atten Disord 14(2):109–120, 2010 20495160

Groenman AP, Oosterlaan J, Rommelse N, et al: Substance use disorders in adolescents with attention deficit hyperactivity disorder: a 4-year follow-up study. Addiction 108(8):1503–1511, 2013 23506232

Hall KM, Irwin MM, Bowman KA, et al: Illicit use of prescribed stimulant medication among college students. J Am Coll Health 53(4):167–174, 2005 15663065

Hammerness P, Petty C, Faraone SV, et al: Do stimulants reduce the risk for alcohol and substance use in youth with ADHD? A secondary analysis of a prospective, 24-month open-label study of osmotic-release methylphenidate. J Atten Disord Dec 20, 2012 23264367 [Epub ahead of print]

Hammerness P, Joshi G, Doyle R, et al: Do stimulants reduce the risk for cigarette smoking in youth with attention-deficit hyperactivity disorder? A prospective, long-term, open-label study of extended-release methylphenidate. J Pediatr 162(1):22–27, 2013 22878114

Hartsough CS, Lambert NM: Pattern and progression of drug use among hyperactives and controls: a prospective short-term longitudinal study. J Child Psychol Psychiatry 28(4):543–553, 1987 3654806

Heil SH, Holmes HW, Bickel WK, et al: Comparison of the subjective, physiological, and psychomotor effects of atomoxetine and methylphenidate in light drug users. Drug Alcohol Depend 67(2):149–156, 2002 12095664

Humphreys KL, Eng T, Lee SS: Stimulant medication and substance use outcomes: a meta-analysis. JAMA Psychiatry 70(7):740–749, 2013 23754458

Jacobsen LK, Krystal JH, Mencl WE, et al: Effects of smoking and smoking abstinence on cognition in adolescent tobacco smokers. Biol Psychiatry 57(1):56–66, 2005 15607301

Jardin B, Looby A, Earleywine M: Characteristics of college students with attention-deficit hyperactivity disorder symptoms who misuse their medications. J Am Coll Health 59(5):373–377, 2011 21500055

Johnson BA, Cloninger CR, Roache JD, et al: Age of onset as a discriminator between alcoholic subtypes in a treatment-seeking outpatient population. Am J Addict 9(1):17–27, 2000 10914290

Kaminer Y, Connor DF, Curry JF, et al: Treatment of comorbid adolsecent cannabis use and major depressive disorder. Psychiatry 5(9):34–39, 2008 2687084

Khantzian EJ: The self-medication hypothesis of substance use disorders: a reconsideration and recent applications. Harv Rev Psychiatry 4(5):231–244, 1997 9385000

Konstenius M, Jayaram-Lindstrom N, Guterstam J, et al: Methylphenidate for attention deficit hyperactivity disorder and drug relapse in criminal offenders with substance dependence: a 24-week randomized placebo-controlled trial. Addiction 109(3):440–449, 2014 24118269

Kousha M, Shahrivar Z, Alaghband-Rad J: Substance use disorder and ADHD: is ADHD a "specific" risk factor? J Atten Disord 16(4):325–332, 2011 22127397

Lee SS, Humphreys KL, Flory K, et al: Prospective association of childhood attention-deficit/hyperactivity disorder (ADHD) and substance use and abuse/dependence: a meta-analytic review. Clin Psychol Rev 31(3):328–341, 2011 21382538

Levin FR, Evans SM, Brooks DJ, et al: Treatment of methadone-maintained patients with adult ADHD: double-blind comparison of methylphenidate, bupropion and placebo. Drug Alcohol Depend 81(2):137–148, 2006 16102908

Levin FR, Evans SM, Brooks DJ, et al: Treatment of cocaine dependent treatment seekers with adult ADHD: double-blind comparison of methylphenidate and placebo. Drug Alcohol Depend 87(1):20–29, 2007 16930863

Lichtenstein P, Halldner L, Zetterqvist J, et al: Medication for attention deficit-hyperactivity disorder and criminality. N Engl J Med 367(21):2006–2014, 2012 23171097

Low KG, Gendaszek AE: Illicit use of psychostimulants among college students: a preliminary study. Psychol Health Med 7(3):283–287, 2002

Mannuzza S, Klein RG, Konig PH, et al: Hyperactive boys almost grown up, IV: criminality and its relationship to psychiatric status. Arch Gen Psychiatry 46(12):1073–1079, 1989 2589922

McAweeney M, Rogers NL, Huddleston C, et al: Symptom prevalence of ADHD in a community residential substance abuse treatment program. J Atten Disord 13(6):601–608, 2010 19365086

McCabe SE, Boyd CJ: Sources of prescription drugs for illicit use. Addict Behav 30(7):1342–1350, 2005 16022931

McCabe SE, West BT: Medical and nonmedical use of prescription stimulants: results from a national multicohort study. J Am Acad Child Adolesc Psychiatry 52(12):1272–1280, 2013 24290460

McCabe SE, Teter CJ, Boyd CJ: The use, misuse and diversion of prescription stimulants among middle and high school students. Subst Use Misuse 39(7):1095–1116, 2004 15387205

McCabe SE, Teter CJ, Boyd CJ: Medical use, illicit use, and diversion of abusable prescription drugs. J Am Coll Health 54(5):269–278, 2006 16539219

McCabe SE, West BT, Teter CJ, et al: Characteristics associated with the diversion of controlled medications among adolescents. Drug Alcohol Depend 118(2–3):452–458, 2011 21665384

McRae-Clark AL, Carter RE, Killeen TK, et al: A placebo-controlled trial of atomoxetine in marijuana-dependent individuals with attention deficit hyperactivity disorder. Am J Addict 19(6):481–489, 2010 20958842

Merikangas KR, He JP, Burstein M, et al: Lifetime prevalence of mental disorders in U.S. adolescents: results from the National Comorbidity Survey Replication—Adolescent Supplement (NCS-A). J Am Acad Child Adolesc Psychiatry 49(10):980–989, 2010 20855043

Merikangas KR, He JP, Burstein M, et al: Service utilization for lifetime mental disorders in U.S. adolescents: results of the National Comorbidity Survey-Adolescent Supplement (NCS-A). J Am Acad Child Adolesc Psychiatry 50(1):32–45, 2011 21156268

Philipsen A, Richter H, Peters J, et al: Structured group psychotherapy in adults with attention deficit hyperactivity disorder: results of an open multicentre study. J Nerv Ment Dis 195(12):1013–1019, 2007 18091195

Poulin C: From attention-deficit/hyperactivity disorder to medical stimulant use to the diversion of prescribed stimulants to non-medical stimulant use: connecting the dots. Addiction 102(5):740–751, 2007 17506151

Rabiner DL, Anastopoulos AD, Costello EJ, et al: The misuse and diversion of prescribed ADHD medications by college students. J Atten Disord 13(2):144–153, 2009 19448150

Riggs P: Multi-site of OROS-MPH for ADHD in substance abusing adolescents. Presented at the 56th Annual Meeting of the American Academy of Child and Adolescent Psychiatry, Honolulu, Hawaii, October 2009

Riggs PD, Winhusen T, Davies RD, et al: Randomized controlled trial of osmotic-release methylphenidate with cognitive-behavioral therapy in adolescents with attention-deficit/hyperactivity disorder and substance use disorders. J Am Acad Child Adolesc Psychiatry 50(9):903–914, 2011 21871372

Safren SA, Otto MW, Sprich S, et al: Cognitive-behavioral therapy for ADHD in medication-treated adults with continued symptoms. Behav Res Ther 43(7):831–842, 2005 15896281

Schmitz M, Denardin D, Laufer Silva T, et al: Smoking during pregnancy and attention-deficit/hyperactivity disorder, predominantly inattentive type: a case-control study. J Am Acad Child Adolesc Psychiatry 45(11):1338–1345, 2006 17075356

Schubiner H, Saules KK, Arfken CL, et al: Double-blind placebo-controlled trial of methylphenidate in the treatment of adult ADHD patients with comorbid cocaine dependence. Exp Clin Psychopharmacol 10(3):286–294, 2002 12233989

Sepúlveda DR, Thomas LM, McCabe SE, et al: Misuse of prescribed stimulant medication for ADHD and associated patterns of substance use: preliminary analysis among college students. J Pharm Pract 24(6):551–560, 2011 22095577

Silva N Jr, Szobot CM, Shih MC, et al: Searching for a neurobiological basis for self-medication theory in ADHD comorbid with substance use disorders: an in vivo study of dopamine transporters using 99mTc-TRODAT-1 SPECT. Clin Nucl Med 39(2):e129–e134, 2014 23856832

Szobot CM, Rohde LA, Bukstein O, et al: Is attention-deficit/hyperactivity disorder associated with illicit substance use disorders in male adolescents? A community-based case-control study. Addiction 102(7):1122–1130, 2007 17567400

Teter CJ, McCabe SE, Boyd CJ, et al: Illicit methylphenidate use in an undergraduate student sample: prevalence and risk factors. Pharmacotherapy 23(5):609–617, 2003 12741435

Teter CJ, McCabe SE, Cranford JA, et al: Prevalence and motives for illicit use of prescription stimulants in an undergraduate student sample. J Am Coll Health 53(6):253–262, 2005 15900989

Teter CJ, McCabe SE, LaGrange K, et al: Illicit use of specific prescription stimulants among college students: prevalence, motives, and routes of administration. Pharmacotherapy 26(10):1501–1510, 2006 16999660

Thurstone C, Riggs PD, Salomonsen-Sautel S, et al: Randomized, controlled trial of atomoxetine for attention-deficit/hyperactivity disorder in adolescents with substance use disorder. J Am Acad Child Adolesc Psychiatry 49(6):573–582, 2010 20494267

Upadhyaya HP, Rose K, Wang W, et al: Attention-deficit/hyperactivity disorder, medication treatment, and substance use patterns among adolescents and young adults. J Child Adolesc Psychopharmacol 15(5):799–809, 2005 16262596

Upadhyaya HP, Kroutil LA, Deas D, et al: Stimulant formulation and motivation for nonmedical use of prescription attention-deficit/hyperactivity disorder medications in a college-aged population. Am J Addict 19(6):569–577, 2010 20958854

van de Glind G, Van Emmerik-van Oortmerssen K, Carpentier PJ, et al: The International ADHD in Substance Use Disorders Prevalence (IASP) study: background, methods and study population. Int J Methods Psychiatr Res Sep 11, 2013 24022983 [Epub ahead of print]

van Emmerik-van Oortmerssen K, van de Glind G, van den Brink W, et al: Prevalence of attention-deficit hyperactivity disorder in substance use disorder patients: a meta-analysis and meta-regression analysis. Drug Alcohol Depend 122(1–2):11–19, 2012 22209385

Vansickel AR, Stoops WW, Glaser PE, et al: Methylphenidate increases cigarette smoking in participants with ADHD. Psychopharmacology (Berl) 218(2):381–390, 2011 21590284

Whelan R, Conrod PJ, Poline JB, et al: Adolescent impulsivity phenotypes characterized by distinct brain networks. Nat Neurosci 15(6):920–925, 2012 22544311

White BP, Becker-Blease KA, Grace-Bishop K: Stimulant medication use, misuse, and abuse in an undergraduate and graduate student sample. J Am Coll Health 54(5):261–268, 2006 16539218

Wilens TE: Attention deficit hyperactivity disorder and substance use disorders. Am J Psychiatry 163(12):2059–2063, 2006 17151154

Wilens TE, Decker MW: Neuronal nicotinic receptor agonists for the treatment of attention-deficit/hyperactivity disorder: focus on cognition. Biochem Pharmacol 74(8):1212–1223, 2007 17689498

Wilens TE, Fusillo MW: When ADHD and substance use disorders intersect: relationship and treatment implications. Curr Psychiatry 9(5):408–414, 2007 17915081

Wilens TE, Spencer TJ: Understanding attention-deficit/hyperactivity disorder from childhood to adulthood. Postgrad Med 122(5):97–109, 2010 20861593

Wilens TE, Spencer SJ: Attention-deficit/hyperactivity disorder: lifetime course and strategies for intervention, in The SAGE Handbook of Developmental Disorders. Edited by Howlin P, Charman T, Ghaziuddin M. London, Sage, 2011, pp 263–286

Wilens TE, Biederman J, Mick E, et al: Attention deficit hyperactivity disorder (ADHD) is associated with early onset substance use disorders. J Nerv Ment Dis 185(8):475–482, 1997 9284860

Wilens TE, Faraone S, Biederman J, et al: Does stimulant therapy of attention-deficit/hyperactivity disorder beget later substance abuse? A meta-analytic review of the literature. Pediatrics 11(1):179–185, 2003 12509574

Wilens TE, Gignac M, Swezey A, et al: Characteristics of adolescents and young adults with ADHD who divert or misuse their prescribed medications. J Am Acad Child Adolesc Psychiatry 45(4):408–414, 2006 16601645

Wilens TE, Adamson J, Sgambati S, et al: Do individuals with ADHD self-medicate with cigarettes and substances of abuse? Results from a controlled family study of ADHD. Am J Addict 16 (suppl 1):14–21, quiz 22–23, 2007 17453603

Wilens TE, Adler LA, Adams J, et al: Misuse and diversion of stimulants prescribed for ADHD: a systematic review of the literature. J Am Acad Child Adolesc Psychiatry 47(1):21–31, 2008a 18174822

Wilens TE, Adler LA, Weiss MD, et al: Atomoxetine treatment of adults with ADHD and comorbid alcohol use disorders. Drug Alcohol Depend 96(1–2):145–154, 2008b 18403134

Wilens TE, Adler LA, Tanaka Y, et al: Correlates of alcohol use in adults with ADHD and comorbid alcohol use disorders: exploratory analysis of a placebo-controlled trial of atomoxetine. Curr Med Res Opin 27(12):2309–2320, 2011a 22029549

Wilens TE, Martelon M, Joshi G, et al: Does ADHD predict substance-use disorders? A 10-year follow-up study of young adults with ADHD. J Am Acad Child Adolesc Psychiatry 50(6):543–553, 2011b 21621138

Wilens TE, McKowen J, Kane M: Transitional-aged youth and substance use: teenaged addicts come of age. Contemporary Pediatrics 30(11) 2013

Winhusen TM, Somoza EC, Brigham GS, et al: Impact of attention-deficit/hyperactivity disorder (ADHD) treatment on smoking cessation intervention in ADHD smokers: a randomized, double-blind, placebo-controlled trial. J Clin Psychiatry 71(12):1680–1688, 2010 20492837

Winhusen TM, Lewis DF, Riggs PD, et al: Subjective effects, misuse, and adverse effects of osmotic-release methylphenidate treatment in adolescent substance abusers with attention-deficit/hyperactivity disorder. J Child Adolesc Psychopharmacol 21(5):455–463, 2011 22040190

Yule AM, Wilens TE, Martelon MK, et al: Does exposure to parental substance use disorders increase substance use disorder risk in offspring? A 5-year follow-up study. Am J Addict 22(5):460–465, 2013 23952891

Zulauf CA, Sprich SE, Safren SA, et al: The complicated relationship between attention deficit/hyperactivity disorder and substance use disorders. Curr Psychiatry Rep 16(3):436, 2014 24526271

CHAPTER 6

Depressive Disorders and Substance Use Disorders

John F. Curry, Ph.D., ABPP
Jacqueline Hersh, Ph.D.

Depression can refer to a normal feeling of sadness, a set of symptoms (syndrome), or a psychiatric disorder (Curry 2001). When the term *depression* is used to designate a psychiatric disorder, it encompasses a set of symptoms that occur together, persist for some duration of time, and adversely affect adaptive functioning. The core symptom of a depressive disorder is a disturbance in mood, as reflected in a persistently sad, depressed, blue, or irritable emotional state or in a loss of the capacity for enjoyment or interest. Even within the more restrictive domain of depression as a mood disorder, so-called depression can range from a relatively mild, time-limited reaction following a clear stressful event to a severe, prolonged, or even psychotic episode. In this chapter, we review depressive disorders; these are among the most common psychiatric disorders of adolescence, and therefore they often co-occur with substance abuse in this age range. We also review literature on adolescent substance abuse and syndromal depression that may or may not be part of a depressive disorder. As we note, the diversity across studies in what constitutes depression contributes to some of the existing uncertainty in the field about its impact on substance abuse treatment outcome.

Some adolescents with depressive disorders go on to develop bipolar disorder, when one or more manic or hypomanic episodes occur after an episode of depression. However, because bipolar disorder is covered in Chapter 7, "Bipolar Disorders and Substance Use Disorders," we do not include the topic in the present chapter.

Diagnoses of Depression

Major depressive disorder (MDD) and persistent depressive disorder (dysthymia) may occur in adolescents with drug or alcohol use disorders. In addition, substance-abusing adolescents may experience a subthreshold depression—that is, one in which the full symptom array for MDD or persistent depressive disorder is lacking. Finally, substance abuse itself can lead to a depressive reaction, or a substance-induced depressive disorder.

MDD is characterized by one or more major depressive episodes (MDEs) in the absence of any manic or hypomanic episodes. The symptoms and required duration of an MDE listed in DSM-5 (American Psychiatric Association 2013) (Box 6–1, criteria A–C) are identical to those previously listed in DSM-IV-TR (American Psychiatric Association 2000). An MDE must be at least 2 weeks in duration and is characterized by a significant decline in functioning. The core symptom is either depressed mood or pervasive anhedonia. A total of five symptoms are required to make the diagnosis. In addition to mood disturbance and/or anhedonia, symptoms may include disturbances in appetite or weight; insomnia or hypersomnia; fatigue or low energy; psychomotor agitation or retardation; feelings of worthlessness or inappropriate guilt; trouble thinking, concentrating, or deciding; and morbid or suicidal thoughts or suicidal behavior.

Box 6–1. DSM-5 Criteria for Major Depressive Disorder

A. Five (or more) of the following symptoms have been present during the same 2-week period and represent a change from previous functioning; at least one of the symptoms is either (1) depressed mood or (2) loss of interest or pleasure.
Note: Do not include symptoms that are clearly attributable to another medical condition.

   1. Depressed mood most of the day, nearly every day, as indicated by either subjective report (e.g., feels sad, empty, hopeless) or observation made by others (e.g., appears tearful). (**Note:** In children and adolescents, can be irritable mood.)
   2. Markedly diminished interest or pleasure in all, or almost all, activities most of the day, nearly every day (as indicated by either subjective account or observation).

3. Significant weight loss when not dieting or weight gain (e.g., a change of more than 5% of body weight in a month), or decrease or increase in appetite nearly every day. (**Note:** In children, consider failure to make expected weight gain.)
4. Insomnia or hypersomnia nearly every day.
5. Psychomotor agitation or retardation nearly every day (observable by others, not merely subjective feelings of restlessness or being slowed down).
6. Fatigue or loss of energy nearly every day.
7. Feelings of worthlessness or excessive or inappropriate guilt (which may be delusional) nearly every day (not merely self-reproach or guilt about being sick).
8. Diminished ability to think or concentrate, or indecisiveness, nearly every day (either by subjective account or as observed by others).
9. Recurrent thoughts of death (not just fear of dying), recurrent suicidal ideation without a specific plan, or a suicide attempt or a specific plan for committing suicide.

B. The symptoms cause clinically significant distress or impairment in social, occupational, or other important areas of functioning.
C. The episode is not attributable to the physiological effects of a substance or to another medical condition.

Note: Criteria A–C represent a major depressive episode.

Note: Responses to a significant loss (e.g., bereavement, financial ruin, losses from a natural disaster, a serious medical illness or disability) may include the feelings of intense sadness, rumination about the loss, insomnia, poor appetite, and weight loss noted in Criterion A, which may resemble a depressive episode. Although such symptoms may be understandable or considered appropriate to the loss, the presence of a major depressive episode in addition to the normal response to a significant loss should also be carefully considered. This decision inevitably requires the exercise of clinical judgment based on the individual's history and the cultural norms for the expression of distress in the context of loss.

D. The occurrence of the major depressive episode is not better explained by schizoaffective disorder, schizophrenia, schizophreniform disorder, delusional disorder, or other specified and unspecified schizophrenia spectrum and other psychotic disorders.
E. There has never been a manic episode or a hypomanic episode.
Note: This exclusion does not apply if all of the manic-like or hypomanic-like episodes are substance-induced or are attributable to the physiological effects of another medical condition.

The DSM-5 category of persistent depressive disorder (Box 6–2) includes what was formerly called dysthymic disorder in DSM-IV-TR (American Psychiatric Association 2000) in addition to persistent episodes of MDD. In adolescents, the duration of a persistent depressive episode must be at least 1 year (2 years in adults), during which time at least two additional symptoms are present and the individual has not had a symptom-free period of at least 2 months. The associated symptoms may involve disturbances in appetite, sleep, energy, self-esteem, or concentration or feelings of hopelessness.

Box 6–2. DSM-5 Criteria for Persistent Depressive Disorder

This disorder represents a consolidation of DSM-IV-defined chronic major depressive disorder and dysthymic disorder.

A. Depressed mood for most of the day, for more days than not, as indicated by either subjective account or observation by others, for at least 2 years.

   Note: In children and adolescents, mood can be irritable and duration must be at least 1 year.

B. Presence, while depressed, of two (or more) of the following:

   1. Poor appetite or overeating.
   2. Insomnia or hypersomnia.
   3. Low energy or fatigue.
   4. Low self-esteem.
   5. Poor concentration or difficulty making decisions.
   6. Feelings of hopelessness.

C. During the 2-year period (1 year for children or adolescents) of the disturbance, the individual has never been without the symptoms in Criteria A and B for more than 2 months at a time.

D. Criteria for a major depressive disorder may be continuously present for 2 years.

E. There has never been a manic episode or a hypomanic episode, and criteria have never been met for cyclothymic disorder.

F. The disturbance is not better explained by a persistent schizoaffective disorder, schizophrenia, delusional disorder, or other specified or unspecified schizophrenia spectrum and other psychotic disorder.

G. The symptoms are not attributable to the physiological effects of a substance (e.g., a drug of abuse, a medication) or another medical condition (e.g., hypothyroidism).

H. The symptoms cause clinically significant distress or impairment in social, occupational, or other important areas of functioning.

Note: Because the criteria for a major depressive episode include four symptoms that are absent from the symptom list for persistent depressive disorder (dysthymia), a very limited number of individuals will have depressive symptoms that have persisted longer than 2 years but will not meet criteria for persistent depressive disorder. If full criteria for a major depressive episode have been met at some point during the current episode of illness, they should be given a diagnosis of major depressive disorder. Otherwise, a diagnosis of other specified depressive disorder or unspecified depressive disorder is warranted.

Reprinted from the *Diagnostic and Statistical Manual of Mental Disorders*, 5th Edition. Arlington, VA, American Psychiatric Association, 2013. Used with permission. Copyright © 2013 American Psychiatric Association.

A number of substances, including alcohol, hallucinogens, opioids, inhalants, and stimulants, have been associated with induced depressive disorders (American Psychiatric Association 2013). As with other depressive disorders, those induced by substances are characterized by a prominent core symptom of either depressed mood or anhedonia. DSM-5 indicates that such a diagnosis should not be made if there is evidence that the depressive syndrome preceded the substance use, has persisted for more than approximately 1 month after cessation of substance intoxication or substance withdrawal symptoms, or otherwise appears to be independent of substance use, as in the case of recurrent depressive episodes that were not substance induced.

Epidemiology of Depression

Depression is one of the more common psychiatric disorders of adolescence. In the National Comorbidity Survey Replication–Adolescent Supplement (Merikangas et al. 2010), lifetime diagnoses of MDD or dysthymia characterized 11.7% of the sample, a lifetime prevalence rate greater than that for any single anxiety disorder other than specific phobia (19.3%), almost as great as that for the most common disruptive behavior disorder, oppositional defiant disorder (12.6%), and almost identical to the rate for any substance use disorder (SUD) (11.4%).

It is well established that depression is more common among adolescents than among children and more common in adolescent (and adult) females than males. In the Great Smoky Mountains Study, an epidemiological project in western North Carolina, involving children ages 9–13 years, the 3-month prevalence of MDD was only 0.03%, whereas prevalence rates of dysthymic disorder and subsyndromal depression were 0.13% and 1.42%, respectively. Over longitudinal follow-up of this sample, 3-month prevalence of any depression diagnosis increased with age, exceeding 3.0% by age 15 or 16 (Costello et al. 2003). In a meta-analysis of 26 epidemiological studies of children born between 1965 and 1996, Costello et al. (2006) reported a general (current or recent) prevalence estimate of 2.8% for those under age 13, rising to 5.6% for those ages 13–18. Prevalence was 5.9% for females ages 13–18 versus 4.6% for males of the same age.

Depression has a variable course. Some individuals experience only a single episode, others have recurrent episodes, and a few experience chronic depression. In a review of studies on MDD over the life span, Kovacs (1996) found that the vast majority (90%–95%) of clinic-referred child or adolescent MDD patients were experiencing their initial episode when they entered treatment. Rates of recovery from the treated episode reached about 70% by 1 year and about 85% by 2 years. Thus, a very large majority of young people with clinically identified MDD recover from their index episode, but a small proportion experience chronic depression. However, even successfully treated MDD is characterized by a high risk of recurrence, with about 50% of individuals of combined child-adolescent samples having a second episode within 3 years.

Another perspective on the course of depression comes from the Oregon Adolescent Depression Project (OADP), involving nonreferred high school students. In the OADP, 1,709 adolescents ages 14–18 from nine high schools completed an initial evaluation, including a diagnostic interview, with 88% returning for a second assessment approximately 1 year later. At the initial assessment, point prevalence was 2.57% for MDD and 0.53% for dysthymic disorder, whereas at 1-year follow-up, the point prevalence was 3.12% for MDD and 0.13% for dysthymic disorder (Lewinsohn et al. 1993). Lifetime prevalence rates were 18.48% for MDD and 3.22% for dysthymic disorder at the initial assessment, higher than the rates reported in the more recent National Comorbidity Survey Replication–Adolescent Supplement, reviewed in the first paragraph of this section (Merikangas et al. 2010). Analyses of recovery and recurrence indicated that 12% of recovered adolescents had a recurrence in 1 year, rising to 33% by 4 years.

When OADP participants reached age 24, they were recruited again for a telephone assessment, and data were reported for 767 subjects (Lewinsohn et al. 1999). Those who had developed bipolar disorder during adolescence ($n=13$) and those who had dysthymic disorder but never an MDE ($n=15$) were excluded from these analyses. Findings showed that almost half (45%) of those with an adolescent episode of MDD had another episode during young adulthood—a rate that was greater than the comparable rates for those who had initially presented with an adjustment disorder with depressed mood (34.2%), a nonaffective disorder (28.2%), or no diagnosed disorder (18.5%).

Another important course-related aspect is episode duration. In the community-based OADP, median adolescent MDD episode duration was only 8 weeks, but the range was 2–520 weeks. It is unlikely that adolescents with very brief episodes of MDD come to clinical attention. Kovacs (1996) reported that in clinically referred cases, the median episode duration for child-onset MDD was 36 weeks, whereas that for child-onset dysthymic disorder was 4 years. In the Treatment for Adolescents with Depression Study (TADS), the sample of moderately to severely depressed adolescents had been in an MDE for a median time period of 40 weeks when these adolescents entered the study (March et al. 2004).

Depressive episode duration and its great variability have received inadequate attention in the literature on treatment of substance-abusing youths. As reviewed in the section "Impact of Comorbid Depression on Substance Abuse Treatment," it is currently unclear how comorbid depression at baseline affects the outcome of substance abuse treatment and whether depression itself needs to be a target of treatment in these comorbid cases. One barrier to understanding these questions has been the failure to take into account the natural course of depression as an episodic disorder.

Etiology of Depression

Neurobiological Factors

A meta-analysis of twin studies found that genes account for approximately 37% of the variance in depression, implying that depression is moderately heritable (Kring et al. 2010; Sullivan et al. 2000). These results suggest that adolescents whose biological parents experienced depression are at a higher risk of developing depression themselves. Studies of neurotransmitters suggest that receptor sensitivity to serotonin and dopamine may play a role in depressive symptoms (Kring et al. 2010). Imaging studies show elevated activity in the amygdala and diminished activity as well as diminished volume in the prefrontal cortex, anterior cingulate, and hippocampus among people with depression. This combination may reflect higher emotional reactivity accompanied by a decreased ability to plan when experiencing increased emotions.

Additional research has shown that depression may also be associated with an overactive hypothalamic-pituitary-adrenocortical axis, leading to high cortisol levels (Kring et al. 2010).

Cognitive Factors

Cognitive theories of depression highlight the role of negative dysfunctional thoughts and attributions in the development and maintenance of depression. Beck (1967) asserted that depression is associated with negative views of the self, world, and future—the *negative triad.* He also proposed that through life experiences, depressed individuals develop *negative schemas*—unconscious beliefs that shape how they understand the world—and that these negative schemas become activated whenever a depressed individual is in a situation similar to the ones that led to the development of his or her negative schema (e.g., peer rejection).

Other research emphasizes the role of attributional style in depression (Abramson et al. 1978). When experiencing negative events, people vulnerable to depression are more likely to attribute their cause to internal (self), stable (permanent), and global (broad) factors rather than to external, unstable, and specific or limited factors. Global and stable attributions can foster feelings of hopelessness marked by the belief that nothing can be done to change the situation (Abramson et al. 1989).

Social and Behavioral Factors

Behavioral theories of depression underscore how maladaptive actions and coping strategies can contribute to depression. For instance, rumination, which is a coping response more common in females than males, is marked by passively, repeatedly focusing on the negative event, thus worsening mood (Nolen-Hoeksema 1987). Social skills deficits, poor problem-solving skills, and excessive reassurance seeking have also been shown to predict depression (Kring et al. 2010).

Integrative Theories

A prominent early theoretical paper by Akiskal and McKinney (1973) emphasized the integration of multiple theories, noting that depressive behaviors are best understood as a convergence of multiple levels of analysis with several factors contributing to the development of depression leading to a final common neurophysiological pathway. This approach is consistent with the contemporary model of developmental psychopathology that is now applied to depression and other disorders over the life span.

Depression Comorbid With SUDs

Armstrong and Costello (2002) reviewed the prevalence of comorbid mental health diagnoses in community adolescents who used or abused substances. Their literature review indicated that depression was present in approximately 5% of non-substance-using adolescents, rising to between 11% and 32% among adolescents with an SUD. Across studies, the median rate of comorbid depression among those with an SUD was 18.8%. Depression was the second most frequent comorbid disorder, following the disruptive behavior disorders, especially conduct disorder.

Rates of comorbid depression are, as expected, even higher in clinical samples, with rates ranging from 24% to 50% across studies (Bukstein et al. 1992; Diamond et al. 2006). The combination of depression and SUD is associated with a number of negative clinical features. Episodes of depression are prolonged in those with this comorbid condition (Baker et al. 2007). Compared to SUD-only adolescents, those with comorbid depression show more substance-related problems and impaired quality of life (Lubman et al. 2007). Treatment outcome is often less favorable for these adolescents with comorbid depression (Grella et al. 2001), and risk of suicidal behavior is greater (Goldston 2004). Depressed suicide attempters with alcohol use disorder are more impulsive and make attempts that are more lethal than those without alcohol use disorder (Sher et al. 2007).

The developmental sequence of onset of depression and onset of substance use and abuse appears to be complex, with no single pattern. Clinical studies generally report that the comorbid depression occurred prior to the onset of the SUD (Armstrong and Costello 2002). Community studies are more mixed, with some showing this same pattern (Rohde et al. 1996) but others showing the reverse sequence (Brook et al. 1998). One of the most intriguing studies in this regard was conducted within the Great Smoky Mountain Study. The investigators (Costello et al. 1999) found that initial symptoms of psychiatric disorder, including depression, often preceded the first use of a substance. Substance use initiation was then followed by development of a diagnosed psychiatric disorder, and then in turn by a diagnosed SUD.

More recent evidence about one possible sequence of depression and SUDs comes from the 5-year follow-up study of adolescents who participated in TADS (Curry et al. 2012). None of these adolescents with MDD had SUD at entry into TADS. Of 192 follow-up study participants, 49 (25.5%) developed either an alcohol or drug use (primarily marijuana) disorder, or both, over the 5-year period subsequent to short-term treatment. Having had a positive short-term response to depression treatment predicted a lower rate of subsequent drug use disorder but was unrelated to onset of alcohol use disorder. Either drug or alcohol disorder was predicted by greater involvement in substance use and by the presence of additional comorbid disorders at baseline. Among the adolescents or young adults who experienced both a recurrence of MDD and onset of an alcohol or drug use disorder, the alcohol or drug use disorder preceded recurrent MDD in almost every case. Thus, it is important to advise adolescents who recover from MDD that development of an alcohol or drug problem could significantly raise their risk for recurrence of MDD.

Impact of Comorbid Depression on Substance Abuse Treatment

Comorbidity, including depression, may affect SUD treatment outcome. In a large sample of adolescents receiving drug or alcohol abuse treatment, comorbidity in general was associated with greater failure to maintain abstinence (Grella et al. 2001). In a 5-year follow-up of delinquent youths with SUD who were treated with multisystemic therapy, those with a comorbid psychiatric disorder tended to fare more poorly than the others across multiple domains, including mental health, physical health, and criminal behavior (Clingempeel et al. 2008). Internalizing psychopathology (anxiety and depression) at baseline predicted later internalizing distress and also more aggressive behavior and crime. In another study, both externalizing (aggression, disruptive behavior) and internalizing symptoms at the outset of brief motivational and cognitive-behavioral SUD treatment predicted more substance-related problems 3 months after treatment (Becker et al. 2012). Comorbid depression at the outset of SUD treatment, or after treatment ends, has also been associated with higher rates of SUD relapse (Cornelius et al. 2004; McCarthy et al. 2005). These studies (excluding Cornelius et al. 2004) assessed syndromal depression or mixed internalizing symptoms rather than depressive disorders specifically.

Nevertheless, the impact of baseline depression on SUD treatment retention or outcome is not uniformly negative across studies. Theoretically, internal distress, including depression, could lead either to hopelessness, anhedonia, and treatment dropout or to heightened motivation to change. Hersh et al. (2014) reviewed 13 adolescent SUD treatment studies that included a specific assessment of baseline depression (syndrome or disorder) but did not include depression as a treatment target. Two of the studies investigated retention, 10 investigated outcome, and one investigated both. The kinds of treatments offered were highly variable, ranging from brief outpatient intervention to day treatment to a sequential decreasing intensity model of outpatient care. Depression at baseline was found to have highly variable effects on treatment retention, in part depending on additional comorbid conditions. Likewise, the studies of treatment outcome were highly variable, with some showing no impact of baseline depression and others showing either a positive or negative effect. Overall, this review suggests a need for investigators to specify at baseline the type, severity, and duration of depression and to take into account both demographic factors (e.g., gender) and additional comorbidity in order to understand the impact of depression on adolescent SUD treatment. In addition, ongoing, frequent assessment of depression is required in order to understand the course of depression during and after SUD treatment.

Assessment

At present, no biological or laboratory tests have been deemed suitable for use in the assessment of depression. Therefore, assessment is based on clinical data collected through interviews, clinician-completed rating scales, and adolescent- or parent-report measures. Having an adolescent complete a self-report symptom checklist may reveal whether there is a set of current symptoms consistent with a syndrome of depression, but assessment of duration and functional impairment to establish the presence of a mood disorder requires more detailed interviewing, with attention to onset, duration, severity, and degree of change from the person's usual level of functioning. Rather than present an exhaustive list of available measures, we illustrate these assessment methods with selected prototypical examples.

Diagnostic Interview

The diagnostic interview is the core assessment tool for adolescent depression. Despite its somewhat misleading title and odd designation for adolescents, the most frequently used interview in adolescent depression treatment research has been the Schedule for Affective Disorders and Schizophrenia for School-Age Children–Present and Lifetime Version (K-SADS-PL; Kaufman et al. 1997). The interview title is historical, as it represents a downward extension of the then-current gold standard adult diagnostic interview. The K-SADS-PL does indeed provide excellent, comprehensive coverage of all possible subtypes of depression, but its reach extends well beyond affective and psychotic disorders to include anxiety, disruptive behavior, and eating and substance abuse disorders. It is compatible with both DSM-IV and its predecessor. Interrater and test-retest reliability ($\kappa=0.90$) for diagnoses of MDD is excellent, and concurrent validity is supported by significant correlations with both self-report and parent-report measures.

The K-SADS-PL is designed to be completed by a trained clinician. It uses a semistructured method, with suggested prompts and probes to be selected by the clinician. The respondent's answers are then evaluated by the clinician to determine whether they meet criteria for a probable or definite symptom. The interview is designed with an initial screening portion that reviews the most salient symptoms of each disorder to be assessed. If the respondent indicates no salient symptoms of a given disorder, further inquiry about that disorder is omitted.

The interview starts with an unstructured portion to develop rapport and to obtain background information, chief complaints, and reasons for coming to the clinic or research project. Both during this section of the interview and after completing diagnostic modules, the clinician needs to assess and, as needed, revise the timeline for onset and offset of each disorder. The unstructured section provides the opportunity to evaluate potential reasons for the adolescent's depression, such as precipitating events; social, familial, and academic context; and the other variables that clinicians typically assess in a standard clinical interview. Omitting this section can lead to an impressive account of symptomatic phenomenology in the absence of any idea of why the teenager became depressed!

We prefer to begin the interview with both the adolescent and parent together, unless there is an unusual degree of conflict or alienation between them, and then to move into individual administration of the full symptom-oriented interview, first with the adolescent and then with the parent. Discrepancies can be expected, especially about symptoms that are primarily internal and relatively easy to mask from observers, including parents. Clinicians may resolve these using their own judgment or may opt for a final interview section with both parties to attempt to reach consensus.

Clinician Rating Scales

Whereas the diagnostic interview can determine presence of a depressive disorder and any comorbid disorders, as well as their onset, sequence, and offset, such interviews are limited in determining current severity of symptoms. To assess severity and change, especially before, during, and after treatment, clinician rating scales are more useful. The prototype of such a scale in the area of adolescent depression is the Children's Depression Rating Scale–Revised (CDRS-R; Poznanski and Mokros 1996). The CDRS-R consists of 14 items that are evaluated on the basis of separate adolescent and parent interviews, along with three observational items—facial affect, speech, and activity level—that are completed by the clinician on the basis of interaction with the adolescent. The interview items are arranged in a sequence designed to move from less difficult discussion topics (school performance, recreational activities) to more difficult ones (morbid or suicidal ideation). Like the K-SADS-PL, the CDRS-R is semistructured, so that the clinician inquires about a symptom area and then evaluates whether and to what degree of severity the respondent's answer suggests current symptomatology. The time frame for symptom severity is typically the past week, and each item is rated on a seven- or five-point scale. Thus, the CDRS-R is sensitive to change over short periods of time. It has been used in the recent major studies of adolescent depression treatment, including TADS (March et al. 2004), in which the interrater reliability of the scale was excellent (the intraclass correlation coefficient was 0.95).

Self-Report Scales

Whereas clinician-completed rating scales are the gold standard for severity assessment, self-report scales are far easier to administer, because they take only minutes on the part of the clinician. Self-report scales are often used as secondary outcome measures in adolescent depression treatment studies and can be readily used as a comorbidity measure in substance abuse treatment studies. One advantage of self-report methods is that they can be used repeatedly to track change. One of the most commonly used self-report scales is the Beck Depression Inventory–Second Edition (BDI-II; Beck et al. 1996). The BDI-II consists of 21 items, each rated on a scale from 0 to 3, which ask about specific symptoms over the past 2 weeks. Therefore, like the CDRS-R, it is sensitive to change over relatively short periods of time. It has excellent internal consistency reliability in adolescent samples ($\alpha=0.92$; Steer et al. 1998) and has been used in clinical trials for adolescent depression (e.g., Diamond et al. 2010).

Supplemental Assessment Methods

Despite their advantages, the measures discussed in the subsections "Diagnostic Interview," "Clinician Rating Scales," and "Self-Report

Scales" do not measure either the psychopathology or the biology of depression. Thus, investigators interested in causes of depression or in mechanisms of change addressed by depression treatments will supplement them with theoretically relevant measures. In the psychological realm, these may include measures of the cognitive, behavioral, or interpersonal factors implicated in the etiology of depression (e.g., automatic thoughts, attributional style, pleasant activities); general personality processes (e.g., neuroticism, introversion, self-efficacy, problem-solving ability); or contextual factors, assessing social or familial variables (e.g., social or family support, expressed emotion). Likewise, in the biological realm, measures of family history of psychiatric disorders, stress reactivity, or biological measures (e.g., sleep markers) may be of interest to investigators seeking to understand critical mechanisms underlying depression.

Treatment of Adolescent Depression

At present, there are three evidence-based psychotherapies—cognitive-behavioral therapy (CBT), interpersonal psychotherapy, and attachment-based family therapy—for adolescent depression (Curry 2014), as well as two medications—fluoxetine and escitalopram—that have been approved by the U.S. Food and Drug Administration for adolescent MDD (Centers for Medicare and Medicaid Services 2013). CBT has the most support in the psychotherapy literature, having proven superior to wait-list (Clarke et al. 1999) and to two alternative psychotherapy (Brent et al. 1997) conditions. Interpersonal psychotherapy has proven superior to wait list, clinical management, and school counseling as usual (Mufson et al. 1999, 2004). The most recent entry into the evidence-based depression psychotherapy category is attachment-based family therapy, which has proven superior to partial wait list and to usual care (Diamond et al. 2002, 2010). Finally, the combination of CBT plus fluoxetine was the most efficacious intervention in TADS, surpassing pill placebo and each of the monotherapies in short-term efficacy with youths having moderate to severe depression (March et al. 2004).

The severity and duration of the index episode of depression need to be taken into account when interpreting the psychotherapy treatment literature. Some psychotherapy studies included mildly depressed youths or those with less than a full MDE. Others, including Brent et al.'s (1997) study and TADS, involved almost entirely moderately to severely depressed youths with significant functional impairment and relatively prolonged episodes.

Approaches to Treating Comorbid Depression and SUD in Adolescents

As reviewed in various chapters in this volume, there are a number of effective psychotherapeutic interventions for adolescent substance use disorders. The strongest evidence base exists for systemic family treatment models (e.g., multisystemic therapy, functional family therapy (FFT), multidimensional family therapy), CBT, and brief motivational interventions (e.g., motivational enhancement therapy [MET]). Becker and Curry (2008) describe these models and analyze their supportive evidence.

Quite reasonably, treatment developers who want to address comorbid depression and substance abuse among adolescents have drawn from the existing treatments for each of these two disorders. Rather than provide a comprehensive review of all such efforts, we give examples that illustrate each of the general or overall strategies that have been used with these adolescents with comorbid conditions. Five general approaches to the treatment of comorbid disorders have been identified to date (Curry 2014):

1. Treating only the primary disorder
2. Using a combined treatment to target both disorders
3. Using sequential treatment to target first one and then the other disorder
4. Selecting a modular treatment consisting of components that target aspects of each disorder
5. Using a common process treatment that targets psychological or biological processes common to the two disorders

In the case of comorbid adolescent depression and substance abuse, we are aware of examples of the first, second, and third of these potential approaches. The modular and common process approaches have been used with other comorbid combinations, such as depression and conduct problems (Chorpita et al. 2013) or depression and anxiety (Weersing et al. 2008), and theoretically could be applied to depression and substance abuse in the future. In the following subsections, we review examples of the first three general approaches.

Primary Disorder Treatment

The approach of treating the primary disorder has been tested more by incidental secondary analyses than in hypothesis-driven studies. In other words, we are not aware of substance abuse treatment studies that set out to test explicitly whether adolescent depression responds to treatment targeting only substance abuse. However, a number of substance abuse studies have measured depression before and either during or after treatment, enabling researchers to determine after the fact the extent to which depression changed during substance abuse treatment.

Riggs et al. (1995) assessed delinquent, substance-dependent adolescents who entered a residential treatment program. The authors found that depression symptoms did not decrease after 4 weeks of abstinence associated with involvement in the program, suggesting that it may be necessary to target depression directly to have an impact on it. In contrast, Hawke et al. (2008) administered diagnostic interviews to 50 adolescents who entered an outpatient CBT program for alcohol and other SUDs. One year later, the interview was repeated. Depression diagnoses declined significantly from pretreatment to 1-year follow-up, even though the depression was never explicitly targeted during treatment. Although these results suggest that substance abuse treatment might effectively address depression, they are limited by lack of a nontreated control group, to control for effects of time, and by the very long amount of time between assessments. Given the episodic nature of depression and the median length of an MDE, a good deal of recovery would be expected over a 1-year time period.

A recent study by Arias et al. (2014) involved a secondary analysis of the Cannabis Youth Treatment (CYT) study (Dennis et al. 2004) to determine whether depression symptom severity at study entry was reduced with substance abuse treatment alone. In the CYT study, adolescents received one of five active treatments: multidimensional family therapy, MET/CBT-5 (two MET sessions followed by three CBT sessions), MET/CBT-12 (two MET sessions followed by 10 CBT sessions), Family Support Network, or Adolescent Community Reinforcement Approach. Depression was assessed with a structured diagnostic interview that yielded symptom severity scores and diagnoses, with assessments completed at baseline and then 3, 6, 9, and 12 months later. Even without treatment addressing depression, there was a linear decline in depression severity regardless of treatment arm. It is also of interest to note that in this study, higher depression at baseline was correlated with higher motivation for treatment.

In summary, evidence suggests that at least for some depressed adolescents, substance abuse treatment alone is associated with improvement in comorbid depression. The reasons for this finding are not clear.

It is possible that nonspecific factors in the substance abuse psychotherapy, such as the therapeutic alliance, empathy, accurate identification of the adolescent's internal experience, or the installation of hopefulness via active intervention, account for this result. It is also possible that some of the skills developed by adolescents in substance abuse treatment, such as self-monitoring, problem solving, or seeking of social support, generalize and thereby account for the improvement in mood. Finally, it may be that characteristics of depressive episodes, such as their severity, type, or median duration, account for the improvement.

Combined Treatment

The second general approach to treatment for comorbid conditions is combined treatment. In this model, adolescents experiencing two disorders receive treatment that targets both disorders, through either a combination of psychotherapies or a combination of psychotherapy plus medication. Given the available evidence-based treatments for adolescent depression, both psychotherapy and medication have been used in combined treatment for depressed substance abusers. An example of a combined psychotherapy study is the pilot study of Family and Coping Skills therapy by Curry et al. (2003). Thirteen adolescents with both an SUD and a depressive disorder received combined family and group CBT targeting both disorders. The CBT was skills based, targeting factors known to be associated with either disorder. For example, family sessions addressed parental monitoring of adolescent behavior and the use of appropriate consequences. Adolescent group sessions addressed self-monitoring of mood and substance use, increasing pleasant non-substance-related activities, and restructuring of cognitions related to depression and substance use. Both family and group sessions addressed communication and problem solving. Using a pretest to posttest design, the pilot study showed improvements in both frequency of substance use and severity of depressive symptoms.

In a well-designed randomized controlled clinical trial, Esposito-Smythers et al. (2011) used a combined and integrated treatment approach with 40 adolescents who abused substances and who were suicidal. Many also met criteria for a depressive disorder. The combined treatment was individual and family therapy, as well as case management. Treatment proved superior to an enhanced, community treatment as usual, in which participants were assisted in accessing community-based care and the study team provided assessment results to help the community providers. Those adolescents who received the combined treatment had fewer heavy drinking days and marijuana use days, although no fewer drinking days. They made fewer suicide attempts and used fewer inpatient or emergency department services.

Psychotherapy for substance abuse has also been combined with medication for depression in a combined treatment model. Cornelius et al. (2009) treated 50 adolescents ages 15–20 who had comorbid MDD and an alcohol use disorder. All subjects received MET and CBT that targeted both alcohol abuse and depression. Half received fluoxetine, and the other half received placebo. Results showed no differential effects for fluoxetine, but overall the group had significant declines in both alcohol use and depressive symptoms. Subsequently, Cornelius et al. (2011) reported results of a 2-year follow-up evaluation in which they compared alcohol and depression symptoms in adolescents who had received MET/CBT versus naturalistic care, as well as those who received fluoxetine versus placebo. The MET/CBT was associated with improvements in both domains, whereas the medication had no significant treatment effect.

A major study of combined treatment was conducted by Riggs et al. (2007). They recruited 126 adolescents with a current SUD and current major depression, as well as a lifetime diagnosis of conduct disorder. All subjects received CBT for substance abuse. Half were randomly assigned to receive fluoxetine for depression, and the other half were randomly assigned to receive placebo. After 16 weeks of treatment, fluoxetine surpassed placebo on one measure of depression (CDRS-R) but not on a global measure of treatment response. Substance use frequency decreased in both groups, but on clean urine drug screens, the placebo group actually surpassed the fluoxetine group. The authors concluded that the CBT, despite its emphasis on substance abuse, may have also contributed to efficacious treatment of depression. It is interesting to note that remission of depression was associated with reduced substance use in this sample, regardless of treatment arm, and that non-remission was associated with lack of change in substance use. Furthermore, the efficacy of fluoxetine did not emerge until week 13 of treatment, which is far later than the typical point of separation between effects of fluoxetine and placebo in depressed-only subjects (Emslie et al. 1997). Finally, even in this highly comorbid group of adolescents, approximately 28% of participants had depression response to treatment by week 4, whether they were receiving fluoxetine or placebo, again suggesting some impact on mood of the CBT targeting substance abuse.

Sequential Treatment

The third approach to treatment for comorbid disorders is sequential treatment. This model was recently tested by Rohde et al. (2014) with adolescents who had an SUD and a depression diagnosis. Two well-established treatments were used in varying sequence: FFT for substance abuse (Waldron et al. 2001) and the cognitive-behavioral Adolescent Coping With Depression (CWD-A) course (Clarke et al. 1999). One hundred seventy adolescents received up to 24 treatment sessions over 20 weeks. One-third received FFT followed by the CWD-A course, one-third received the reverse sequence, and the final third received a coordinated version of the two treatments. Depression severity decreased in all three groups, with no differential effects between groups. Overall, substance use outcomes were better in the FFT followed by CWD-A course condition than in coordinated treatment, with the CWD-A course followed by FFT condition falling in an intermediate range. However, for the subgroup of adolescents with full MDD at baseline, the CWD-A course followed by FFT was superior on substance use outcomes. Of note, the improvements in depression occurred early in the treatment regardless of sequence. Further attendance in the second treatment received was generally lower than in the first treatment received, regardless of sequence. It is also noteworthy that the coordinated treatment in no case surpassed either of the two sequenced treatments, suggesting that simultaneous targeting of two disorders may weaken the effect of treatment for either condition.

Summary and Future Directions

A depressive syndrome and/or disorder is frequently comorbid with alcohol or drug use disorders in adolescents. Depression in these adolescents may present as a full MDD, a persistent dysthymia, or a set of associated symptoms. Community studies generally support the notion that substance abuse precedes the onset of comorbid disorders, but the opposite sequence can occur, especially in clinical samples, and more fine-grained analyses suggest a potential cyclical pattern in which substance use can lead to depressive symptoms, which are then followed by SUD and depressive disorders.

Providers of adolescent substance abuse treatment may then be faced with an array of possible comorbidity pictures. These would include adolescents in whom depression preceded SUD, those in whom depression followed SUD, and those in whom depression was caused or exacerbated by SUD. Libby et al. (2005) assessed 126 youths with SUD, major depression, and conduct disorder who participated in the combined fluoxetine and CBT study (Riggs et al. 2007) reviewed in subsection

"Combined Treatment." Comparisons were made between those in whom depression preceded substance abuse and those in whom substance abuse preceded depression. In this sample, almost 70% experienced depression first. There were relatively few demographic or clinical differences between the two groups, however. Those who experienced MDD first were, on average, younger and more likely to have a diagnosis of cannabis dependence. Otherwise, the authors noted remarkable similarity between the two groups on measures of substance dependence and problem severity. Although this is only a single study of a seriously impaired sample, it suggests that treatment planning cannot yet be enhanced by determining which disorder came first.

Other implications of the literature reviewed in this chapter suggest future directions for research and for clinical intervention. By assessing depression not only at entry into substance abuse treatment but also during and immediately after treatment, researchers can determine the types and severity levels of depressive conditions that are likely to respond to substance abuse treatment alone. By analyzing those conditions, researchers can then determine who among the adolescents with comorbid disorders needs treatment that also targets depression. These questions suggest the utility of adaptive treatment designs for research, whereby depression treatment is delivered only to those still in need of it after some period of substance abuse treatment.

As noted in the section "Approaches to Treating Comorbid Depression and SUD in Adolescents," there are five models for treating comorbid conditions. To our knowledge, not all of them have been attempted with depressed substance-abusing youths. Specifically, we are not aware of attempts to apply the modular or common process approaches to these comorbid conditions. Combined treatments are generally intensive, falling between regular outpatient care and intensive outpatient or day treatment, with more than one session per week and/or considerable case management. It is possible that this model will prove to be quite efficacious, but it may be suitable only for the more impaired or complicated outpatient cases. Sequential treatment is lengthy, and results of a recent study (Rohde et al. 2014) suggest a tendency for attendance to drop off at the time of the second treatment. Given that depression improved in this study regardless of treatment sequence, whereas substance abuse improvement was more variable, the study's findings could provide further evidence that at least some depressions respond to psychotherapy targeting substance abuse. It is possible that treatment research results with depressed substance-abusing adolescents could be clarified if those youths whose depressive symptoms responded relatively quickly to substance abuse treatment were then excluded from further depression treatment. In other words, the impact of depression treatment for these youths would be clearer if such treatment were given only to those in need of it. In a sense, this situation is analogous to the placebo lead-in method used in some antidepressant medication studies: adolescents whose depression responds to an initial trial with placebo are excluded from the randomized comparison of active drug to placebo. Rather than a placebo lead-in method, however, an adaptive treatment design might be quite useful with depressed substance-abusing adolescents. In such a design, all participants receive substance abuse treatment, but only those who are still depressed after a certain period of time receive additional depression treatment. Empirical research is needed to determine whether this approach will be effective.

Attempts to use modular and common process approaches to comorbid depression and substance abuse are also warranted. Particularly given the favorable results for modular treatment of the challenging comorbidity of depression and conduct disorder in young people (Chorpita et al. 2013), it seems appropriate to design and test such interventions for adolescents with depression and substance abuse. These approaches are potentially less complicated or lengthy than combination or sequential treatment. Modular treatment uses an overall model, such as CBT, and applies treatment components that match the needs of the individual. Elements of CBT for depression and elements of CBT for substance abuse would be selected and applied according to an algorithm that would guide treatment and prevent drift. The common process approach is perhaps more challenging for depression and substance abuse than for other comorbid conditions to which it has been applied, because this comorbidity is "heterotypic" (like depression and conduct disorder) rather than "homotypic" (like depression and anxiety).

Finally, the development and testing of more effective medications for moderate to severe adolescent depression would enhance the ability of researchers and clinicians to develop effective approaches for use with depressed substance-abusing adolescents.

KEY POINTS

- Depression is one of the most common psychiatric disorders of adolescence and the second most common comorbid disorder with adolescent substance use disorders.

- Depression is far more prevalent among adolescents who use substances than among those who do not.

- Substance-abusing adolescents should be assessed for comorbid depression using interview and self-report methods.

- Cognitive-behavioral therapy and certain antidepressant medications are efficacious treatments for adolescent depression.

- Combined or sequential treatment for both depression and substance use disorders may be effective for adolescents with both disorders.

References

Abramson LY, Seligman ME, Teasdale JD: Learned helplessness in humans: critique and reformulation. J Abnorm Psychol 87(1):49–74, 1978 649856

Abramson LY, Metalsky GI, Alloy LB: Hopelessness depression: a theory-based subtype of depression. Psychol Rev 96(2):358–372, 1989

Akiskal HS, McKinney WT Jr: Depressive disorders: toward a unified hypothesis. Science 182(4107):20–29, 1973 4199732

American Psychiatric Association: Diagnostic and Statistical Manual of Mental Disorders, 4th Edition, Text Revision. Washington, DC, American Psychiatric Association, 2000

American Psychiatric Association: Diagnostic and Statistical Manual of Mental Disorders, 5th Edition. Arlington, VA, American Psychiatric Association, 2013

Arias AJ, Burleson JA, Kaminer Y, et al: Examining the relationship between depression and alcohol use in youth being treated for a cannabis use disorder. Poster presented at the 37th Annual Research Society on Alcoholism Meeting, Bellevue, WA, June 2014

Armstrong TD, Costello EJ: Community studies on adolescent substance use, abuse, or dependence and psychiatric comorbidity. J Consult Clin Psychol 70(6):1224–1239, 2002 12472299

Baker KD, Lubman DI, Cosgrave EM, et al: Impact of co-occurring substance use on 6 month outcomes for young people seeking mental health treatment. Aust NZ J Psychiatry 41(11):896–902, 2007 17924242

Beck AT: Depression: Clinical, Experimental and Theoretical Aspects. New York, Harper & Row, 1967

Beck AT, Steer R, Brown G: The Beck Depression Inventory, 2nd Edition. San Antonio, TX, Psychological Corporation, 1996

Becker SJ, Curry JF: Outpatient interventions for adolescent substance abuse: a quality of evidence review. J Consult Clin Psychol 76(4):531–543, 2008 18665683

Becker SJ, Stein GL, Curry JF, et al: Ethnic differences among substance-abusing adolescents in a treatment dissemination project. J Subst Abuse Treat 42(3):328–336, 2012 22000324

Brent DA, Holder D, Kolko D, et al: A clinical psychotherapy trial for adolescent depression comparing cognitive, family, and supportive therapy. Arch Gen Psychiatry 54(9):877–885, 1997 9294380

Brook JS, Cohen P, Brook DW: Longitudinal study of co-occurring psychiatric disorders and substance use. J Am Acad Child Adolesc Psychiatry 37(3):322–330, 1998 9519638

Bukstein OG, Glancy LJ, Kaminer Y: Patterns of affective comorbidity in a clinical population of dually diagnosed adolescent substance abusers. J Am Acad Child Adolesc Psychiatry 31(6):1041–1045, 1992 1429402

Centers for Medicare and Medicaid Services: Antidepressant Medications: Use in Pediatric Patients. Baltimore, MD, Centers for Medicare and Medicaid Services, August 2013

Chorpita BF, Weisz JR, Daleiden EL, et al: Long-term outcomes for the Child STEPs randomized effectiveness trial: a comparison of modular and standard treatment designs with usual care. J Consult Clin Psychol 81(6):999–1009, 2013 23978169

Clarke GN, Rohde P, Lewinsohn PM, et al: Cognitive-behavioral treatment of adolescent depression: efficacy of acute group treatment and booster sessions. J Am Acad Child Adolesc Psychiatry 38(3):272–279, 1999 10087688

Clingempeel WG, Britt SC, Henggeler SW: Beyond treatment effects: comorbid psychopathologies and long-term outcomes among substance-abusing delinquents. Am J Orthopsychiatry 78(1):29–36, 2008 18444724

Cornelius JR, Maisto SA, Martin CS, et al: Major depression associated with earlier alcohol relapse in treated teens with AUD. Addict Behav 29(5):1035–1038, 2004 15219354

Cornelius JR, Bukstein OG, Wood DS, et al: Double-blind placebo-controlled trial of fluoxetine in adolescents with comorbid major depression and an alcohol use disorder. Addict Behav 34(10):905–909, 2009 19321268

Cornelius JR, Douaihy A, Bukstein OG, et al: Evaluation of cognitive behavioral therapy/motivational enhancement therapy (CBT/MET) in a treatment trial of comorbid MDD/AUD adolescents. Addict Behav 36(8):843–848, 2011 21530092

Costello EJ, Erkanli A, Federman E, et al: Development of psychiatric comorbidity with substance abuse in adolescents: effects of timing and sex. J Clin Child Psychol 28(3):298–311, 1999 10446679

Costello EJ, Mustillo S, Erkanli A, et al: Prevalence and development of psychiatric disorders in childhood and adolescence. Arch Gen Psychiatry 60(8):837–844, 2003 12912767

Costello EJ, Erkanli A, Angold A: Is there an epidemic of child or adolescent depression? J Child Psychol Psychiatry 47(12):1263–1271, 2006 17176381

Curry JF: Childhood depression, in International Encyclopedia of the Social and Behavioral Sciences. Edited by Smelser NJ, Baltes PB. Oxford, UK, Elsevier, 2001, pp 1705–1709

Curry JF: Future directions in research on psychotherapy for adolescent depression. J Clin Child Adolesc Psychol 43(3):510–526, 2014 24730421

Curry JF, Wells KC, Lochman JE, et al: Cognitive-behavioral intervention for depressed, substance-abusing adolescents: development and pilot testing. J Am Acad Child Adolesc Psychiatry 42(6):656–665, 2003 12921473

Curry J, Silva S, Rohde P, et al: Onset of alcohol or substance use disorders following treatment for adolescent depression. J Consult Clin Psychol 80(2):299–312, 2012 22250853

Dennis M, Godley SH, Diamond G, et al: The Cannabis Youth Treatment (CYT) study: main findings from two randomized trials. J Subst Abuse Treat 27(3):197–213, 2004 15501373

Diamond G, Reis BF, Diamond GM, et al: Attachment-based family therapy for depressed adolescents: a treatment development study. J Am Acad Child Adolesc Psychiatry 41(10):1190–1196, 2002 12364840

Diamond G, Panichelli-Mindel SM, Shera D, et al: Psychiatric syndromes in adolescents with marijuana abuse and dependency in outpatient treatment. J Child Adolesc Subst Abuse 15(4):37–54, 2006

Diamond G, Wintersteen MB, Brown GK, et al: Attachment-based family therapy for adolescents with suicidal ideation: a randomized controlled trial. J Am Acad Child Adolesc Psychiatry 49(2):122–131, 2010 20215934

Emslie GJ, Rush AJ, Weinberg WA, et al: A double-blind, randomized, placebo-controlled trial of fluoxetine in children and adolescents with depression. Arch Gen Psychiatry 54(11):1031–1037, 1997 9366660

Esposito-Smythers C, Spirito A, Kahler CW, et al: Treatment of co-occurring substance abuse and suicidality among adolescents: a randomized trial. J Consult Clin Psychol 79(6):728–739, 2011 22004303

Goldston DB: Conceptual issues in understanding the relationship between suicidal behavior and substance use during adolescence. Drug Alcohol Depend 76(suppl):S79–S91, 2004 15555819

Grella CE, Hser YI, Joshi V, et al: Drug treatment outcomes for adolescents with comorbid mental and substance use disorders. J Nerv Ment Dis 189(6):384–392, 2001 11434639

Hawke JM, Kaminer Y, Burke R, et al: Stability of comorbid psychiatric diagnosis among youths in treatment and aftercare for alcohol use disorders. Subst Abus 29(2):33–41, 2008 19042322

Hersh J, Curry JF, Kaminer Y: What is the impact of comorbid depression on adolescent substance abuse treatment? Subst Abus 35(4):364–375, 2014 25157785

Kaufman J, Birmaher B, Brent D, et al: Schedule for Affective Disorders and Schizophrenia for School-Age Children-Present and Lifetime Version (K-SADS-PL): initial reliability and validity data. J Am Acad Child Adolesc Psychiatry 36(7):980–988, 1997 9204677

Kovacs M: Presentation and course of major depressive disorder during childhood and later years of the life span. J Am Acad Child Adolesc Psychiatry 35(6):705–715, 1996 8682751

Kring AM, Johnson SL, Davison GC, et al: Abnormal Psychology, 11th Edition. Hoboken, NJ, Wiley, 2010

Lewinsohn PM, Hops H, Roberts RE, et al: Adolescent psychopathology, I: prevalence and incidence of depression and other DSM-III-R disorders in high school students. J Abnorm Psychol 102(1):133–144, 1993 8436689

Lewinsohn PM, Rohde P, Klein DN, et al: Natural course of adolescent major depressive disorder, I: continuity into young adulthood. J Am Acad Child Adolesc Psychiatry 38(1):56–63, 1999 9893417

Libby AM, Orton HD, Stover SK, et al: What came first, major depression or substance use disorder? Clinical characteristics and substance use comparing teens in a treatment cohort. Addict Behav 30(9):1649–1662, 2005 16098679

Lubman DI, Allen NB, Rogers N, et al: The impact of co-occurring mood and anxiety disorders among substance-abusing youth. J Affect Disord 103(1–3):105–112, 2007 17291589

March J, Silva S, Petrycki S, et al: Fluoxetine, cognitive-behavioral therapy, and their combination for adolescents with depression: Treatment for Adolescents with Depression Study (TADS) randomized controlled trial. JAMA 292(7):807–820, 2004 15315995

McCarthy DM, Tomlinson KL, Anderson KG, et al: Relapse in alcohol- and drug-disordered adolescents with comorbid psychopathology: changes in psychiatric symptoms. Psychol Addict Behav 19(1):28–34, 2005 15783275

Merikangas KR, He JP, Burstein M, et al: Lifetime prevalence of mental disorders in U.S. adolescents: results from the National Comorbidity Survey Replication—Adolescent Supplement (NCS-A). J Am Acad Child Adolesc Psychiatry 49(10):980–989, 2010 20855043

Mufson L, Weissman MM, Moreau D, et al: Efficacy of interpersonal psychotherapy for depressed adolescents. Arch Gen Psychiatry 56(6):573–579, 1999 10359475

Mufson L, Dorta KP, Wickramaratne P, et al: A randomized effectiveness trial of interpersonal psychotherapy for depressed adolescents. Arch Gen Psychiatry 61(6):577–584, 2004 15184237

Nolen-Hoeksema S: Sex differences in unipolar depression: evidence and theory. Psychol Bull 101(2):259–282, 1987 3562707

Poznanski E, Mokros H: Children's Depression Rating Scale–Revised Manual. Los Angeles, CA, Western Psychological Services, 1996

Riggs PD, Baker S, Mikulich SK, et al: Depression in substance-dependent delinquents. J Am Acad Child Adolesc Psychiatry 34(6):764–771, 1995 7608050

Riggs PD, Mikulich-Gilbertson SK, Davies RD, et al: A randomized controlled trial of fluoxetine and cognitive behavioral therapy in adolescents with major depression, behavior problems, and substance use disorders. Arch Pediatr Adolesc Med 161(11):1026–1034, 2007 17984403

Rohde P, Lewinsohn PM, Seeley JR: Psychiatric comorbidity with problematic alcohol use in high school students. J Am Acad Child Adolesc Psychiatry 35(1):101–109, 1996 8567601

Rohde P, Waldron HB, Turner CW, et al: Sequenced versus coordinated treatment for adolescents with comorbid depressive and substance use disorders. J Consult Clin Psychol 82(2):342–348, 2014 24491069

Sher L, Sperling D, Stanley BH, et al: Triggers for suicidal behavior in depressed older adolescents and young adults: do alcohol use disorders make a difference? Int J Adolesc Med Health 19(1):91–98, 2007 17458328

Steer RA, Kumar G, Ranieri WF, et al: Use of the Beck Depression Inventory-II with adolescent psychiatric outpatients. J Psychopathol Behav Assess 20(2):127–135, 1998

Sullivan PF, Neale MC, Kendler KS: Genetic epidemiology of major depression: review and meta-analysis. Am J Psychiatry 157(10):1552–1562, 2000 11007705

Waldron HB, Slesnick N, Brody JL, et al: Treatment outcomes for adolescent substance abuse at 4- and 7-month assessments. J Consult Clin Psychol 69(5):802–813, 2001 11680557

Weersing VR, Gonzalez A, Campo JV, et al: Brief behavioral therapy for pediatric anxiety and depression: piloting an integrated treatment approach. Cogn Behav Pract 15:129–139, 2008

CHAPTER 7

Bipolar Disorders and Substance Use Disorders

Anne Duffy, M.D., M.Sc., FRCPC
Maryam Nemati, M.A., CCC

A wealth of evidence supports an association between substance misuse and risk of mood disorders (Levin and Hennessy 2004). The most commonly misused substances in both the general population and patients with mood disorders including bipolar disorder are cannabis and alcohol. Cannabis is considered a gateway drug that leads to an increased risk of polysubstance dependence. Furthermore, exposure to cannabis during adolescence has been strongly and specifically associated with the subsequent risk of developing schizophrenia and psychotic mania, as well as reducing the age at onset (De Hert et al. 2011). These associations may be related to the accelerated neurobiological development that is taking place during adolescence (Paus et al. 2008).

However, most adolescents who are exposed to or regularly use alcohol and/or cannabis do not develop psychosis or psychotic mood disorders. It appears that exposure to substances in adolescence requires the interaction of other causal factors to result in psychiatric illness. In patients with established bipolar disorder (see Box 7–1), there is some evidence of a temporal sequence of substance use related to the polarity of the episodes and the course of illness (Baethge et al. 2005, 2008). Nonetheless, the relationship between mood disorders and substance use is complex. There are likely different causal pathways leading to substance use in subgroups of vulnerable high-risk individuals and different factors maintaining substance use in subgroups of patients with established illness.

Box 7–1. DSM-5 Criteria for Bipolar I Disorder (Excerpts)

Manic Episode

A. A distinct period of abnormally and persistently elevated, expansive, or irritable mood and abnormally and persistently increased goal-directed activity or energy, lasting at least 1 week and present most of the day, nearly every day (or any duration if hospitalization is necessary).

B. During the period of mood disturbance and increased energy or activity, three (or more) of the following symptoms (four if the mood is only irritable) are present to a significant degree and represent a noticeable change from usual behavior:

1. Inflated self-esteem or grandiosity.
2. Decreased need for sleep (e.g., feels rested after only 3 hours of sleep).
3. More talkative than usual or pressure to keep talking.
4. Flight of ideas or subjective experience that thoughts are racing.
5. Distractibility (i.e., attention too easily drawn to unimportant or irrelevant external stimuli), as reported or observed.
6. Increase in goal-directed activity (either socially, at work or school, or sexually) or psychomotor agitation (i.e., purposeless non-goal-directed activity).
7. Excessive involvement in activities that have a high potential for painful consequences (e.g., engaging in unrestrained buying sprees, sexual indiscretions, or foolish business investments).

Hypomanic Episode

A. A distinct period of abnormally and persistently elevated, expansive, or irritable mood and abnormally and persistently increased activity or energy, lasting at least 4 consecutive days and present most of the day, nearly every day.

B. During the period of mood disturbance and increased energy and activity, three (or more) of the following symptoms (four if the mood is only irritable) have persisted, represent a noticeable change from usual behavior, and have been present to a significant degree:

1. Inflated self-esteem or grandiosity.
2. Decreased need for sleep (e.g., feels rested after only 3 hours of sleep).
3. More talkative than usual or pressure to keep talking.
4. Flight of ideas or subjective experience that thoughts are racing.

5. Distractibility (i.e., attention too easily drawn to unimportant or irrelevant external stimuli) as reported or observed (i.e., purposeless non-goal-directed activity).
6. Increase in goal-directed activity (either socially, at work or school, or sexually) or psychomotor agitation.
7. Excessive involvement in activities that have a high potential for painful consequences (e.g., engaging in unrestrained buying sprees, sexual indiscretions, or foolish business investments).

The overarching observation is that substance use is associated with worsened outcomes in vulnerable youths and patients across all measurable domains, including clinical, functional, and quality-of-life domains (Khalsa et al. 2008; Nery et al. 2014; Strakowski et al. 2000; Treuer and Tohen 2010). Although substance use is neither necessary nor sufficient to explain the development of psychotic and bipolar disorders, it is definitely a major risk factor and complicating influence and therefore should be an intensive target of preventive and early intervention efforts (Arseneault et al. 2004).

Strength and Impact of the Association Between Bipolar and Comorbid SUDs

Both community-based and clinical studies have reported very high rates of lifetime substance use disorders (SUDs) in patients meeting criteria for bipolar disorder. For example, in a naturalistic study by Stephens et al. (2014), of 103 adolescents with first-episode mania (FEM), 49 (48%) either had an SUD at baseline or developed one during the follow-ups; 24% of the adolescents who did not have a history of SUD at baseline developed one during follow-up. The Epidemiologic Catchment Area study reported that 46.2% of patients with bipolar I disorder had a lifetime history of alcohol use disorder and 40.7% had a drug use disorder, compared to 13.5% and 6.1%, respectively, in the general population (Regier et al. 1990). Furthermore, over 40% of bipolar patients with an alcohol use disorder had a history of other drug use disorders. Similarly, in the National Comorbidity Survey, bipolar patients had several-fold elevated rates of alcohol and drug use disorders and were 8.4 times more likely to have a lifetime drug dependency compared to the general population (Kessler et al.

1997). In a comprehensive review of lifetime rates of SUD in bipolar patients, Cassidy et al. (2001) estimated that across studies using different methods, the lifetime rates of SUD in bipolar patients were in excess of 30%. Rates of lifetime SUD are higher for patients with bipolar disorder than for patients with unipolar disorder. For example, the Epidemiologic Catchment Area study reported a 16.5% lifetime rate of alcohol abuse and 18% lifetime rate of drug abuse for unipolar patients (Regier et al. 1990). Generally, rates of major mood disorders have been increasing and age at onset decreasing over the past century (Chengappa et al. 2003; Klerman 1976; Klerman and Weissman 1989). Interestingly, at the same time, there has been a progressive increase in the rate of SUD in affectively ill patients admitted to the hospital for the first time (Minnai et al. 2006). Specifically, annual rates of comorbid SUD and mood disorder increased continuously over a 25-year period and were associated with younger age at onset and younger age at first hospitalization (Minnai et al. 2006). These findings suggest that among other factors, increasing substance use in vulnerable individuals may contribute to the increasing rate of mood disorders and reduced age at onset.

Typically, but not always, rates of SUD are reportedly more common among males than among females in both community and clinical studies of bipolar patients, paralleling the difference noted in the general population. There is also a strong and consistent association between alcohol use and the use of other drugs. Specifically, a lifetime history of alcohol use disorder has been reported to increase the odds of a drug use disorder by approximately twofold; similarly, a drug use disorder has been reported to increase the odds of an alcohol use disorder by approximately threefold (Cassidy et al. 2001). Although alcohol use disorders are historically the most prevalent form of SUD, evidence suggests that cannabis is becoming the most common substance of misuse in younger populations of patients with bipolar disorder (Strakowski and DelBello 2000; Strakowski et al. 2007).

Clearly, substance use has a strong and clinically important association with bipolar disorder. Patients with comorbid bipolar and substance use disorders are at increased risk of worsened outcomes, including increased hospitalizations, worsened quality of remission, higher recurrence rates, poorer physical health, higher indices of morbidity and mortality, higher suicide rates, lower socioeconomic status, higher rates of unemployment and school dropout, and lower global functioning and quality of life (Cassidy et al. 2001; De Hert et al. 2011; Heffner et al. 2008; Khalsa et al. 2008; Levin and Hennessy 2004; Meier et al. 2012; Strakowski et al. 2000; Treuer and Tohen 2010). Worsened outcomes likely reflect a combination of direct deleterious effects of the substance use on brain development and the primary disease pathophysiology (Ashton 2001), as well as indirect deleterious effects related to poor adherence to treatment and other aspects of health and lifestyle choices (e.g., less exercise, poor diet, medical decline) (Levin and Hennessy 2004).

Nature of the Association Between Bipolar Disorders and SUDs

The nature of the association between exposure to substances on the one hand and development of psychosis or mania on the other is an issue of intense interest and importance. Overall, there is a modest association (twofold increased risk) in the general population between cannabis use in adolescence and risk of psychotic spectrum disorders in adulthood (Arseneault et al. 2004). A Swedish cohort study reported a sixfold increased risk of schizophrenia 15 years later in adolescents who were heavy cannabis users at age 18 (i.e., those who used more than 50 times) (Andréasson et al. 1987). However, more than 50% of these adolescent heavy cannabis users met lifetime criteria for psychiatric disorder at age 18, reducing the adjusted risk of subsequent schizophrenia to 2.3-fold. Furthermore, only 3% of heavy cannabis users developed schizophrenia. In the Dunedin, New Zealand, birth cohort study, cannabis users (using three or more times) by ages 15 and 18 had an increased risk of psychotic symptoms at age 26, even after controlling for antecedent psychotic symptoms at age 11 (Arseneault et al. 2002). The effect was stronger for earlier cannabis use (at age 15). However, the association fell short of significance when the outcome was schizophreniform disorder. As pointed out by Arseneault et al. (2002), the population-attributable fraction (estimation of the number of cases that would be eliminated in the population by removal of cannabis use from the New Zealand population aged 15 years) is 8%: "In other words, removal of cannabis use from the New Zealand population aged 15 years would have led to an 8% reduction in the incidence of schizophrenia in that population" (Arseneault et al. 2004, p. 115).

Studies of patients with FEM have reported very high rates of substance use preceding or contiguous with the first activated episode. Baethge et al. (2005) reported that 33% of FEM patients admitted to the hospital met criteria for SUDs, the majority of which were diagnosed as substance dependence. After 24 months of follow-up, the rate of

SUDs rose to 39%. Interestingly, cannabis-dependent patients spent more time in manic states, whereas alcohol-dependent patients spent more time in the depressed state. Compared with bipolar patients without SUD, bipolar polysubstance users had worse outcomes and tended to be younger, less educated, and more likely to have a family history of psychiatric illness and mixed states. Similarly, bipolar substance users are at increased risk for suicide, poor medication adherence, and poor overall functioning compared with bipolar patients without SUD (Stephens et al. 2014).

Baethge et al. (2008) subsequently delved further into the association between substance use and polarity of episodes in patients with bipolar disorder. Specifically, they observed that in patients with bipolar disorder, cannabis use preceded or occurred at the same time as manic episodes, whereas alcohol use preceded or occurred at the same time as depressive episodes. This observation suggested that there was some specificity in the association between substance use and polarity of episodes in patients with established illness.

Tobacco smoking is two to three times more common in patients with bipolar disorder than in the general population and has been associated with an increased risk of other SUDs and worsened outcome in patients with bipolar disorder (Baethge et al. 2009). In a study of FEM inpatients, Heffner et al. (2008) reported that 36% of adolescent FEM patients were current smokers, with a mean age of 13 years at onset of smoking. Cigarette smoking at hospitalization was associated with a significantly increased risk of either a cannabis or alcohol use disorder over the 12-month follow-up period (odds ratio=16.62). Therefore, in addition to the well-established detrimental effects of smoking on physical health, smoking in adolescents with bipolar disorder may be a risk factor for the subsequent development of other SUDs.

Although exposure to substances early in development appears to be a risk factor for subsequent psychosis and mania, the majority of adolescents who use cannabis or other substances do not develop psychiatric disorders. Therefore, as discussed by Arseneault et al. (2004), it is most likely that substance use is one risk factor that interacts with other risk factors in vulnerable individuals.

Some clues come from the fact that bipolar disorder and schizophrenia are heritable diseases. Caspi et al. (2005) reported evidence from the Dunedin birth cohort longitudinal study data of an interaction between genetic vulnerability and exposure to cannabis in adolescence and increased risk of psychosis. Specifically, the authors showed that carriers of the catechol O-methyltransferase (COMT) valine allele were most likely to manifest psychotic symptoms and schizophreniform disorder in adulthood if they used cannabis in adolescence. This gene × environment interaction was not seen in homozygous carriers of the COMT methionine allele. Other evidence, as reviewed by Ashton (2001), addresses the overlapping biological pathways implicated in both cannabis use and psychosis.

SUDs and the Association With Early Clinical Stages of Bipolar Disorder

Increasingly, longitudinal high-risk studies have established that both bipolar disorder and psychotic spectrum disorders onset years before the full-threshold illness is clinically apparent. Specifically, early neurodevelopmental problems and psychological and behavioral changes precede the onset of full-blown psychosis (Cannon et al. 1997, 2002; Murray et al. 2004), and anxiety and circadian disturbances manifest years before the onset of bipolar mood episodes (Duffy 2010; Duffy et al. 2014). Therefore, it may be that substance use in high-risk individuals is associated and interacts with the early clinical stages of emerging disorder.

In an ongoing Canadian longitudinal study of the offspring of parents with well-characterized bipolar disorders (high-risk offspring), a significantly higher risk of SUDs was found in high-risk offspring compared with matched control subjects (offspring of well parents). Furthermore, the hazard of SUD in the high-risk offspring was earlier, peaking between ages 14 and 18 years (Duffy et al. 2012). The cumulative risk of SUDs in high-risk offspring increased with progression of illness development. High exposure and duration of exposure to active parental illness during the first decade of life were independently and significantly associated with a higher risk of SUD (S. Doucette, E. Levy, G. Flowerdew, et al., Early environmental and biological predictors of mood disorder in a well characterized Canadian sample of offspring of a bipolar parent, unpublished manuscript, 2015). Research findings also suggest that adolescents with bipolar disorder who have experienced trauma (emotional or physical) and/or psychotic symptoms are at higher risk of developing SUD compared with bipolar patients with no history of trauma or psychotic symptoms (Stephens et al. 2014).

Summary and Future Directions

Clearly, exposure to tobacco, alcohol, cannabis, and other substances should be avoided during an accelerated and critical period of neurodevelopment such as adolescence. This is particularly important for vulnerable adolescents who have other risk factors or are in the early clinical stages of psychiatric illness development. The accruing evidence has direct implications for public health policy and targeted high-risk intervention. Specifically, it would be important to legislatively prohibit the use of such deleterious substances until adulthood and to support this with effective educational material targeting adolescents and their parents. Furthermore, there should be evidence-based prevention and early intervention programs for youths at risk because of familial and clinical factors of developing schizophrenia and bipolar disorder; these programs should incorporate and study the effectiveness of specific treatment focusing on substance use in this population.

Many of the educational and psychotherapeutic interventions for youths with bipolar disorder are extrapolated from adult studies, although whether these are effective or evidence-based approaches is unclear. Systematic investigation of preventive and early intervention programs in bipolar youths is needed, specifically in regard to preventing substance use and the impact on a variety of clinical and functional outcomes.

There is a dearth of evidence with regard to substance use prevention and early intervention in youths who are at high risk because of familial factors and/or who are in the early clinical stages of developing bipolar disorder. Clearly, this is a prime high-risk subgroup to target and in which to study the effectiveness of psychoeducational and therapeutic approaches to preventing substance misuse. This would also be an ideal population in which to investigate the nature of the association between the use of certain substances at various stages in illness development and genetically sensitive causal pathways, which might then lead to more specific and novel intervention targets (see Figure 7–1).

KEY POINTS

- Although substance use is neither necessary nor sufficient to explain the development of psychotic and bipolar disorders, it is definitely a major risk factor and therefore should be a target of early intervention efforts.

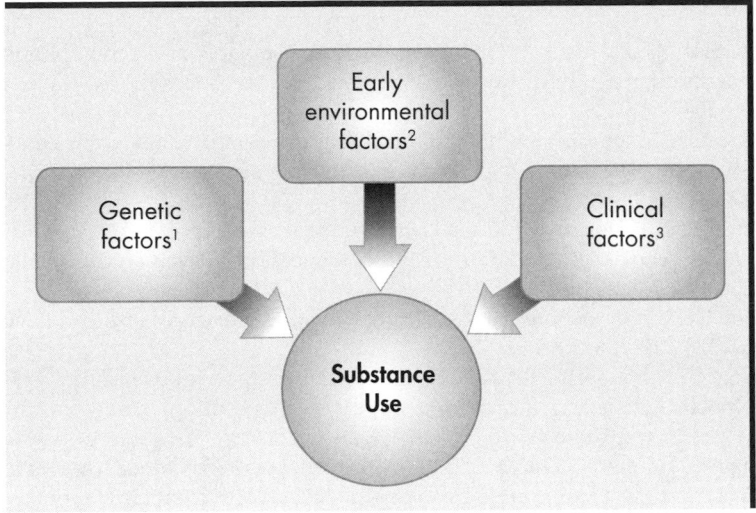

FIGURE 7–1.   Substance use in youths at high risk of developing bipolar disorder.

[1]Genetic factors that interact with other risk factors.
[2]Early adversity—includes exposure to active parental illness.
[3]Early clinical stages of bipolar disorder.

- Exposure to cannabis during adolescence has been strongly and specifically associated with the subsequent risk of developing schizophrenia and psychotic mania.

- Longitudinal studies suggest that both bipolar disorder and psychotic spectrum disorders onset years before the full-threshold illness is clinically apparent. Therefore, it may be that substance use in high-risk individuals is associated with the early clinical stages of emerging disorder.

- It is important to legislatively prohibit the use of deleterious substances until adulthood and to support this with effective educational material targeting adolescents and their parents.

- Evidence-based prevention and early intervention programs are needed for youths at risk of developing schizophrenia and bipolar disorder; these programs need to study the effectiveness of specific treatment modules focusing on substance use in this population.

References

Andréasson S, Allebeck P, Engström A, et al: Cannabis and schizophrenia: a longitudinal study of Swedish conscripts. Lancet 2(8574):1483–1486, 1987 2892048

Arseneault L, Cannon M, Poulton R, et al: Cannabis use in adolescence and risk for adult psychosis: longitudinal prospective study. BMJ 325(7374):1212–1213, 2002 12446537

Arseneault L, Cannon M, Witton J, et al: Causal association between cannabis and psychosis: examination of the evidence. Br J Psychiatry 184:110–117, 2004 14754822

Ashton CH: Pharmacology and effects of cannabis: a brief review. Br J Psychiatry 178:101–106, 2001 11157422

Baethge C, Baldessarini RJ, Khalsa HM, et al: Substance abuse in first-episode bipolar I disorder: indications for early intervention. Am J Psychiatry 162(5):1008–1010, 2005 15863809

Baethge C, Hennen J, Khalsa HM, et al: Sequencing of substance use and affective morbidity in 166 first-episode bipolar I disorder patients. Bipolar Disord 10(6):738–741, 2008 18837869

Baethge C, Tondo L, Lepri B, et al: Coffee and cigarette use: association with suicidal acts in 352 Sardinian bipolar disorder patients. Bipolar Disord 11(5):494–503, 2009 19624388

Cannon M, Jones P, Gilvarry C, et al: Premorbid social functioning in schizophrenia and bipolar disorder: similarities and differences. Am J Psychiatry 154(11):1544–1550, 1997 9356562

Cannon M, Caspi A, Moffitt TE, et al: Evidence for early-childhood, pan-developmental impairment specific to schizophreniform disorder: results from a longitudinal birth cohort. Arch Gen Psychiatry 59(5):449–456, 2002 11982449

Caspi A, Moffitt TE, Cannon M, et al: Moderation of the effect of adolescent-onset cannabis use on adult psychosis by a functional polymorphism in the catechol-O-methyltransferase gene: longitudinal evidence of a gene X environment interaction. Biol Psychiatry 57(10):1117–1127, 2005 15866551

Cassidy F, Ahearn EP, Carroll BJ: Substance abuse in bipolar disorder. Bipolar Disord 3(4):181–188, 2001 11552957

Chengappa KN, Kupfer DJ, Frank E, et al: Relationship of birth cohort and early age at onset of illness in a bipolar disorder case registry. Am J Psychiatry 160(9):1636–1642, 2003 12944339

De Hert M, Wampers M, Jendricko T, et al: Effects of cannabis use on age at onset in schizophrenia and bipolar disorder. Schizophr Res 126(1–3):270–276, 2011 20674280

Duffy A: The early natural history of bipolar disorder: what we have learned from longitudinal high-risk research. Can J Psychiatry 55(8):477–485, 2010 20723275

Duffy A, Horrocks J, Milin R, et al: Adolescent substance use disorder during the early stages of bipolar disorder: a prospective high-risk study. J Affect Disord 142(1–3):57–64, 2012 22959686

Duffy A, Horrocks J, Doucette S, et al: The developmental trajectory of bipolar disorder. Br J Psychiatry 204(2):122–128, 2014 24262817

Heffner JL, DelBello MP, Fleck DE, et al: Cigarette smoking in the early course of bipolar disorder: association with ages-at-onset of alcohol and marijuana use. Bipolar Disord 10(7):838–845, 2008 19032716

Kessler RC, Crum RM, Warner LA, et al: Lifetime co-occurrence of DSM-III-R alcohol abuse and dependence with other psychiatric disorders in the National Comorbidity Survey. Arch Gen Psychiatry 54(4):313–321, 1997 9107147

Khalsa HM, Salvatore P, Hennen J, et al: Suicidal events and accidents in 216 first-episode bipolar I disorder patients: predictive factors. J Affect Disord 106(1–2):179–184, 2008 17614135

Klerman GL: Age and clinical depression: today's youth in the twenty-first century. J Gerontol 31(3):318–323, 1976 1270767

Klerman GL, Weissman MM: Increasing rates of depression. JAMA 261(15):2229–2235, 1989 2648043

Levin FR, Hennessy G: Bipolar disorder and substance abuse. Biol Psychiatry 56(10):738–748, 2004 15556118

Meier MH, Caspi A, Ambler A, et al: Persistent cannabis users show neuropsychological decline from childhood to midlife. Proc Natl Acad Sci USA 109(40):E2657–E2664, 2012 22927402

Minnai GP, Tondo L, Salis P, et al: Secular trends in first hospitalizations for major mood disorders with comorbid substance use. Int J Neuropsychopharmacol 9(3):319–326, 2006 16316480

Murray RM, Sham P, Van Os J, et al: A developmental model for similarities and dissimilarities between schizophrenia and bipolar disorder. Schizophr Res 71(2–3):405–416, 2004 15474912

Nery FG, Miranda-Scippa A, Nery-Fernandes F, et al: Prevalence and clinical correlates of alcohol use disorders among bipolar disorder patients: results from the Brazilian Bipolar Research Network. Compr Psychiatry 55(5):1116–1121, 2014 24746528

Paus T, Keshavan M, Giedd JN: Why do many psychiatric disorders emerge during adolescence? Nat Rev Neurosci 9(12):947–957, 2008 19002191

Regier DA, Farmer ME, Rae DS, et al: Comorbidity of mental disorders with alcohol and other drug abuse: results from the Epidemiologic Catchment Area (ECA) study. JAMA 264(19):2511–2518, 1990 2232018

Stephens JR, Heffner JL, Adler CM, et al: Risk and protective factors associated with substance use disorders in adolescents with first-episode mania. J Am Acad Child Adolesc Psychiatry 53(7):771–779, 2014 24954826

Strakowski SM, DelBello MP: The co-occurrence of bipolar and substance use disorders. Clin Psychol Rev 20(2):191–206, 2000 10721497

Strakowski SM, DelBello MP, Fleck DE, et al: The impact of substance abuse on the course of bipolar disorder. Biol Psychiatry 48(6):477–485, 2000 11018221

Strakowski SM, DelBello MP, Fleck DE, et al: Effects of co-occurring cannabis use disorders on the course of bipolar disorder after a first hospitalization for mania. Arch Gen Psychiatry 64(1):57–64, 2007 17199055

Treuer T, Tohen M: Predicting the course and outcome of bipolar disorder: a review. Eur Psychiatry 25(6):328–333, 2010 20444581

CHAPTER 8

Anxiety Disorders and Substance Use Disorders

Jessica J. Black, Ph.D.
Tammy Chung, Ph.D.
Duncan B. Clark, M.D., Ph.D.

Adolescence is a dynamic period for the emergence of anxiety and substance use disorders (SUDs) because both disorders typically have an onset and peak between ages 12 and 25 years (Kessler et al. 2005). Anxiety disorders are among the most common psychiatric disorders for adolescents, and they are prevalent among adolescents with SUDs (Clark et al. 1994). The different types of anxiety disorders vary in relation to the perceived threats, related fearful or anxious behaviors, and associated cognitive processes. Research supports a strong relationship between some anxiety disorders and SUDs (e.g., social anxiety and alcohol), although there is little to no support of an association between other anxiety disorders and SUDs (e.g., specific phobia and alcohol) (Blumenthal et al. 2011).

This research was supported by National Institute on Alcohol Abuse and Alcoholism grant T32 AA07453, awarded to J.J. Black, Ph.D.; and grant K02 AA018195, awarded to T. Chung, Ph.D.; and National Institute on Alcohol Abuse and Alcoholism grant R01 AA016482 and National Institute on Drug Abuse grant P50 DA05605, awarded to D.B. Clark, M.D., Ph.D.

We begin this chapter by outlining the features of DSM-5 (American Psychiatric Association 2013) anxiety disorders. We then review the etiology of the most common anxiety disorders. We discuss the role of anxiety disorders in relation to a clinical course of SUD, referencing epidemiological data and theoretical models of anxiety and SUD comorbidity. Within this framework, important protective and resilience factors are noted. We cover best assessment practices and discuss evidence-based treatments and then conclude by providing recommendations for future research.

Features and Diagnosis of Anxiety Disorders

Anxiety disorders are characterized by excessive *fear*—the emotional response to a real or perceived threat—and/or *anxiety*—the anticipation of a future threat—along with engagement in associated fear- or anxiety-related behaviors. DSM-5 includes the following anxiety disorders: separation anxiety disorder, selective mutism, specific phobia, social anxiety disorder (SAD [social phobia]), panic disorder, agoraphobia, and generalized anxiety disorder (GAD) (American Psychiatric Association 2013). With the recent transition from DSM-IV-TR (American Psychiatric Association 2000) to DSM-5, the classification of anxiety disorders has changed somewhat. Perhaps most notable is that posttraumatic stress disorder is now classified among the trauma- and stressor-related disorders (and is discussed in this text in Chapter 9, "Posttraumatic Stress Disorder and Substance Use Disorders"). Obsessive-compulsive disorder also is no longer included among the anxiety disorders; it is listed in DSM-5 among obsessive-compulsive and related disorders. Another change is that both separation anxiety disorder and selective mutism are now included with the DSM-5 anxiety disorders rather than being grouped in the section called "Other Disorders of Infancy, Childhood, or Adolescence." The prevalence rates discussed in the following paragraphs were obtained from DSM-5.

Separation anxiety disorder is defined as the experiencing of anxiety about separation from the home or from attachment figures in excess of what would be expected given an individual's developmental level (Box 8–1). The prevalence of separation anxiety disorder declines after age 12 and is estimated to be 1.6% among adolescents, occurring equally among males and females.

Box 8–1. DSM-5 Criteria for Separation Anxiety Disorder

A. Developmentally inappropriate and excessive fear or anxiety concerning separation from those to whom the individual is attached, as evidenced by at least three of the following:

1. Recurrent excessive distress when anticipating or experiencing separation from home or from major attachment figures.

2. Persistent and excessive worry about losing major attachment figures or about possible harm to them, such as illness, injury, disasters, or death.

3. Persistent and excessive worry about experiencing an untoward event (e.g., getting lost, being kidnapped, having an accident, becoming ill) that causes separation from a major attachment figure.

4. Persistent reluctance or refusal to go out, away from home, to school, to work, or elsewhere because of fear of separation.

5. Persistent and excessive fear of or reluctance about being alone or without major attachment figures at home or in other settings.

6. Persistent reluctance or refusal to sleep away from home or to go to sleep without being near a major attachment figure.

7. Repeated nightmares involving the theme of separation.

8. Repeated complaints of physical symptoms (e.g., headaches, stomachaches, nausea, vomiting) when separation from major attachment figures occurs or is anticipated.

B. The fear, anxiety, or avoidance is persistent, lasting at least 4 weeks in children and adolescents and typically 6 months or more in adults.

C. The disturbance causes clinically significant distress or impairment in social, academic, occupational, or other important areas of functioning.

D. The disturbance is not better explained by another mental disorder, such as refusing to leave home because of excessive resistance to change in autism spectrum disorder; delusions or hallucinations concerning separation in psychotic disorders; refusal to go outside without a trusted companion in agoraphobia; worries about ill health or other harm befalling significant others in generalized anxiety disorder; or concerns about having an illness in illness anxiety disorder.

Reprinted from the *Diagnostic and Statistical Manual of Mental Disorders*, 5th Edition. Arlington, VA, American Psychiatric Association, 2013. Used with permission. Copyright © 2013 American Psychiatric Association.

Selective mutism is a rare disorder with usual onset before age 5 (Box 8–2). Children presenting with symptoms consistent with selective mutism fail to speak in some situations in which speech is expected but demonstrate the ability to speak in other situations (e.g., in the home). Selective mutism may be accompanied by SAD, with symptoms of selective mutism remitting in adolescence and social anxiety commonly persisting.

Box 8–2. DSM-5 Criteria for Selective Mutism

A. Consistent failure to speak in specific social situations in which there is an expectation for speaking (e.g., at school) despite speaking in other situations.

B. The disturbance interferes with educational or occupational achievement or with social communication.

C. The duration of the disturbance is at least 1 month (not limited to the first month of school).

D. The failure to speak is not attributable to a lack of knowledge of, or comfort with, the spoken language required in the social situation.

E. The disturbance is not better explained by a communication disorder (e.g., childhood-onset fluency disorder) and does not occur exclusively during the course of autism spectrum disorder, schizophrenia, or another psychotic disorder.

Reprinted from the *Diagnostic and Statistical Manual of Mental Disorders*, 5th Edition. Arlington, VA, American Psychiatric Association, 2013. Used with permission. Copyright © 2013 American Psychiatric Association.

Specific phobia is the excessive fear or anxiety about a specific object or situation, which then causes a person to avoid the feared stimuli or to endure intense distress (Box 8–3). Among adolescents, the estimated prevalence of specific phobia is 16%.

Box 8–3. DSM-5 Criteria for Specific Phobia

A. Marked fear or anxiety about a specific object or situation (e.g., flying, heights, animals, receiving an injection, seeing blood).

   Note: In children, the fear or anxiety may be expressed by crying, tantrums, freezing, or clinging.

B. The phobic object or situation almost always provokes immediate fear or anxiety.

C. The phobic object or situation is actively avoided or endured with intense fear or anxiety.

D. The fear or anxiety is out of proportion to the actual danger posed by the specific object or situation and to the sociocultural context.

E. The fear, anxiety, or avoidance is persistent, typically lasting for 6 months or more.

F. The fear, anxiety, or avoidance causes clinically significant distress or impairment in social, occupational, or other important areas of functioning.

G. The disturbance is not better explained by the symptoms of another mental disorder, including fear, anxiety, and avoidance of situations associated with panic-like symptoms or other incapacitating symptoms (as in agoraphobia); objects or situations related to obsessions (as in obsessive-compulsive disorder); reminders of traumatic events (as in posttraumatic stress disorder); separation from home or attachment figures (as in separation anxiety disorder); or social situations (as in social anxiety disorder).

Reprinted from the *Diagnostic and Statistical Manual of Mental Disorders*, 5th Edition. Arlington, VA, American Psychiatric Association, 2013. Used with permission. Copyright © 2013 American Psychiatric Association.

Social anxiety disorder is characterized by extreme preoccupation with being humiliated or embarrassed in social or performance situations, resulting in intense discomfort in or avoidance of social situations (Box 8–4). The yearly prevalence rates for SAD are around 7% for adolescents. Social anxiety rates are higher among females than males, especially during adolescence.

Box 8–4. DSM-5 Criteria for Social Anxiety Disorder

A. Marked fear or anxiety about one or more social situations in which the individual is exposed to possible scrutiny by others. Examples include social interactions (e.g., having a conversation, meeting unfamiliar people), being observed (e.g., eating or drinking), and performing in front of others (e.g., giving a speech).

Note: In children, the anxiety must occur in peer settings and not just during interactions with adults.

B. The individual fears that he or she will act in a way or show anxiety symptoms that will be negatively evaluated (i.e., will be humiliating or embarrassing; will lead to rejection or offend others).

C. The social situations almost always provoke fear or anxiety.

Note: In children, the fear or anxiety may be expressed by crying, tantrums, freezing, clinging, shrinking, or failing to speak in social situations.

D. The social situations are avoided or endured with intense fear or anxiety.

E. The fear or anxiety is out of proportion to the actual threat posed by the social situation and to the sociocultural context.

F. The fear, anxiety, or avoidance is persistent, typically lasting for 6 months or more.

G. The fear, anxiety, or avoidance causes clinically significant distress or impairment in social, occupational, or other important areas of functioning.
H. The fear, anxiety, or avoidance is not attributable to the physiological effects of a substance (e.g., a drug of abuse, a medication) or another medical condition.
I. The fear, anxiety, or avoidance is not better explained by the symptoms of another mental disorder, such as panic disorder, body dysmorphic disorder, or autism spectrum disorder.
J. If another medical condition (e.g., Parkinson's disease, obesity, disfigurement from burns or injury) is present, the fear, anxiety, or avoidance is clearly unrelated or is excessive.

Reprinted from the *Diagnostic and Statistical Manual of Mental Disorders*, 5th Edition. Arlington, VA, American Psychiatric Association, 2013. Used with permission. Copyright © 2013 American Psychiatric Association.

Panic disorder involves the experience of recurrent unexpected brief periods of intense fear accompanied by physical symptoms, causing the person to worry about future attacks or to modify his or her behaviors to accommodate anticipated attacks (Box 8–5). Again, females are more likely to meet criteria for panic attacks than are males; the 12-month prevalence rates for adolescents are 2%–3%.

Box 8–5.   DSM-5 Criteria for Panic Disorder

A. Recurrent unexpected panic attacks. A panic attack is an abrupt surge of intense fear or intense discomfort that reaches a peak within minutes, and during which time four (or more) of the following symptoms occur:

Note: The abrupt surge can occur from a calm state or an anxious state.

1. Palpitations, pounding heart, or accelerated heart rate.
2. Sweating.
3. Trembling or shaking.
4. Sensations of shortness of breath or smothering.
5. Feelings of choking.
6. Chest pain or discomfort.
7. Nausea or abdominal distress.
8. Feeling dizzy, unsteady, light-headed, or faint.
9. Chills or heat sensations.
10. Paresthesias (numbness or tingling sensations).
11. Derealization (feelings of unreality) or depersonalization (being detached from oneself).
12. Fear of losing control or "going crazy."
13. Fear of dying.

Note: Culture-specific symptoms (e.g., tinnitus, neck soreness, headache, uncontrollable screaming or crying) may be seen. Such symptoms should not count as one of the four required symptoms.

B. At least one of the attacks has been followed by 1 month (or more) of one or both of the following:

1. Persistent concern or worry about additional panic attacks or their consequences (e.g., losing control, having a heart attack, "going crazy").
2. A significant maladaptive change in behavior related to the attacks (e.g., behaviors designed to avoid having panic attacks, such as avoidance of exercise or unfamiliar situations).

C. The disturbance is not attributable to the physiological effects of a substance (e.g., a drug of abuse, a medication) or another medical condition (e.g., hyperthyroidism, cardiopulmonary disorders).

D. The disturbance is not better explained by another mental disorder (e.g., the panic attacks do not occur only in response to feared social situations, as in social anxiety disorder; in response to circumscribed phobic objects or situations, as in specific phobia; in response to obsessions, as in obsessive-compulsive disorder; in response to reminders of traumatic events, as in posttraumatic stress disorder; or in response to separation from attachment figures, as in separation anxiety disorder).

Reprinted from the *Diagnostic and Statistical Manual of Mental Disorders,* 5th Edition. Arlington, VA, American Psychiatric Association, 2013. Used with permission. Copyright © 2013 American Psychiatric Association.

Agoraphobia involves marked fear or anxiety about two or more of a wide range of situations and often includes a fear of inability to escape danger or to receive the necessary help (Box 8–6). For example, a person with agoraphobia may fear using public transportation and also fear being outside the home. Approximately 1.7% of adolescents suffer from agoraphobia, with incidence rates peaking in late adolescence and early adulthood.

Box 8–6. DSM-5 Criteria for Agoraphobia

A. Marked fear or anxiety about two (or more) of the following five situations:

1. Using public transportation (e.g., automobiles, buses, trains, ships, planes).
2. Being in open spaces (e.g., parking lots, marketplaces, bridges).
3. Being in enclosed places (e.g., shops, theaters, cinemas).
4. Standing in line or being in a crowd.
5. Being outside of the home alone.

B. The individual fears or avoids these situations because of thoughts that escape might be difficult or help might not be available in the event of developing panic-like symptoms or other incapacitating or embarrassing symptoms (e.g., fear of falling in the elderly; fear of incontinence).

C. The agoraphobic situations almost always provoke fear or anxiety.

D. The agoraphobic situations are actively avoided, require the presence of a companion, or are endured with intense fear or anxiety.

E. The fear or anxiety is out of proportion to the actual danger posed by the agoraphobic situations and to the sociocultural context.

F. The fear, anxiety, or avoidance is persistent, typically lasting for 6 months or more.

G. The fear, anxiety, or avoidance causes clinically significant distress or impairment in social, occupational, or other important areas of functioning.

H. If another medical condition (e.g., inflammatory bowel disease, Parkinson's disease) is present, the fear, anxiety, or avoidance is clearly excessive.

I. The fear, anxiety, or avoidance is not better explained by the symptoms of another mental disorder—for example, the symptoms are not confined to specific phobia, situational type; do not involve only social situations (as in social anxiety disorder); and are not related exclusively to obsessions (as in obsessive-compulsive disorder), perceived defects or flaws in physical appearance (as in body dysmorphic disorder), reminders of traumatic events (as in posttraumatic stress disorder), or fear of separation (as in separation anxiety disorder).

Note: Agoraphobia is diagnosed irrespective of the presence of panic disorder. If an individual's presentation meets criteria for panic disorder and agoraphobia, both diagnoses should be assigned.

Reprinted from the *Diagnostic and Statistical Manual of Mental Disorders,* 5th Edition. Arlington, VA, American Psychiatric Association, 2013. Used with permission. Copyright © 2013 American Psychiatric Association.

Generalized anxiety disorder is characterized by worry about numerous events or activities to a degree that is excessive in relation to the actual likelihood or impact of the anticipated events or activities (Box 8–7). Persons with GAD find it difficult to control their worries, and their GAD-related thoughts often interfere with their daily functioning. Prevalence of GAD is 0.9% among U.S. adolescents, with females twice as likely as males to experience GAD.

Box 8–7.   DSM-5 Criteria for Generalized Anxiety Disorder

A. Excessive anxiety and worry (apprehensive expectation), occurring more days than not for at least 6 months, about a number of events or activities (such as work or school performance).

B. The individual finds it difficult to control the worry.

C. The anxiety and worry are associated with three (or more) of the following six symptoms (with at least some symptoms having been present for more days than not for the past 6 months):

Note: Only one item is required in children.

1. Restlessness or feeling keyed up or on edge.
2. Being easily fatigued.
3. Difficulty concentrating or mind going blank.
4. Irritability.
5. Muscle tension.
6. Sleep disturbance (difficulty falling or staying asleep, or restless, unsatisfying sleep).

D. The anxiety, worry, or physical symptoms cause clinically significant distress or impairment in social, occupational, or other important areas of functioning.

E. The disturbance is not attributable to the physiological effects of a substance (e.g., a drug of abuse, a medication) or another medical condition (e.g., hyperthyroidism).

F. The disturbance is not better explained by another mental disorder (e.g., anxiety or worry about having panic attacks in panic disorder, negative evaluation in social anxiety disorder [social phobia], contamination or other obsessions in obsessive-compulsive disorder, separation from attachment figures in separation anxiety disorder, reminders of traumatic events in posttraumatic stress disorder, gaining weight in anorexia nervosa, physical complaints in somatic symptom disorder, perceived appearance flaws in body dysmorphic disorder, having a serious illness in illness anxiety disorder, or the content of delusional beliefs in schizophrenia or delusional disorder).

Generally, females are more likely than males to suffer from anxiety disorders. The most prevalent anxiety disorder among adolescents is SAD, followed by panic disorder, agoraphobia, separation anxiety disorder, and GAD. Although we discuss the association between all anxiety disorders and SUDs, we focus on SAD, panic disorder, and GAD because these three disorders have the highest rates of comorbidity with SUDs (Kushner et al. 2000).

Etiology of Anxiety Disorders and Transition to a Clinical Course of SUD

This section reviews three primary models of the etiology and nature of the association between anxiety disorders and SUDs: 1) the influence of anxiety disorders on SUDs, 2) the influence of SUDs on anxiety disorders, and 3) shared vulnerabilities for both disorders (Kushner et al. 2000). Then we discuss the co-occurrence of SAD, panic disorder, and GAD with SUDs, providing evidence to support the different theoretical models.

Etiological Models of the Association Between Anxiety Disorder and SUD

The first model, that anxiety precedes SUD—referenced in short here as anxiety → SUD—has gained increasing support in recent years. The conceptual framework for anxiety influencing the onset of SUDs is largely based on the self-medication hypothesis, the stress-dampening model, and social learning theory (Blane and Leonard 1987). The self-medication hypothesis and stress-dampening model are similar theories, both of which posit that SUDs arise when persons repeatedly and inappropriately use substances to cope with distressing affective states (Blane and Leonard 1987). For example, among individuals with anxiety, alcohol consumption may be expected to reduce anxiety, leading some individuals with problematic anxiety to consume alcohol and develop alcohol-related problems. Social learning theory proposes that SUDs result from a combination of high positive use expectancies, low negative use expectancies, and low refusal self-efficacy related to high-risk substance use situations (Blane and Leonard 1987). For example, an anxious person may expect substance use to act as a social facilitator and to decrease anxious feelings and may be less confident about his or her ability to refuse substances.

The second model—referenced in short as SUDs → anxiety—theorizes that SUDs might facilitate the development of anxiety disorders because of chronic substance use and/or withdrawal resulting in anxiety symptoms (Kushner et al. 2000). Heightened anxiety is a key symptom of withdrawal in many SUDs and can persist long after physical symptoms of withdrawal have subsided. Many adolescents are often in the early stages of substance use, characterized by fewer physiological symptoms, suggesting that this model may be more likely to be observed in adults or individuals with more heavy and chronic substance use.

The last theoretical model proposes that there are shared vulnerabilities for both disorders. For example, children of fathers with SUD have an increased risk for SUD and anxiety disorders (Clark et al. 1997b). Adolescents at risk for SUD, as determined by having at least one parent with SUD, may be hypersensitive to fear stimuli. Specifically, a functional magnetic resonance imaging study that compared youths with a family history of SUD to healthy control subjects found that youths with a positive family history had increased amygdala activation during an affect-laden faces task, suggesting hypersensitivity to fear stimuli (Thatcher et al. 2014). A possible mechanism for a shared vulnerability to SUD and anxiety disorder may be patterns of psychopathology in the parents. Also, there is a tendency for men with SUD to marry and mate with women with anxiety disorders (Clark et al. 2004). Through such assortative mating, parents may transmit a propensity for both anxiety and SUD.

Social Anxiety Disorder and SUD Comorbidity

Generally, there is strong support that SAD is associated with SUDs. SAD is frequently the primary or preceding disorder, particularly in relation to alcohol problems (Tomlinson and Brown 2012). The average age at onset is 14 years for SAD and 23 years for alcohol use disorder.

Social Anxiety Disorder → Alcohol Use Disorder

Because SAD typically precedes SUDs among comorbid individuals, SAD has been hypothesized to contribute to the onset of SUDs. Examination of adolescents in psychiatric or substance use treatment provides support for this model. Social anxiety preceded substance involvement 65%–100% of the time, and the average time between onset of social anxiety and substance use involvement was 2 years (Tomlinson and Brown 2012). In addition, endorsement of coping-related motives for substance use among youths with social anxiety suggests that social anxiety precedes substance use. In support of this, heightened social anxiety was associated with coping-related drinking motives in youth (Blumenthal et al. 2010). SAD was specifically related to coping-related drinking motives in a longitudinal study of youth (Windle and Windle 2012) and in studies of college students (Schry and White 2013). In summary, research indicates that some adolescents with social anxiety drink to cope with negative affect, which is in line with the similar stress-dampening model and self-medication hypothesis (Tomlinson and Brown 2012).

SUD → Social Anxiety Disorder and Shared Vulnerabilities

The evidence supporting the concept that SUD leads to SAD is weak. It is possible that engaging in embarrassing behaviors while intoxicated can increase sensitivity to negative evaluation in social situations (Crawford and Novak 2013), but there is little evidence suggesting that this leads to SAD. Likewise, few data support a shared vulnerabilities model of SUD and SAD.

Panic Disorder and SUD Comorbidity

Compared with other anxiety disorders, panic disorder is most strongly associated with SUDs, and data suggest that those with panic disorder are more likely to seek treatment than those with co-occurring SAD or a specific phobia (Grant et al. 2004). A systematic review of the adult literature on the association between panic disorder and SUD found support for all three theoretical models; that is, panic disorder both preceded and followed SUD, and individuals with panic disorder and SUD had shared vulnerabilities (Cosci et al. 2007). Little is known, however, about the nature of the association between panic disorder and SUD in youths. This gap in knowledge may exist because panic disorder typically has an onset during young adulthood, although adolescents may experience a panic attack without meeting full syndrome criteria. Some cross-sectional research does support an association between panic symptoms and higher rates of alcohol and cigarette use among adolescent girls (mean age of 13.5 years; Hayward et al. 1997).

Panic Disorder → SUD

Similarly, youths in late adolescence with panic disorder reported higher rates of substance use than average, a finding that was interpreted as supporting a model in which panic disorder is associated with the onset of SUDs (Valentiner et al. 2004). In contrast, some work suggests that adolescent panic disorder is *negatively* associated with cigarette smoking in adulthood (Goodwin et al. 2013); this negative association suggests that panic disorder may be protective against cigarette use in some adolescents. The adult literature provides clearer support for the possible influence of panic disorder on SUDs. For example, a prospective study of adults indicated that panic disorder was associated with a modestly higher risk for SUD onset (Kinley et al. 2011).

SUD → Panic Disorder

Research with adolescents provides some evidence to support a model in which substance use increases risk for panic symptoms and disorder. For example, in a longitudinal study, nicotine dependence increased the risk for onset of panic disorder; however, panic disorder did not increase the risk for nicotine dependence or smoking (Isensee et al. 2003).

Similarly, cross-sectional research indicated that an adolescent's alcohol use history was uniquely associated with panic symptomatology—both retrospective self-report of panic and physiological reactivity to an in-laboratory hyperventilation task (Blumenthal et al. 2012). It is important to keep in mind that Blumenthal et al.'s (2012) results based on self-report are limited by possible retrospective recall bias. Evidence from the adult literature also supports SUD as a preceding factor for panic disorder. For example, analysis of data from a large epidemiological study found that smoking predicted the onset of panic disorder (Johnston et al. 2011).

Shared Vulnerabilities

Family studies support shared vulnerabilities for panic disorder and SUDs, particularly alcohol use disorders. In a large community sample of adults, Goodwin et al. (2011) found that compared with participants with first-degree relatives without panic disorder, participants with first-degree relatives with panic disorder had significantly higher odds of having an alcohol use disorder. Similar studies with clinical populations from various countries have also found increased risk of alcohol use disorder among those with first-degree relatives with panic disorder (Merikangas et al. 1998). Davids et al. (2002) found that patients with comorbid panic disorder and alcohol use disorder were more likely to have parents with subthreshold panic symptoms. Although results support familial risk for panic disorder and SUD comorbidity, the mechanisms underlying shared vulnerabilities remain unclear.

General Anxiety Disorder and SUD Comorbidity

An association between GAD and SUDs has been clearly demonstrated. An estimated 50% of people with GAD meet criteria for a lifetime SUD (Alegria et al. 2010). The dearth of support for specific mechanisms linking GAD and SUD limits the conceptual formulation. Also, studies on adolescent GAD and SUD are scarce.

General Anxiety Disorder → SUD

In a study by Smith and Book (2010), GAD occurred prior to alcohol use disorder 67% of the time among adults in substance use treatment. Research with clinical samples suggests that GAD may exacerbate problematic substance use and increase treatment resistance. In another adult treatment study, presence of GAD predicted substance dependence onset at 12-month follow-up (Compton et al. 2003). In line with the self-medication hypothesis and the stress-dampening model, individuals with GAD reported using substances as a means of self-medication at higher rates than individuals with other anxiety disorders (Robinson et al. 2009).

SUD → General Anxiety Disorder and Shared Vulnerabilities

In community samples, SUD onset typically precedes GAD, suggesting that SUD may promote GAD symptoms (Alegria et al. 2010). Using a prospective design, Bruce et al. (2005) examined the natural course of anxiety and other psychiatric disorders among adults over a 12-year period and found that SUD significantly diminished GAD recovery.

Little is known about the shared vulnerabilities for GAD and SUDs. More research is needed because etiological evidence is very limited and preliminary models suggest a combination of genetics and environmental stressors.

Conclusions

Support for a particular theoretical model of the association between anxiety disorder and SUD varies by anxiety disorder. Most pertinent research indicates that SAD contributes to SUDs. Once adolescents with SAD are continually exposed to substance use in social situations, typically in mid- to late adolescence, coping motives for use, positive use expectancies, and poor refusal self-efficacy are important risk factors for SUD. For panic disorder, there is some support for SUD leading to panic symptoms and for shared vulnerabilities. Neurobiological changes resulting from substance use may place persons at higher risk for panic disorder (e.g., Johnston et al. 2011). Family studies also suggest that there may be strong genetic factors and/or familial experiences at play in the comorbid relationship between panic and SUDs. Given that the relationship between GAD and SUDs has been researched the least, it is not surprising that findings are mixed on a theoretical model of how these disorders are related to one another. Overall, research focusing on adolescence is limited, especially mechanism research, which limits confidence in any conceptual model when applied to youths with a comorbid anxiety disorder and SUD.

Assessments and Interventions

Assessment

The insidious, chronic nature of anxiety disorders reinforces the need for accurate assessment. The American Academy of Child and Adolescent Psychiatry (Connolly et al. 2007) recommends assessing anxiety as part of the psychiatric evaluation of adolescents. Several assessment instruments designed specifically for adolescents are available. There are a few factors to keep in mind when assessing adolescent anxiety. First, symptoms should be viewed in light of developmental considerations. For example, adolescents are likely to worry about social competence and school performance (Vasey et al. 1994). Second, many adolescents with anxiety present with affect-related physical symptoms, such as headaches or fatigue. When the etiology of somatic symptoms is uncertain, diagnostic consultation with the adolescent's primary care physician is advised. Third, accurate assessment requires inquiry about anxiety symptoms and related functioning in all domains of the adolescent's life (school, extracurricular activities, social activities, home, etc.) rather than one milieu (e.g., home). Finally, owing to the recent transition from DSM-IV-TR to DSM-5, many assessment instruments have not yet been adapted to DSM-5 diagnostic criteria; consequently, information gleaned from such measures should be interpreted cautiously.

Patients with anxiety disorders commonly present in medical settings. Use of screening measures can alleviate some of the burden of identifying psychiatric disorders during medical visits because health care providers are often under strict time constraints. Screening measures are also advantageous in psychiatric or SUD programs, because anxiety disorders may be neglected in the context of other problems during intake, which can then limit treatment efficacy (Clark et al. 1995). The 41-item Screen for Child Anxiety Related Emotional Disorders (SCARED; Birmaher et al. 1997) and the 38-item Spence Children's Anxiety Scale (SCAS; Spence 1998) are two validated screening instruments; the SCARED and SCAS have both a youth version and a parent's report version (Birmaher et al. 1997; Nauta et al. 2004).

Systematic interview methods allow for more comprehensive assessment of anxiety symptoms and can improve diagnostic accuracy. Semistructured interviews afford flexibility in the wording and presentation of questions and involve interviewer judgment regarding the clinical significance of symptoms reported. This approach is advantageous when clinically experienced and thoroughly trained interviewers are available. When anxiety is expected to be the cardinal disorder, the Anxiety Disorders Interview Schedule (ADIS) is a useful semistructured interview option for assessing anxiety, mood, and externalizing DSM-IV (American Psychiatric Association 1994) disorders based on parent and child input (Silverman et al. 2001). The ADIS has been demonstrated to have acceptable psychometric properties (Silverman et al.

2001). Another well-validated semistructured interview is the widely used Schedule for Affective Disorders and Schizophrenia for School-Age Children–Present and Lifetime Version (K-SADS-PL; Kaufman et al. 1997). The K-SADS-PL includes all youth psychiatric disorders according to the DSM-IV criteria (Kaufman et al. 1997) and is freely accessible on the Internet for clinical or research uses. Pertinent to the population of adolescents who use substances is the Child Semi-Structured Assessment for the Genetics of Alcoholism, Adolescent version (C-SSAGA-A; Bucholz et al. 1994), which is designed to distinguish substance-induced syndromes from independent symptoms of mood, anxiety, psychotic, and personality disorders. It is important to note that although the C-SSAGA-A has been validated in adult populations, psychometric studies of the adolescent version (ages 13–17) are limited.

When time, resource, or feasibility limitations conflict with the use of semistructured interviews, structured interviews are an acceptable alternative. Structured interview administration follows the exact wording of questions and decision trees, with minimal latitude for variation in administration or interpretation of responses. Some structured diagnostic interviews may be computer administered. For example, the National Survey on Drug Use and Health administers a structured diagnostic interview via computer to determine DSM-IV psychiatric diagnoses, including anxiety disorders and SUDs. This approach has been extensively evaluated, and results are comparable to interviewer-administered methods (Harford et al. 2005).

In addition to brief screening measures and diagnostic interviews, instruments with graded severity ratings play an important role in adolescent anxiety assessment. Graded severity ratings can increase sensitivity to change in symptoms and may catch subclinical symptoms that are problematic and/or prodromal symptoms that can be targeted for prevention. For example, SCARED scores can be used as a broad change indicator (Clark et al. 1995). Deciding on a global assessment of anxiety or an assessment of a specific anxiety disorder can guide assessors as to what adolescent-validated severity-graded measure is best. For example, the Hamilton Anxiety Rating Scale (HARS; Clark and Donovan 1994) and the State-Trait Anxiety Inventory for Children (STAIC; Kirisci et al. 1996) can assess global anxiety among adolescents. For the assessment of SAD, the Social Phobia and Anxiety Inventory for Adolescents (SPAI; see also Clark et al. 1997a) can be used, and for the assessment of GAD, the Penn State Worry Questionnaire for Children (PSWQ-C; Chorpita et al. 1997) is a possible choice.

Intervention

A multimodal approach, including psychoeducation, consultation, and treatment, is recommended for the treatment of adolescent anxiety disorders. Specifically, the patient and family can be provided with educational information about the disorder. Consultation with school officials and medical providers can be used to supplement assessment and to coordinate treatment. Evidence-based behavioral interventions and pharmacotherapy can be selected based on the patient's needs. Approaches that integrate anxiety treatment into substance use treatment programs have led to better substance use outcomes in adults (Kushner et al. 2005); however, delivering two separate treatment protocols rather than one integrated treatment program has also been shown to overwhelm adult clients. A search in PubMed (archive of biomedical and life sciences journal [primarily] literature at the U.S. National Institutes of Health's National Library of Medicine) and PsycINFO (American Psychological Association abstracting and indexing database devoted to peer-reviewed literature in the behavioral sciences and mental health) using keywords such as "youth," "adolescents," "anxiety," "substance use," "substance use treatment," and "anxiety treatment" yielded limited results on integrated adolescent treatments. One brief pilot intervention for socially anxious adolescent or young adult drinkers has shown promising efficacy (as described by Black et al. 2012).

Anxiety could potentially serve as a catalyst for adolescents to abstain from substance use. For example, Smith and Tran (2007) found that among hazardous drinkers in late adolescence (median age of 19 years), those with elevated global anxiety reported an increased readiness to change drinking behaviors. Treating anxiety at a young age has been shown to result in decreased substance involvement at long-term follow-up (Kendall et al. 2004). However, less is known about the effects of substance use treatment on adolescent anxiety outcomes. Evidence from the adult literature suggests that standard substance use treatment does not directly decrease anxiety. Among adults with high trait anxiety and comorbid alcohol use disorder who had successfully completed detoxification and participated in 3 weeks of alcohol use treatment, no substantial decrease in trait anxiety was found at 6-month follow-up (Driessen et al. 2001). Furthermore, increased trait anxiety was associated with relapse to alcohol use (Driessen et al. 2001). In sum, examination of the adult and adolescent literature on treating each disorder separately reveals that treating anxiety in isolation may somewhat improve SUD outcomes;

however, treating SUD in isolation was not found to reduce anxiety, and anxiety may be an important relapse-related variable.

Given that there is no known widely accepted effective protocol for the simultaneous treatment of anxiety and SUDs among adolescents, we cover effective treatments for SUDs and for anxiety disorders separately.

Substance Use

Psychosocial interventions are generally preferred over pharmacological interventions for initial adolescent SUD treatment. In the treatment of adolescent substance use, it is also important to have realistic outcome expectations because most adolescents return to using shortly after treatment completion (Cornelius et al. 2003). With regard to specific adolescent SUD treatment modality, no one treatment has been found to be superior to another (Waldron and Turner 2008). In a large clinical trial for adolescent substance use, the Cannabis Youth Treatment study (Dennis et al. 2004), the researchers compared the effectiveness of five evidence-based treatments: cognitive-behavioral therapy (CBT), multidimensional family therapy, Family Support Network, Adolescent Community Reinforcement Approach, and motivational enhancement therapy (which includes personalized feedback plus motivational interviewing). Dennis et al. (2004) found no single intervention to be more effective than another. However, individual differences or personality factors may render one treatment more appropriate for a particular adolescent. For example, matching youths from families with dysfunctional communication with multidimensional family therapy and youths with externalizing disorders with contingency management may be beneficial. Generally, however, factors that are common to adolescent SUD treatments, such as goal setting or strong therapeutic rapport, may better account for positive change in adolescent substance use than methods that are unique to particular forms of treatment, such as family therapy versus CBT (Black and Chung 2014).

Anxiety Disorders

CBT is the gold-standard behavioral treatment for adolescent anxiety disorders. Long-term follow-up from a large, multisite randomized clinical trial, the Child/Adolescent Anxiety Multimodal Study (CAMS), indicates that CBT results in long-term gains (Ginsburg et al. 2014). Youths in the CAMS with more severe anxiety, heightened caregiver stress, and a cardinal diagnosis of separation anxiety disorder were more likely to have worse outcomes (Compton et al. 2014). Interestingly, random assignment to CBT, sertraline (a selective serotonin reuptake inhibitor [SSRI]), or CBT plus sertraline resulted in similar overall positive effects at 6-year follow-up compared with placebo (Ginsburg et al. 2014). However, examination of specific disorders indicated small differences between treatment conditions: participants with SAD had better outcomes with sertraline than CBT, whereas participants with GAD had better outcomes with CBT than sertraline (Compton et al. 2014). These findings highlight the need to adjust CBT based on the adolescent's primary anxiety disorder. Hannesdottir and Ollendick (2007) argued that adolescents with SAD or panic disorder may benefit from supplementing CBT with emotion regulation skills. Given the pervasive worry or excessive concern about potential future threats inherent to GAD, studies on the efficacy and effectiveness of mindfulness practice on adolescent GAD may be beneficial. Mindfulness involves training oneself to focus on the present moment without judgment. Adult randomized controlled studies of mindfulness have shown promising results in reducing GAD symptoms. Also, a randomized clinical trial of mindfulness for adolescents has shown positive effects on anxiety (Biegel et al. 2009).

Existing research supports SSRIs, including sertraline, fluoxetine, fluvoxamine, and paroxetine, as the medications of choice for treating adolescent anxiety disorder (Kodish et al. 2011). SSRIs are preferred because of demonstrated effectiveness and increased safety compared with other drug classes. For example, tricyclic antidepressants are associated with greater risk of arrhythmia (irregular heart beat) and hazardous overdose. Among individuals with SUDs or a history of SUDs, use of benzodiazepines is typically advised against given their addiction potential (Clark 2012).

See Table 8–1 for a review of assessment and treatment for anxiety and adolescent SUDs.

Summary and Future Directions

Adolescence encompasses the typical developmental time window for onset of SUD and anxiety disorders. Some anxiety disorders, particularly SAD, panic disorder, and GAD, are more prevalent than others among individuals with SUDs. Comorbidity is associated with a more chronic, severe, and treatment-resistant SUD course. The implications of this comorbidity call for more research on SUDs and anxiety during adolescence, including studies to advance the understanding of etiologies as well as methods to improve prevention and treatment.

TABLE 8–1. Assessment and treatment outline for anxiety and adolescent substance use disorders

Assessment: anxiety and SUDs

General considerations	Assess symptoms in developmental context; assess lifetime and current behavior, including "change points" (onset and offset)	Assess symptoms and functioning in multiple domains (e.g., school, home); consult with teachers and health care providers
	Assess possible physical symptoms that might be due to anxiety or substance use	Distinguish substance-induced from independent anxiety symptoms
Measures		
Interviews	Semistructured	Anxiety Disorders Interview Schedule (ADIS); Schedule for Affective Disorders and Schizophrenia for School-Age Children–Present and Lifetime Version (K-SADS-PL); Child Semi-Structured Assessment for the Genetics of Alcoholism, Adolescent version (C-SSAGA-A)
	Structured	Diagnostic Interview Schedule for Children (DISC; Shaffer et al. 2000)
Screening tools	Substance use	Alcohol Screening and Brief Intervention for Youth: A Practitioner's Guide (NIAAA) (Johnston et al. 2011), questions about frequency of using tobacco and drugs
	Global anxiety	Screen for Child Anxiety Related Emotional Disorders (SCARED); Hamilton Anxiety Rating Scale (HARS); State-Trait Anxiety Inventory for Children (STAIC)
	Specific anxiety disorder	Social Phobia and Anxiety Inventory for Adolescents (SPAI); Penn State Worry Questionnaire for Children (PSWQ-C)

TABLE 8–1. Assessment and treatment outline for anxiety and adolescent substance use disorders *(continued)*

Treatment: stabilize SUD, then address anxiety

Psychoeducation and psychotherapy	SUDs	Provide psychoeducation on SUDs and anxiety CBT; MET; family therapy
	Anxiety disorders	CBT
Pharmacotherapy	Anxiety disorders	SSRIs; avoid benzodiazepines because of potential for misuse

Note. Research on integrated SUD and anxiety treatments for adolescents is lacking.
CBT=cognitive-behavioral therapy; MET=motivational enhancement therapy; NIAAA=National Institute on Alcohol Abuse and Alcoholism; SSRI=selective serotonin reuptake inhibitor; SUD=substance use disorder.

There is no universal conceptual model for anxiety and SUDs. Support for a particular model varies by anxiety disorder. At present, most research supports SAD → SUDs, SUDS → panic disorder, and shared vulnerabilities → panic disorder and SUDs; findings on GAD and SUDs have been mixed. In general, more adolescent studies are needed. Conceptual models are also limited by type of substance examined, because most research has focused on alcohol use. The existing theoretical models regarding anxiety and SUD are rather simplistic. An important step to move the field forward may be the development and testing of more complex theoretical models that account for the type of substance, stage of substance involvement, developmental stage, and specific anxiety disorder.

Although evidence from adult studies suggests that integrating anxiety treatment into substance use treatment results in better outcomes, studies on integrated adolescent treatments are lacking. Research on adolescent substance use treatment indicates that no one treatment is more effective than another. Instead, factors common across treatment modalities (e.g., strong therapeutic rapport) may account for positive outcomes. Research on youth anxiety treatment has largely shown CBT to be effective. With regard to psychotropic medication for adolescents with anxiety and SUDs, SSRIs are the drug class of choice. Future studies on integrated treatment of adolescent anxiety and SUDs are recommended.

In summary, adolescence is an optimal developmental period for addressing anxiety disorder and SUD prevention and treatment. The assessment of anxiety disorders is recommended when substance use is a concern. Conceptual models of adolescent anxiety and SUDs could be enhanced by considering developmental stage, anxiety disorder, and substance type. Studies on integrated treatments for co-occurring anxiety disorder and SUD in adolescents are recommended. Until integrated treatment approaches are developed and shown to be effective, utilization of the empirically supported behavioral treatments and pharmacotherapy for each separate disorder is advised. Delaying treatment could result in more severe anxiety and SUD outcomes, with both disorders becoming more difficult to treat.

KEY POINTS

- Both anxiety and substance use disorders (SUDs) typically have an onset during adolescence.

- Assessment of anxiety disorders is recommended when adolescent substance use is of concern because of the potential for worse SUD outcomes if anxiety is not addressed.

- Cognitive-behavioral therapy, family therapy, and motivational enhancement therapy are all evidence-based interventions with similar outcomes for adolescent SUDs.

- Cognitive-behavioral therapy is the recommended evidence-based behavioral intervention for adolescent anxiety.

- Selective serotonin reuptake inhibitors are the recommended pharmacotherapy for adolescents with anxiety and SUDs.

References

Alegria AA, Hasin DS, Nunes EV, et al: Comorbidity of generalized anxiety disorder and substance use disorders: results from the National Epidemiologic Survey on Alcohol and Related Conditions. J Clin Psychiatry 71(9):1187–1195, quiz 1252–1253, 2010 20923623

American Psychiatric Association: Diagnostic and Statistical Manual of Mental Disorders, 4th Edition. Washington, DC, American Psychiatric Association, 1994

American Psychiatric Association: Diagnostic and Statistical Manual of Mental Disorders, 4th Edition, Text Revision. Washington, DC, American Psychiatric Association, 2000

American Psychiatric Association: Diagnostic and Statistical Manual of Mental Disorders, 5th Edition. Arlington, VA, American Psychiatric Association, 2013

Biegel GM, Brown KW, Shapiro SL, et al: Mindfulness-based stress reduction for the treatment of adolescent psychiatric outpatients: a randomized clinical trial. J Consult Clin Psychol 77(5):855–866, 2009 19803566

Birmaher B, Khetarpal S, Brent D, et al: The Screen for Child Anxiety Related Emotional Disorders (SCARED): scale construction and psychometric characteristics. J Am Acad Child Adolesc Psychiatry 36(4):545–553, 1997 9100430

Black JJ, Chung T: Mechanisms of change in adolescent substance use treatment: how does treatment work? Subst Abus 35(4):344–351, 2014 24901750

Black JJ, Tran GQ, Goldsmith AA, et al: Alcohol expectancies and social self-efficacy as mediators of differential intervention outcomes for college hazardous drinkers with social anxiety. Addict Behav 37(3):248–255, 2012 22112424

Blane HT, Leonard KE (eds): Psychological Theories of Drinking and Alcoholism (The Guilford Alcohol Studies Series). New York, Guilford, 1987

Blumenthal H, Leen-Feldner EW, Frala JL, et al: Social anxiety and motives for alcohol use among adolescents. Psychol Addict Behav 24(3):529–534, 2010 20853939

Blumenthal H, Leen-Feldner EW, Badour CL, et al: Anxiety psychopathology and alcohol use among adolescents: a critical review of the empirical literature and recommendations for future research. J Exp Psychopathol 2(3):318–353, 2011 23243493

Blumenthal H, Leen-Feldner EW, Knapp AA, et al: Alcohol use history and panic-relevant responding among adolescents: a test using a voluntary hyperventilation challenge. Psychol Addict Behav 26(4):683–692, 2012 22369219

Bruce SE, Yonkers KA, Otto MW, et al: Influence of psychiatric comorbidity on recovery and recurrence in generalized anxiety disorder, social phobia, and panic disorder: a 12-year prospective study. Am J Psychiatry 162(6):1179–1187, 2005 15930067

Bucholz KK, Cadoret R, Cloninger CR, et al: A new, semi-structured psychiatric interview for use in genetic linkage studies: a report on the reliability of the SSAGA. J Stud Alcohol 55(2):149–158, 1994 8189735

Chorpita BF, Tracey SA, Brown TA, et al: Assessment of worry in children and adolescents: an adaptation of the Penn State Worry Questionnaire. Behav Res Ther 35(6):569–581, 1997 9159982

Clark DB: Pharmacotherapy for adolescent alcohol use disorder. CNS Drugs 26(7):559–569, 2012 22676261

Clark DB, Donovan JE: Reliability and validity of the Hamilton Anxiety Rating Scale in an adolescent sample. J Am Acad Child Adolesc Psychiatry 33(3):354–360, 1994 8169180

Clark DB, Smith MG, Neighbors BD, et al: Anxiety disorders in adolescence: characteristics, prevalence and comorbidities. Clin Psychol Rev 14(2):113–137, 1994

Clark DB, Bukstein OG, Smith MG, et al: Identifying anxiety disorders in adolescents hospitalized for alcohol abuse or dependence. Psychiatr Serv 46(6):618–620, 1995 7641008

Clark DB, Feske U, Masia CL, et al: Systematic assessment of social phobia in clinical practice. Depress Anxiety 6(2):47–61, 1997a 9451546

Clark DB, Moss HB, Kirisci L, et al: Psychopathology in preadolescent sons of fathers with substance use disorders. J Am Acad Child Adolesc Psychiatry 36(4):495–502, 1997b 9100424

Clark DB, Cornelius J, Wood DS, et al: Psychopathology risk transmission in children of parents with substance use disorders. Am J Psychiatry 161(4):685–691, 2004 15056515

Compton SN, Peris TS, Almirall D, et al: Predictors and moderators of treatment response in childhood anxiety disorders: results from the CAMS trial. J Consult Clin Psychol 82(2):212–224, 2014 24417601

Compton WM III, Cottler LB, Jacobs JL, et al: The role of psychiatric disorders in predicting drug dependence treatment outcomes. Am J Psychiatry 160(5):890–895, 2003 12727692

Connolly SD, Bernstein GA; Work Group on Quality Issues: Practice parameter for the assessment and treatment of children and adolescents with anxiety disorders. J Am Acad Child Adolesc Psychiatry 46(2):267–283, 2007 17242630

Cornelius JR, Maisto SA, Pollock NK, et al: Rapid relapse generally follows treatment for substance use disorders among adolescents. Addict Behav 28(2):381–386, 2003 12573689

Cosci F, Schruers KRJ, Abrams K, et al: Alcohol use disorders and panic disorder: a review of the evidence of a direct relationship. J Clin Psychiatry 68(6):874–880, 2007 17592911

Crawford LA, Novak KB: The effects of public self-consciousness and embarrassability on college student drinking: evidence in support of a protective self-presentational model. J Soc Psychol 153(1):109–122, 2013 23421009

Davids E, Müller MJ, Rollmann N, et al: Syndrome profiles in alcoholism and panic disorder with or without agoraphobia: an explorative family study. Prog Neuropsychopharmacol Biol Psychiatry 26(6):1079–1087, 2002 12452529

Dennis M, Godley SH, Diamond G, et al: The Cannabis Youth Treatment (CYT) study: main findings from two randomized trials. J Subst Abuse Treat 27(3):197–213, 2004 15501373

Driessen M, Meier S, Hill A, et al: The course of anxiety, depression and drinking behaviours after completed detoxification in alcoholics with and without co-morbid anxiety and depressive disorders. Alcohol Alcohol 36(3):249–255, 2001 11373263

Ginsburg GS, Becker EM, Keeton CP, et al: Naturalistic follow-up of youths treated for pediatric anxiety disorders. JAMA Psychiatry 71(3):310–318, 2014 24477837

Goodwin RD, Lipsitz JD, Keyes K, et al: Family history of alcohol use disorders among adults with panic disorder in the community. J Psychiatr Res 45(8):1123–1127, 2011 21334007

Goodwin RD, Perkonigg A, Höfler M, et al: Mental disorders and smoking trajectories: a 10-year prospective study among adolescents and young adults in the community. Drug Alcohol Depend 130(1–3):201–207, 2013 23375557

Grant BF, Stinson FS, Dawson DA, et al: Prevalence and co-occurrence of substance use disorders and independent mood and anxiety disorders: results from the National Epidemiologic Survey on Alcohol and Related Conditions. Arch Gen Psychiatry 61(8):807–816, 2004 15289279

Hannesdottir DK, Ollendick TH: The role of emotion regulation in the treatment of child anxiety disorders. Clin Child Fam Psychol Rev 10(3):275–293, 2007 17705098

Harford TC, Grant BF, Yi HY, et al: Patterns of DSM-IV alcohol abuse and dependence criteria among adolescents and adults: results from the 2001 National Household Survey on Drug Abuse. Alcohol Clin Exp Res 29(5):810–828, 2005 15897727

Hayward C, Killen JD, Kraemer HC, et al: Assessment and phenomenology of nonclinical panic attacks in adolescent girls. J Anxiety Disord 11(1):17–32, 1997 9131879

Isensee B, Wittchen HU, Stein MB, et al: Smoking increases the risk of panic: findings from a prospective community study. Arch Gen Psychiatry 60(7):692–700, 2003 12860773

Johnston LD, O'Malley PM, Bachman JG, et al: Monitoring the Future National Survey Results on Adolescent Drug Use: Overview of Key Findings. Ann Arbor, Institute for Social Research, University of Michigan, 2011

Jamal M, Does AJ, Penninx BW, et al: Age at smoking onset and the onset of depression and anxiety disorders. Nicotine Tob Res 13(9):809–819, 2011 21543549

Kaufman J, Birmaher B, Brent D, et al: Schedule for Affective Disorders and Schizophrenia for School-Age Children—Present and Lifetime Version (K-SADS-PL): initial reliability and validity data. J Am Acad Child Adolesc Psychiatry 36(7):980–988, 1997 9204677

Kendall PC, Safford S, Flannery-Schroeder E, et al: Child anxiety treatment: outcomes in adolescence and impact on substance use and depression at 7.4-year follow-up. J Consult Clin Psychol 72(2):276–287, 2004 15065961

Kessler RC, Berglund P, Demler O, et al: Lifetime prevalence and age-of-onset distributions of DSM-IV disorders in the National Comorbidity Survey Replication. Arch Gen Psychiatry 62(6):593–602, 2005 15939837

Kinley DJ, Walker JR, Enns MW, et al: Panic attacks as a risk for later psychopathology: results from a nationally representative survey. Depress Anxiety 28(5):412–419, 2011 21400640

Kirisci L, Clark DB, Moss HB: Reliability and validity of the State-Trait Anxiety Inventory for Children in an adolescent sample: confirmatory factor analysis and item response theory. J Child Adolesc Subst Abuse 5:57–69, 1996

Kodish I, Rockhill C, Ryan S, et al: Pharmacotherapy for anxiety disorders in children and adolescents. Pediatr Clin North Am 58(1):55–72, x, 2011 21281848

Kushner MG, Abrams K, Borchardt C: The relationship between anxiety disorders and alcohol use disorders: a review of major perspectives and findings. Clin Psychol Rev 20(2):149–171, 2000 10721495

Kushner MG, Abrams K, Thuras P, et al: Follow-up study of anxiety disorder and alcohol dependence in comorbid alcoholism treatment patients. Alcohol Clin Exp Res 29(8):1432–1443, 2005 16131851

Merikangas KR, Stevens DE, Fenton B, et al: Co-morbidity and familial aggregation of alcoholism and anxiety disorders. Psychol Med 28(4):773–788, 1998 9723135

Nauta MH, Scholing A, Rapee RM, et al: A parent-report measure of children's anxiety: psychometric properties and comparison with child-report in a clinic and normal sample. Behav Res Ther 42(7):813–839, 2004 15149901

Robinson J, Sareen J, Cox BJ, et al: Self-medication of anxiety disorders with alcohol and drugs: results from a nationally representative sample. J Anxiety Disord 23(1):38–45, 2009 18571370

Schry AR, White SW: Understanding the relationship between social anxiety and alcohol use in college students: a meta-analysis. Addict Behav 38(11):2690–2706, 2013 23906724

Shaffer D, Fisher P, Lucas C, et al: NIMH Diagnostic Interview Schedule for Children, Version IV (NIMH DISC-IV): description, differences from previous versions, and reliability of some common diagnoses. J Am Acad Child Psychiatry 39(1):28–38, 2000 10638065

Silverman WK, Saavedra LM, Pina AA: Test-retest reliability of anxiety symptoms and diagnoses with the Anxiety Disorders Interview Schedule for DSM-IV: Child and Parent Versions. J Am Acad Child Adolesc Psychiatry 40(8):937–944, 2001 11501694

Smith JP, Book SW: Comorbidity of generalized anxiety disorder and alcohol use disorders among individuals seeking outpatient substance abuse treatment. Addict Behav 35(1):42–45, 2010 19733441

Smith JP, Tran GQ: Does negative affect increase change readiness among college hazardous drinkers? Addict Behav 32(10):2281–2285, 2007 17317023

Spence SH: A measure of anxiety symptoms among children. Behav Res Ther 36(5):545–566, 1998 9648330

Thatcher DL, Pajtek S, Tarter R, et al: Amygdala activation and emotional processing in adolescents at risk for substance use disorders. J Child Adolesc Subst Abuse 23(3):200–204, 2014 24748761

Tomlinson KL, Brown SA: Self-medication or social learning? A comparison of models to predict early adolescent drinking. Addict Behav 37(2):179–186, 2012 22055793

Valentiner DP, Mounts NS, Deacon BJ: Panic attacks, depression and anxiety symptoms, and substance use behaviors during late adolescence. J Anxiety Disord 18(5):573–585, 2004 15275940

Vasey M, Crnic K, Carter W: Worry in childhood: a developmental perspective. Cognit Ther Res 18(6):529–549, 1994

Waldron HB, Turner CW: Evidence-based psychosocial treatments for adolescent substance abuse. J Clin Child Adolesc Psychol 37(1):238–261, 2008 18444060

Windle M, Windle RC: Testing the specificity between social anxiety disorder and drinking motives. Addict Behav 37(9):1003–1008, 2012 22626889

CHAPTER 9

Posttraumatic Stress Disorder and Substance Use Disorders

Julian D. Ford, Ph.D.
Josephine M. Hawke, Ph.D.

Growing recognition of the extent of exposure to psychological trauma and the prevalence of psychobiological impairment involving posttraumatic stress reactions (including but not limited to posttraumatic stress disorder [PTSD]) among individuals with substance use disorders (SUDs) has prompted clinicians and programs to use trauma-focused assessments and interventions or to adapt existing ones that are focused on SUDs (Ford 2013b). Adolescence is a developmental period during which use and abuse of substances as well as exposure to traumatic stressors and onset of PTSD are common and potentially debilitating, with adverse sequelae that can last a lifetime (Ford 2011b, 2012; Kaminer et al. 2011). In this chapter, we describe and review the current literature on the prevalence of trauma exposure and PTSD and associated internalizing and externalizing psychiatric disorders among substance-using adolescents, as well as assessment and treatment approaches for comorbid PTSD and SUDs among adolescents.

Exposure to Traumatic Stressors in Adolescence and Childhood

Traumatic stressors are events that are threats to individuals' survival; these may occur with or without direct physical injury or trauma (Ford 2009). The types of events that qualify as traumatic stressors, according to DSM-5 (American Psychiatric Association 2013), include actual or threatened physical and sexual assaults, abuse, or injury; witnessing severe violence or death (or learning about this occurring to a close family member or friend); and "experiencing repeated or extreme exposure to aversive details of [these types of] traumatic event(s) (e.g., first responders collecting human remains; police officers repeatedly exposed to details of child abuse)" (p. 271). Experiences involving the unexpected or premature death of a primary caregiver fit this definition, but it is not clear whether abandonment by a caregiver—which can have profound adverse effects on child development and adolescent and adult functioning (D'Andrea et al. 2012) and may lead to added trauma exposure or adversities such as multiple out-of-home placements (Ford et al. 2009)—constitutes a traumatic stressor. "Betrayal traumas" (Freyd 1997) that do not involve death, or the threat of death or severe physical injury, such as emotional abuse and childhood neglect, also do not technically constitute traumatic stressors, despite clearly constituting serious risks to child health and development (D'Andrea et al. 2012).

With regard to the prevalence of exposure to traumatic stressors among adolescents in the U.S. population, two epidemiological studies of nationally representative samples of adolescents (Kilpatrick et al. 2003; McLaughlin et al. 2013) found that between 50% and 62% of youths had been exposed to at least one traumatic event in their lives. The median age at first-reported exposure to potentially traumatic events varied from the earliest childhood years for intrafamilial violence; to latency for serious accidents, illness, and disasters; to mid-adolescence for community violence and traumatic loss. An epidemiological study of adolescents and young adults in Germany (Perkonigg et al. 2000) reported much lower, but still substantial, prevalence estimates for trauma exposure (26% among males, 18% among females), whereas an epidemiological study of children and adolescents in two more economically impoverished countries in Africa (Seedat et al. 2004) estimated trauma exposure as much higher (80%).

Exposure to interpersonal victimization often begins early in childhood (Briggs-Gowan et al. 2010a, 2010b). Most cases of kidnapping and roughly half of cases of physical abuse by a caregiver or witnessing of intimate partner violence were reported by adolescents to have begun before they were age 8 years (McLaughlin et al. 2013). This evidence of frequent early onset of intrafamilial traumas replicates results of a prior study that assessed infants and toddlers younger than age 4 years (Briggs-Gowan et al. 2010a, 2010b). Adolescents at greatest risk for traumatic stressor exposure were those not living in two-parent biological families. This finding is consistent with data from prior research showing that separation from biological parent(s), exposure to interparental conflict, the stresses of single parenting, the absence of a secure attachment bond with caregivers, and out-of-home (e.g., foster, adoptive, or institutional) placements put children and adolescents at risk for exposure to traumatic stressors (Herrenkohl et al. 2008; Stein et al. 2013) as well as for developing SUDs (Ford et al. 2010).

Substance-using adolescents are more likely than other teens to report histories of exposure to traumatic stressors (Kaminer et al. 2011). Giaconia et al. (2000) estimated that more than half (55.5%) of adolescents with SUD had experienced at least one traumatic stressor in their lifetimes. Clark et al. 1997) reported that adolescents with alcohol abuse or dependence were 6–12 times more likely to have histories of physical maltreatment and 18–21 times more likely to report histories of sexual abuse than adolescents with no substance use problems. Substance-abusing youths also often report exposure to multiple types of traumatic stressors, including life-threatening accidents, childhood physical and sexual abuse, and witnessing of community or domestic violence, as well as adversities associated with vulnerability to traumatic exposure, including abandonment and parental drug use or mental illness (Hawke et al. 2000, 2003, 2009).

Studies based on clinical samples of adolescents in treatment for alcohol and other substance use disorders report similarly high prevalence of trauma exposure. Estimates of lifetime prevalence range from 39% to 86% for boys and 59% to 92% for girls, depending on the breadth of trauma exposure assessed (Grella and Joshi 2003; Hawke et al. 2009; Jaycox et al. 2004). Hawke et al. (2009) found that 90% of adolescents in outpatient treatment reported exposure to any trauma, 49% reported exposure to interpersonal violence (including physical assaults), and 19% reported being sexually abused. In a national study of 803 adolescents in programs for the treatment of alcohol and substance use disorders, Grella and Joshi (2003) reported that 39% of males and 59% of females acknowledged having histories of physical and sexual abuse. Hawke et al. (2000) estimated that between 24% of boys and 64% of girls in a sample of 938 adolescents in residential drug treatment had histories of sexual abuse victimization. In addition, complex exposures to multiple types of traumatic stressors involving interpersonal violence and loss are prevalent among substance-using adolescents. On average, these youths report between seven and nine different traumas over their lifetimes, often involving both multiple types of events and multiple occurrences (Crimmins et al. 2000; Hawke et al. 2009; Jaycox et al. 2004).

Posttraumatic Stress Disorder

According to DSM-5, PTSD involves a profile of symptoms reflective of persistent and impairing stress reactions following exposure to one or more traumatic stressors (Box 9–1). A number of important changes have been made in the operational definition of criteria for PTSD in DSM-5 compared with DSM-IV (American Psychiatric Association 1994), and these changes have important implications for researchers and clinicians working with adolescents with SUDs. First, the entry criterion (A) for PTSD, exposure to a traumatic stressor, no longer includes the second DSM-IV requirement (A2) that the person feel extreme fear, helplessness, or horror during or soon after the event(s). The A2 criterion was eliminated because research demonstrated that almost all individuals who meet the symptom criteria for PTSD (described in the following paragraphs) also recall experiencing this subjective sense of intense shock, and it is impossible to discern clinically or scientifically whether this recollection of past reactions is accurate or partially or fully a by-product of the current PTSD symptoms (Brewin et al. 2009; Kilpatrick et al. 2009). Importantly, the emotional impact of experiencing traumatic stressors was not lost in the DSM-5 PTSD operationalization because it is captured by newly added symptom items.

Box 9–1.   DSM-5 Criteria for Posttraumatic Stress Disorder

Posttraumatic Stress Disorder

Note: The following criteria apply to adults, adolescents, and children older than 6 years. For children 6 years and younger, see corresponding criteria below.

A. Exposure to actual or threatened death, serious injury, or sexual violence in one (or more) of the following ways:

   1. Directly experiencing the traumatic event(s).

   2. Witnessing, in person, the event(s) as it occurred to others.

3. Learning that the traumatic event(s) occurred to a close family member or close friend. In cases of actual or threatened death of a family member or friend, the event(s) must have been violent or accidental.

4. Experiencing repeated or extreme exposure to aversive details of the traumatic event(s) (e.g., first responders collecting human remains; police officers repeatedly exposed to details of child abuse).

   Note: Criterion A4 does not apply to exposure through electronic media, television, movies, or pictures, unless this exposure is work related.

B. Presence of one (or more) of the following intrusion symptoms associated with the traumatic event(s), beginning after the traumatic event(s) occurred:

1. Recurrent, involuntary, and intrusive distressing memories of the traumatic event(s).

   Note: In children older than 6 years, repetitive play may occur in which themes or aspects of the traumatic event(s) are expressed.

2. Recurrent distressing dreams in which the content and/or affect of the dream are related to the traumatic event(s).

   Note: In children, there may be frightening dreams without recognizable content.

3. Dissociative reactions (e.g., flashbacks) in which the individual feels or acts as if the traumatic event(s) were recurring. (Such reactions may occur on a continuum, with the most extreme expression being a complete loss of awareness of present surroundings.)

   Note: In children, trauma-specific reenactment may occur in play.

4. Intense or prolonged psychological distress at exposure to internal or external cues that symbolize or resemble an aspect of the traumatic event(s).

5. Marked physiological reactions to internal or external cues that symbolize or resemble an aspect of the traumatic event(s).

C. Persistent avoidance of stimuli associated with the traumatic event(s), beginning after the traumatic event(s) occurred, as evidenced by one or both of the following:

1. Avoidance of or efforts to avoid distressing memories, thoughts, or feelings about or closely associated with the traumatic event(s).

2. Avoidance of or efforts to avoid external reminders (people, places, conversations, activities, objects, situations) that arouse distressing memories, thoughts, or feelings about or closely associated with the traumatic event(s).

D. Negative alterations in cognitions and mood associated with the traumatic event(s), beginning or worsening after the traumatic event(s) occurred, as evidenced by two (or more) of the following:

1. Inability to remember an important aspect of the traumatic event(s) (typically due to dissociative amnesia and not to other factors such as head injury, alcohol, or drugs).
2. Persistent and exaggerated negative beliefs or expectations about oneself, others, or the world (e.g., "I am bad," "No one can be trusted," "The world is completely dangerous," "My whole nervous system is permanently ruined").
3. Persistent, distorted cognitions about the cause or consequences of the traumatic event(s) that lead the individual to blame himself/herself or others.
4. Persistent negative emotional state (e.g., fear, horror, anger, guilt, or shame).
5. Markedly diminished interest or participation in significant activities.
6. Feelings of detachment or estrangement from others.
7. Persistent inability to experience positive emotions (e.g., inability to experience happiness, satisfaction, or loving feelings).

E. Marked alterations in arousal and reactivity associated with the traumatic event(s), beginning or worsening after the traumatic event(s) occurred, as evidenced by two (or more) of the following:

1. Irritable behavior and angry outbursts (with little or no provocation) typically expressed as verbal or physical aggression toward people or objects.
2. Reckless or self-destructive behavior.
3. Hypervigilance.
4. Exaggerated startle response.
5. Problems with concentration.
6. Sleep disturbance (e.g., difficulty falling or staying asleep or restless sleep).

F. Duration of the disturbance (Criteria B, C, D, and E) is more than 1 month.
G. The disturbance causes clinically significant distress or impairment in social, occupational, or other important areas of functioning.
H. The disturbance is not attributable to the physiological effects of a substance (e.g., medication, alcohol) or another medical condition.

Specify whether:

With dissociative symptoms: The individual's symptoms meet the criteria for posttraumatic stress disorder, and in addition, in response to the stressor, the individual experiences persistent or recurrent symptoms of either of the following:

1. **Depersonalization:** Persistent or recurrent experiences of feeling detached from, and as if one were an outside observer of, one's mental processes or body (e.g., feeling as though one were in a dream; feeling a sense of unreality of self or body or of time moving slowly).

2. **Derealization:** Persistent or recurrent experiences of unreality of surroundings (e.g., the world around the individual is experienced as unreal, dreamlike, distant, or distorted).

Note: To use this subtype, the dissociative symptoms must not be attributable to the physiological effects of a substance (e.g., blackouts, behavior during alcohol intoxication) or another medical condition (e.g., complex partial seizures).

Specify if:

With delayed expression: If the full diagnostic criteria are not met until at least 6 months after the event (although the onset and expression of some symptoms may be immediate).

Posttraumatic Stress Disorder for Children 6 Years and Younger

A. In children 6 years and younger, exposure to actual or threatened death, serious injury, or sexual violence in one (or more) of the following ways:

1. Directly experiencing the traumatic event(s).
2. Witnessing, in person, the event(s) as it occurred to others, especially primary caregivers.

   Note: Witnessing does not include events that are witnessed only in electronic media, television, movies, or pictures.

3. Learning that the traumatic event(s) occurred to a parent or caregiving figure.

B. Presence of one (or more) of the following intrusion symptoms associated with the traumatic event(s), beginning after the traumatic event(s) occurred:

1. Recurrent, involuntary, and intrusive distressing memories of the traumatic event(s).

   Note: Spontaneous and intrusive memories may not necessarily appear distressing and may be expressed as play reenactment.

2. Recurrent distressing dreams in which the content and/or affect of the dream are related to the traumatic event(s).

   Note: It may not be possible to ascertain that the frightening content is related to the traumatic event.

3. Dissociative reactions (e.g., flashbacks) in which the child feels or acts as if the traumatic event(s) were recurring. (Such reactions may occur on a continuum, with the most extreme expression being a complete loss of awareness of present surroundings.) Such trauma-specific reenactment may occur in play.

4. Intense or prolonged psychological distress at exposure to internal or external cues that symbolize or resemble an aspect of the traumatic event(s).

5. Marked physiological reactions to reminders of the traumatic event(s).

C. One (or more) of the following symptoms, representing either persistent avoidance of stimuli associated with the traumatic event(s) or negative alterations in cognitions and mood associated with the traumatic event(s), must be present, beginning after the event(s) or worsening after the event(s):

Persistent Avoidance of Stimuli

1. Avoidance of or efforts to avoid activities, places, or physical reminders that arouse recollections of the traumatic event(s).
2. Avoidance of or efforts to avoid people, conversations, or interpersonal situations that arouse recollections of the traumatic event(s).

Negative Alterations in Cognitions

3. Substantially increased frequency of negative emotional states (e.g., fear, guilt, sadness, shame, confusion).
4. Markedly diminished interest or participation in significant activities, including constriction of play.
5. Socially withdrawn behavior.
6. Persistent reduction in expression of positive emotions.

D. Alterations in arousal and reactivity associated with the traumatic event(s), beginning or worsening after the traumatic event(s) occurred, as evidenced by two (or more) of the following:

1. Irritable behavior and angry outbursts (with little or no provocation) typically expressed as verbal or physical aggression toward people or objects (including extreme temper tantrums).
2. Hypervigilance.
3. Exaggerated startle response.
4. Problems with concentration.
5. Sleep disturbance (e.g., difficulty falling or staying asleep or restless sleep).

E. The duration of the disturbance is more than 1 month.

F. The disturbance causes clinically significant distress or impairment in relationships with parents, siblings, peers, or other caregivers or with school behavior.

G. The disturbance is not attributable to the physiological effects of a substance (e.g., medication or alcohol) or another medical condition.

Specify whether:

With dissociative symptoms: The individual's symptoms meet the criteria for posttraumatic stress disorder, and the individual experiences persistent or recurrent symptoms of either of the following:

1. **Depersonalization:** Persistent or recurrent experiences of feeling detached from, and as if one were an outside observer of, one's mental processes or body (e.g., feeling as though one were in a dream; feeling a sense of unreality of self or body or of time moving slowly).

2. **Derealization:** Persistent or recurrent experiences of unreality of surroundings (e.g., the world around the individual is experienced as unreal, dreamlike, distant, or distorted).

Note: To use this subtype, the dissociative symptoms must not be attributable to the physiological effects of a substance (e.g., blackouts) or another medical condition (e.g., complex partial seizures).

Specify if:

With delayed expression: If the full diagnostic criteria are not met until at least 6 months after the event (although the onset and expression of some symptoms may be immediate).

As shown in Box 9–1, a diagnosis of PTSD requires that the individual exhibit at least one of five potential intrusion (reexperiencing) symptoms (Criterion B), at least one of two potential avoidance symptoms (Criterion C), at least two of seven potential negative alterations in cognitions or mood associated with the traumatic events (Criterion D), and at least two of six potential hyperarousal and reactivity symptoms (Criterion E) (American Psychiatric Association 2013). The intrusive reexperiencing symptoms (Criterion B) include repeated unwanted memories, recurrent frightening dreams (which, in DSM-5, may include affect and/or content related to traumatic events or, for children, may be nightmares "without recognizable content"), flashbacks (i.e., feeling as if the trauma is happening all over again in the present moment, or reenactment of a traumatic experience), or intense psychological distress or physiological reactivity in response to stimuli that resemble or symbolize the traumatic events. Efforts to avoid reminders of traumatic memories (Criterion C) may take the form of avoiding the memories (or related thoughts or feelings) themselves or "external reminders (people, places, conversations, activities, objects, situations) that arouse distressing memories, thoughts, or feelings about or closely associated with the traumatic event(s)" (American Psychiatric Association 2013, p. 271).

In DSM-5, a number of symptoms of emotional numbing (i.e., inability to recognize positive emotions, amnesia about some or all important parts of a traumatic event, feeling detached from relationships, and believing one's life will be cut short—a sense of a foreshortened future) that were grouped together with avoidance in DSM-IV are now placed with new symptoms under the new Criterion D. The added symptoms represent trauma-related beliefs and emotional dysregulation that extend beyond fear and anxiety. Hence, PTSD is no longer grouped in DSM-5 with the anxiety disorders as it was in DSM-III (American Psychiatric Association 1980) and DSM-IV, but it is now in a new diagnostic class called trauma and stressor-related disorders. The newly added symptoms reflect negative changes in beliefs and emotions that began during or worsened after traumatic events (persistent negative beliefs about oneself, distorted blame of self or others for the traumatic events, and emotional distress in the form of anger, guilt, shame, or horror) as well as or instead of fear and anxiety. With these new negative mood and/or cognition symptoms, PTSD now encompasses the trauma-related impairments in self-regulation that hundreds of research studies have shown to be aftereffects of exposure to interpersonal traumatic stressors in childhood (e.g., abuse, violent or sexual victimization, family violence) and in some cases in adulthood as well (e.g., genocide, torture, intimate partner violence) (D'Andrea et al. 2012). These changes in the DSM-5 are particularly relevant to understanding how and why traumatized youth are at risk for SUDs, because the new PTSD dysregulation symptoms are well known to be risk factors for and contributors to the severe and treatment-refractory SUDs (Ford et al. 2008).

PTSD hyperarousal symptoms (DSM-5 Criterion E) include the DSM-III and DSM-IV symptoms of severe sleep difficulties, anger and irritability, concentration problems, scanning the environment for potential threat (hypervigilance), and exaggerated startle responses. To these have been added one expansion of a prior symptom (i.e., verbal or physical aggression as a component of posttraumatic anger problems) and an entirely new symptom, reckless or self-destructive behavior. As with the new negative mood and/or cognition symptoms in Criterion D, PTSD's problems with hyperarousal now include risk factors for SUDs (e.g., impulsivity, disregard of consequences, aggression).

Most children and adolescents who are exposed to traumatic stressors do not develop full PTSD, regardless of their age (Kessler et al. 1995; McLaughlin et al. 2013; Perkonigg et al. 2000). In the recent epidemiological studies of adolescent PTSD, lifetime prevalence of traumatic stressor exposure was above 60%, but PTSD prevalence was estimated as 5% (McLaughlin et al. 2013). Although PTSD may develop in early childhood (Briggs-Gowan et al. 2012), many if not most adolescents who incurred PTSD earlier in childhood are likely to also currently have PTSD, according to the finding that between 3.7% and 6.3% of adolescents met criteria for PTSD in the previous 6 months (Kilpatrick et al. 2003). Moreover, almost half of cases of childhood or adolescent PTSD were found to be chronic, in that they were unremitted at 3- to 4-year prospective follow-up assessments (Perkonigg et al. 2005).

Which adolescents, then, are most vulnerable to developing PTSD? Over and above the risk conferred by trauma exposure per se, the key vulnerability factors identified in epidemiological studies are female gender, exposure to multiple types of trauma, having developed a "fear or distress" disorder prior to exposure to the worst traumatic stressor, and having either a depressive or a substance use disorder (Kilpatrick et al. 2003; McLaughlin et al. 2013). Biological factors have been implicated for vulnerability to developing PTSD. These include brain abnormalities such as reduced size or dysregulation of areas in the brain associated with stress reactivity, memory, self-control, and emotion regulation (Kelly et al. 2013; Kühn and Gallinat 2013; Teicher and Samson 2013); alterations in brain-body reactions to stressors (e.g., dysregulation of the hypothalamic-pituitary-adrenal axis as reflected in elevated or depleted cortisol levels); genetic factors (Guffanti et al. 2013; Sumner et al. 2014; Teicher and Samson 2013; White et al. 2013); and learned vulnerabilities that may involve intergenerational (i.e., parent-to-child) transmission via epigenetic (i.e., changes in genes based on experience; Yehuda et al. 2014) and gene by environment interactions (Xie et al. 2010) mechanisms. Traumatic victimization, especially in childhood, may thus result in psychobiological alterations or exacerbation of preexisting vulnerabilities that may sensitize a child or adolescent and thereby increase susceptibility to developing PTSD (Grasso et al. 2013) and comorbid SUD (Norman et al. 2012).

Although not all youths who are exposed to traumas develop PTSD, many develop posttraumatic stress symptoms that can interfere with their abilities to engage in treatment and recover from addiction. Subthreshold or partial syndromes are more common than full PTSD in both the general population and clinical samples. Subthreshold syndromes can be associated with significant psychosocial impairment (McFarlane 2000). Stevens et al. (2003) found that 54% of a sample of 378 adolescents from four substance abuse treatment programs exhibited posttraumatic stress symptoms. The prevalence of PTSD and posttraumatic stress impairment is higher among clinical samples of substance-using adolescents than among adolescents in the community (Abram et al. 2004, 2007; Brosky and Lally 2004; Carrion and Steiner 2000; Cauffman et al. 1998; Ruchkin et al. 2002), with estimates ranging between 5% and 30%, depending on characteristics of the sample, setting, and criteria used for assessing PTSD. Jaycox et al. (2004) reported that 29% of a sample of adolescents in residential substance use treatment met criteria for current PTSD. Hawke et al. (2009) found that 12.5% of youths in out-patient treatment for SUDs met criteria for full or partial PTSD, defined as having exposure to a traumatic event plus at least one symptom in each of the three DSM-IV PTSD symptom categories.

Empirical evidence indicates that girls are more likely than boys to develop PTSD, as well as internalizing psychiatric disorders that often co-occur with PTSD, such as depression (Tolin and Foa 2006). The higher rates of these disorders in females are in part due to differences in the types of traumas that girls tend to experience. Both community and clinical samples show that girls are more likely than boys to experience sexual abuse. Sexual abuse is most strongly associated with PTSD diagnosis and severity of symptoms (Hawke et al. 2000, 2003; Kessler et al. 1995; Tolin and Foa 2006). Epidemiological findings suggest that the higher rates are not due to girls being more prone than boys to emotionality or affect dysregulation, because female gender was a risk factor independent of the risk conferred by having a "fear or distress" disorder (McLaughlin et al. 2013). Boys, in contrast, report higher rates of community violence and externalizing behavior disorders such as oppositional defiant disorder or problems with overt aggression (Herrenkohl et al. 2008; Stein et al. 2013).

Evidence also indicates that race and cultural factors influence the development and diagnosis of PTSD (Pole et al. 2008); however, the impact of racial or ethnic differences on trauma-related disorders or outcomes is unclear because findings are rarely reported by race or ethnicity. Statistics indicate that rates of exposure to traumas such as childhood maltreatment and community violence are higher among minorities, especially those living in impoverished communities (Pole et al. 2008). Some studies, but not others, find that minorities report higher levels of PTSD symptoms. Lewis-Fernández et al. (2008) found higher rates of PTSD among Hispanics, compared to non-Hispanic whites. Among adjudicated youths, Abram et al. (2004) found no differences in PTSD among African American, Hispanic, and white juvenile delinquents, although the type of trauma exposure varied. Differential rates of exposure, lack of economic resources to avail treatment, and cultural orientations that foster protective factors (e.g., social support networks) have been posited as potential factors associated with racial and ethnic differences in prevalence estimates of PTSD.

Epidemiological findings also shed light on which adolescents are more or less likely to recover from exposure to traumatic stressors and PTSD. Specifically, youths with multiple types of trauma exposure or extreme emotion dysregulation (i.e., bipolar disorder) were less likely than other trauma-exposed youths to recover from PTSD (McLaughlin et al. 2013). More than half of the teens who report any trauma exposure have experienced at least two different types of potentially traumatic stressors (McLaughlin et al. 2013), and 10%–15% have experienced multiple types of traumatic victimization, making them so-called poly-victims (Finkelhor et al. 2005; Ford et al. 2010). Poly-victims have three times the risk of PTSD, double the risk of depression, and—of particular relevance to the current chapter—two to five times the risk of SUDs and involvement in delinquency or with delinquent peers, compared with other youths, including teens who have experienced traumatic stressors but not as extensively as the poly-victims (Ford et al. 2010). In samples of high-risk youths who tend to use substances problematically or have full SUDs, up to 40% are poly-victims who have severe posttraumatic stress and associated internalizing and externalizing problems and emotion dysregulation (Ford et al. 2013c).

The high prevalence estimates of traumatic stressor exposure in childhood and adolescence, particularly for youths who are at risk for or have an SUD, and the correspondingly high prevalence estimates of PTSD and related symptoms among these vulnerable youths suggest that assessment and treatment of adolescent SUDs should take into account the potential complications created by posttraumatic stress. Addressing posttraumatic stress is all the more important because a recent national survey of adults found that the median age at PTSD onset was 23 years (Kessler et al. 2005). Thus, many trauma-exposed adolescents who do not currently have PTSD will develop PTSD in adulthood unless preventive interventions are provided to those at risk. This possibility further underscores the importance of identifying and delivering evidence-based treatment to adolescents with PTSD before they reach adulthood, as well as prevention interventions for children and adolescents who are at risk for PTSD on a selective basis before posttraumatic symptoms emerge or on a targeted basis before posttraumatic symptoms crystallize into a disorder involving serious developmental and psychosocial impairment.

Compared with other types of traumatic stressors, those that are deliberately inflicted or interpersonal in nature tend to be more likely to result in PTSD and a wide range of associated problems with emotion regulation, interpersonal relationships, and psychobiological development (D'Andrea et al. 2012). Exposure to traumas in early childhood, when children are less cognitively developed and more physically dependent on adult caretakers, tends to be associated with dissociative symptoms (Dalenberg et al. 2012). Prolonged exposure to traumatic stressors that adversely affect psychobiological development (e.g., childhood abuse, intimate partner violence, genocide, torture) also tends to produce more severe PTSD, SUD, and comorbid emotional and behavioral problems (D'Andrea et al. 2012; Gola et al. 2012).

PTSD is associated with significant impairment in functioning that in and of itself has the potential to undermine normal developmental trajectories and thwart recovery efforts (Layne et al. 2008). Children and adolescents do not necessarily exhibit symptoms of PTSD in the same manner as adults. The more developmentally mature a child is, the more likely he or she is to exhibit symptoms consistent with PTSD's adult symptomatology. Among substance-using adolescents, variation can be great. The intense emotions of extreme fear, helplessness, and horror associated with PTSD can be exhibited as disorganized or agitated behavior. Traumatized adolescents may be out of touch with their feelings and lack the vocabulary to describe their emotions.

PTSD symptoms may not occur simultaneously and will vary over time: one set of symptoms may be manifested with high frequency in one period, whereas other symptoms predominate during other periods. Adolescents may not make the connection between symptoms (e.g., nightmares) and past events or may minimize symptoms in order to convince adults or peers that they are not affected by traumatic experiences. Compared to adult survivors, adolescents may exhibit more impulsive and aggressive behaviors and engage in more traumatic reenactments (i.e., incorporating aspects of traumatic events into their daily lives) (Ford and Blaustein 2013; Ford et al. 2012a). Behavioral and emotional dyscontrol is more common in adolescents than adults from developmental neuroimaging research, which is consistent with evidence that inhibitory areas of the brain (e.g., the prefrontal cortex) mature later than areas related to stress reactivity (e.g., the amygdala) and reward seeking (e.g., the midbrain). Adolescent substance use problems therefore are more likely when youths attempt to cope with physiologically and psychosocially based distress and impulses that are intensified by PTSD or complex PTSD symptoms such as intrusive reexperiencing, pervasive dysphoria, or hypervigilance (e.g., when youths self-medicate in an effort to regain a tolerable emotional state) (Teicher and Samson 2013).

Factors associated with resilience or recovery (Layne et al. 2008) following exposure to traumatic stressors include early and ongoing helpful social support, noninvolvement in risky or undermining relationships, access to protections and resources that prevent retraumatization, adaptive personality and cognitive characteristics, and an absence of prior psychiatric disorders or substance abuse (both by the person and his or her family) (Milan et al. 2013; Wittchen et al. 2012). These protective factors closely mirror those identified empirically in epidemiological studies on the etiology of SUDs (Harrington et al. 2011). Although the factors associated with preventing versus facilitating recovery from PTSD or SUDs are not identical (Kelly and Greene 2014; Parmenter et al. 2013), they consistently include the creation or strengthening of healthy social bonds and resources as well as psychobiological capacities necessary for adaptive self-regulation (Ford and Blaustein 2013).

Among adolescents, PTSD is associated with a 3.2–14.1 times greater risk of SUD (Chilcoat and Menard 2003). Comorbidity of PTSD and SUD is associated with levels of impairment, poor psychosocial functioning, high substance use relapse rates, and severity of PTSD symptoms (Chilcoat and Menard 2003; Ford et al. 2007). Moreover, PTSD is often triply comorbid with SUDs and mood or anxiety disorders (Crum et al. 2013a, 2013b) and disruptive behavior disorders (Ford 2009; Ford et al. 2012a). These complex multiply co-occurring disorders are particularly likely when youths have experienced poly-victimization (D'Andrea et al. 2012; Finkelhor et al. 2007).

Trauma and PTSD Screening and Assessment in Adolescent SUD Treatment

Inquiry about traumatic stress history and PTSD symptoms should be made routinely in comprehensive intake assessments of adolescents with SUD (Ford et al. 2007). Clinicians may be reticent about asking adolescents direct questions about traumatic experiences for fear of triggering painful emotional reactions and interfering with SUD treatment efforts; however, empirical evidence and clinical consensus do not support such concerns. A systematic screen, performed at intake, of the nature and severity of traumatic stressor exposure(s) and PTSD offers an opportunity to provide youths (and family members) with education about expectable traumatic stress reactions and their adaptive origins (Ford 2013a). Questions about potentially shame-inducing experiences can be difficult to ask and can be emotionally painful for the youth. Consequently, it is essential that clinicians ask the questions in a clinically astute and interpersonally sensitive manner, with a clear communication about the youth's right to decline to answer uncomfortable questions or to end the interview if desired. For the majority of youths, being asked about exposure to traumas is likely to be associated with short-term discomfort only. However, follow-up monitoring of the youth's well-being is advisable, and additional counseling may be indicated.

Clinicians should be on guard throughout the screening and assessment process for any potential safety concerns. The first step is always to ascertain whether the youth is currently 1) being exposed to ongoing traumatic stressors, 2) feeling severely depressed or suicidal, 3) experiencing extreme panic or disorganized thinking, or 4) needing alcohol or drug detoxification. Assessment instruments often contain questions or probes to assess risks of self-harm and/or the potential to harm others. Clinicians need to discuss mandated reporting requirements up front so that both child and parent understand the limits of confidentiality and the consequences of disclosure.

Several instruments are available to assess trauma experiences or PTSD symptoms in children and adolescents. A few comprehensive reviews of screening and assessment tools have been published (Ford 2011a; Ford et al. 2013a; Frueh et al. 2012). No single instrument is accepted as the gold standard for screening or assessment of adolescent traumatic stressor history and PTSD. The available instruments vary in the constructs of trauma assessed, the time required to administer the instruments, and the rigor with which their psychometric properties have been evaluated (Frueh et al. 2012).

Screening typically involves the use of brief psychometrically sound instruments that can be administered quickly to identify adolescents who require further assessment for trauma-related psychopathology. Typically, screening instruments obtain information about trauma exposure and psychiatric symptoms associated with PTSD. Some of the most widely used instruments include the Global Appraisal of Individual Needs–Short Screener (GAIN-SS; Dennis 1999), Traumatic Events Screening Instrument (TESI; Daviss et al. 2000; Ford et al. 2000), University of California at Los Angeles Posttraumatic Stress Disorder Reaction Index (UCLA PTSD RI; Steinberg et al. 2004), and Trauma Symptom Checklist for Children (TSCC; Briere 1996). Anticipating the need for clinical screening of the broader set of PTSD symptoms in DSM-5, Ford et al. (2011) developed a brief clinician-rated scale for PTSD symptoms, the Symptoms of Traumatic Stress Scale for Children, Research Version (SOTS-C-RV), and field-tested it for reliability and validity with children and adolescents (ages 5–17 years) in psychiatric treatment or the juvenile justice system. This scale has single items assessing intrusive reexperiencing, avoidance, emotional numbing, and hyperarousal symptoms. Symptom ratings are made on a seven-point scale with specific operational definitions for not present, normal range, mild, moderate, moderate-severe, severe, and extreme.

Traumatic stress and PTSD assessments generally involve examining relevant history, symptoms, previous and current functioning, and other biopsychosocial factors that may relate to an adolescent's clinical presentation. A thorough assessment can take several hours and should, when possible, obtain data from multiple sources and informants to evaluate the youth's functioning and to reduce the impact of individual biases (Frueh et al. 2012). The Clinician-Administered PTSD Scale for Children and Adolescents (CAPS-CA; Nader et al. 1996) is a widely used diagnostic interview for adolescent PTSD assessment that has been updated for the DSM-5 revision of PTSD (CAPS-5; Weathers et al. 2013).

Assessing the often complex comorbid problems accompanying PTSD may be particularly relevant for substance-using adolescents, given the typical range of behavioral and psychological problems they face. It is important to determine whether an adolescent has been subjected to repeated exposure to multiple types of childhood-onset traumatic stressors. In addition to the reexperiencing, avoidance, hyperarousal, and numbing symptoms of PTSD, complex posttraumatic reactions may include alterations in affect regulation, reduced impulse control, cognitive disturbances, and somatoform disorders (Ford 2011a; Ford et al. 2013b). The Developmental Trauma Disorder Semistructured Interview (DTD-SI) for childhood complex PTSD (Ford 2011b) has been developed and shown to have good psychometrics (i.e., interrater and test-retest reliability; convergent and discriminant validity) in a multisite field trial (Ford et al. 2014), with a replication field trial being conducted between 2014 and 2015.

When working with ethnically diverse adolescents, a clinician should use assessment instruments that are culturally sensitive and validated. Although a variety of widely used instruments have been translated into various languages, much work is still needed to validate trauma screening and assessment instruments with culturally diverse populations. For example, there are Dutch, Norwegian, and Spanish versions of instruments such as the Traumatic Events Screening Inventory–Parent Report Revised (C. G. Ippen, J. Ford, R. Racusin, M. Acker, K. Bosquert, K. Rogers, C. Ellis, J. Schiffman, D. Ribbe, P. Cone, M. Lukovitz, and J. Edwards, 2002, available from Chandra.ghosh@ucsf.edu), and the Harvard Trauma Questionnaire (HTQ; Mollica et al. 1992) has been translated into Cambodian, Laotian, Vietnamese, Bosnian, and Japanese. Although some English-language PTSD instruments have been translated into other languages, not all non-English versions have been evaluated in the translated form; only the Cambodian, Laotian, and Vietnamese versions of the HTQ have been validated in their respective languages (Mollica et al. 1992).

The cultural appropriateness of screening and assessment is another important issue. Key trauma-related constructs are defined within cultural contexts in various ways and with different expressions (e.g., flashbacks may be referred to as "visions," hyperarousal may be called *"ataque de nervios,"* dissociation may be presented as "spirit possession"; Manson 1996). Similarly, the threshold for defining a PTSD reaction as "distressing" or as a problem warranting intervention differs not only across national and cultural groups but also within subgroups (e.g., geographic regions of a country with different subcultures, different religious communities within the same geographic area). As a result, clinicians need to select assessment tools and protocols that are respectful of cultural values or practices and that are meaningful within the youth's cultural context (Frueh et al. 2012).

In summary, a range of screening and assessment tools are available to help clinicians and programs identify adolescents in need of treatment. Screening for both trauma exposure and related PTSD symptoms should be routine at intake, and a comprehensive trauma assessment should be undertaken when warranted. Further research is needed to 1) validate instruments for ethnically diverse populations and 2) develop effective, cost-efficient strategies to identify youths with developmental trauma disorder.

Evidence-Informed Psychotherapy for Adolescents With Comorbid PTSD and SUD

Although relatively little research has been conducted to show the efficacy of trauma-focused interventions with substance-using adolescents, best practices include the use of interventions that have been shown empirically to be effective or to have promise for the treatment of problems associated with the experience of trauma in adolescents (Connor et al. 2014; Smith et al. 2013).

Several cognitive-behavioral approaches to PTSD treatment for adolescents have been found to be efficacious or effective in controlled research studies or have shown promise in open or quasi-experimental field trial evaluations (Connor et al. 2014). Key components of cognitive-behavioral therapies include 1) psychoeducation about traumatic stressors and posttraumatic stress reactions and problematic coping such as by substance use; 2) emotional management skills building that helps youths cope with psychological and physiological distress related to trauma cues; 3) problem-solving skills that help survivors break down problems, identify options for responding to them, and try the skills out in safe settings; and 4) cognitive restructuring that addresses distorted beliefs and cognitive schemas about the self and others and teaches survivors to use self-talk that enhances their ability to manage traumatic stress symptoms. These skills are also fundamental components of sustained recovery from addiction among adolescents (e.g., Byrne and Mazanov 1998; Dawes et al. 2000; Myers et al. 1993; Wagner et al. 1999).

Additionally, some cognitive-behavioral treatments combine prolonged exposure or cognitive processing of traumatic memories and feelings in tolerable doses so that they can be mastered and integrated into a coherent life or self-narrative. The most extensively researched model is trauma-focused cognitive-behavioral therapy (TF-CBT; Cohen et al. 2010, 2011). TF-CBT includes emotion identification, stress inoculation (e.g., breathing, relaxation) techniques, direct discussion of trauma experiences through gradual exposure exercises, cognitive restructuring, psychoeducation, and safety skills building. TF-CBT has been shown to be efficacious for children exposed to sexual abuse, family and community violence, and disasters (de Arellano et al. 2014). The efficacy of TF-CBT with substance-abusing youths (who often display many of the new DSM-5 dysregulation and hyperarousal symptoms) has not been supported in those clinical research trials (Cohen et al. 2010).

Therapies that address the emotional, self-related, and interpersonal dysregulation that is central to the expanded DSM-5 definition of PTSD are needed for traumatized adolescents who are using substances problematically, particularly when they also are heading for or are involved with risky lifestyles and peer groups (e.g., school failure, delinquency, social isolation, self-harm). One example is Trauma Affect Regulation: Guide for Education and Therapy (TARGET; Ford and Hawke 2012; Ford et al. 2012b; Marrow et al. 2012), a psychobiologically based present-centered psychotherapy that addresses affect regulation deficits and automatic stress reactions of survivors of childhood traumatic stressors. TARGET was initially validated with adults in treatment for SUD (Frisman et al. 2008; Ford et al. 2007), and the adolescent adaptation specifically addresses substance use triggers and patterns. Several other promising psychotherapies for adolescents with PTSD and SUD or risky substance use have been developed (Ford and Courtois 2014) or adapted from adult versions (Courtois and Ford 2009), including the Trauma Recovery and Empowerment Model (Ford et al. 2009), the Sanctuary Model (Bloom 2013), Trauma Systems Therapy (Navalta et al. 2013), dialectical behavior therapy (DeRosa and Rathus 2013), attachment, regulation, competency (Ford et al. 2013a), and Structured Psychotherapy for Adolescents Responding to Chronic Stress (Ford et al. 2013d).

Seeking Safety (Najavits 2002) is a multicomponent therapy for groups or individuals that was developed specifically to treat co-occurring PTSD and SUD. Seeking Safety has shown promising results in numerous clinical field trials, with generally comparable positive outcomes to those of comparison therapies such as relapse prevention and multimodal case management (Najavits and Hien 2013). The most consistent findings for Seeking Safety with multiply disadvantaged and poly-victimized adults have been reduction in PTSD symptoms. In a randomized clinical trial with female adolescents in SUD treatment, Seeking Safety's immediate posttreatment (but not 3-month follow-up) outcomes across a range of domains (including SUD risk factors, depression, and somatic/anorexic problems)—but not PTSD symptoms—surpassed those of SUD treatment as usual (Najavits et al. 2006).

Pharmacological Interventions

Pharmacological interventions are often considered as adjunct to psychotherapy for PTSD. Medications can reduce symptoms when impairment disrupts daily functioning or can help a child tolerate emotional pain associated with traumatic memories that may be augmented by psychotherapy (Connor and Meltzer 2006). However, the use of pharmacological interventions with substance-abusing adolescents with comorbid trauma-related disorders can be challenging. Drugs that have abusive potential or that have adverse interactions with drugs of abuse (e.g., stimulants) are not recommended.

Although treating medication-responsive PTSD symptoms may help reduce the severity of associated substance use problems, there is little or no scientific evidence to guide the choice of pharmacological interventions. Several medications have shown promise in treating symptoms associated with PTSD among adults, but no particular drug has emerged as a definitive treatment for PTSD among adolescents. Most controlled studies of the effects of medications for PTSD are derived from the adult literature.

Selective serotonin reuptake inhibitors (SSRIs) are often chosen for treating pediatric PTSD and recommended for treating substance-using adolescents (Connor and Meltzer 2006). To date, studies of the use of SSRIs in childhood and adolescence are primarily small open trials rather than controlled studies. In open-label studies, adolescents with moderate to severe PTSD who were treated with SSRIs experienced significant reductions in overall symptom severity, as well as in intrusive, avoidance, and hyperarousal symptoms (Seedat et al. 2001, 2002). These improvements were consistent with those seen in open trials of SSRIs in adults (van der Kolk et al. 2007). However, in a randomized clinical trial, Cohen et al. (2007) found no evidence of added benefit when an SSRI (sertraline) was combined with TF-CBT for youths ages 10–17 who had histories of sexual abuse. More research on effective strategies for the use of pharmacological interventions in combination with psychotherapies is needed (Connor et al. 2014).

Summary and Future Directions

Despite a number of promising treatment approaches, there continues to be a need for clinical innovation and rigorous scientific research to determine the most effective methods to treat trauma-related disorders among adolescents with SUDs (Najavits and Hien 2013). Cognitive-behavioral interventions that address the range of symptoms associated with DSM-5 or complex PTSD as well as DSM-IV PTSD are particularly relevant for adolescents with SUD, who often have multiple forms of self-regulation problems (Ford et al. 2005). However, there is still relatively little published empirical research on the efficacy of trauma-based interventions with substance-using youths (Najavits and Hien 2013). The most extensively researched interventions, such as TF-CBT, have been developed for child survivors of trauma and do not specifically include content on addiction and recovery issues. Most have not been tested empirically with substance-using youths. Research on the efficacy of trauma-informed interventions with diverse subpopulations of substance-abusing youths with PTSD in different settings is still needed. Adaptations of evidence-based treatment models to address ethnocultural differences are much needed (Hall et al. 2014).

Significant gaps exist in the knowledge base. Empirical evidence is lacking on the prevalence estimates and risk and protective factors for the newly expanded syndrome of PTSD, as well as complex PTSD and developmental trauma disorder, among adolescents in treatment for

SUDs. This is especially true with regard to complex sequelae of exposure to childhood victimization and poly-victimization (e.g., dysregulation of emotions, self, and relationships; D'Andrea et al. 2012; Ford 2005), which put adolescents at risk for (and severely exacerbate) substance use problems. Although integrated treatments that simultaneously address both PTSD and SUDs have been shown to be effective with adult substance users, evidence about their effectiveness with substance-using adolescents is just beginning to emerge. Whether trauma-based interventions work equally well with subgroups of substance-using adolescents (e.g., across ethnic groups, genders, or abusers of different types of drugs) remains to be explored. Finally, little is known about the impact of trauma or symptoms associated with PTSD on treatment process and outcomes.

Nevertheless, resources for clinicians and researchers working with traumatized youths who have substance use problems are increasingly available. The National Child Traumatic Stress Network, authorized and funded by Congress with oversight by the Substance Abuse and Mental Health Services Administration, is a unique infrastructure for the nationwide dissemination of public and professional education and training, as well as evidence-based prevention and treatment models, to serve traumatized children and teens and their families (www.nctsn.org). The National Child Traumatic Stress Network includes a national center colocated at Duke University in Durham, North Carolina, and the University of California, Los Angeles, as well as more than 100 community-based and academic centers, which bring evidence-informed PTSD interventions to thousands of traumatized and at-risk children and adolescents every year. Centers specifically focused on providing technical assistance and training for professionals working with youths who have comorbid traumatic stress and SUDs include the Center for Trauma Recovery and Juvenile Justice in Farmington, Connecticut; the Urban Youth Trauma Center in Chicago, Illinois; and the Adolescent Trauma Training Center in Los Angeles, California.

KEY POINTS

- Posttraumatic stress disorder (PTSD) is a common comorbidity with youth substance use disorders (SUDs).

- PTSD diagnostic criteria in DSM-5 include symptoms not included in DSM-IV that may exacerbate substance use and

SUDs, including reckless behavior and negative core beliefs about self, relationships, and the world.

- Evidence-based treatments that exist for teens with comorbid PTSD and SUDs include Seeking Safety, cognitive-behavioral therapy, and Trauma Affect Regulation: Guide for Education and Therapy (TARGET).

- Evidence-based treatments addressing SUDs can be conducted concurrently with evidence-based PTSD interventions with youths who have co-occurring SUDs and PTSD.

- Treatments of PTSD and SUD share the aim of enhancing teens' basic capacities for self-regulation.

References

Abram KM, Teplin LA, Charles DR, et al: Posttraumatic stress disorder and trauma in youth in juvenile detention. Arch Gen Psychiatry 61(4):403–410, 2004 15066899

Abram KM, Washburn JJ, Teplin LA, et al: Posttraumatic stress disorder and psychiatric comorbidity among detained youths. Psychiatr Serv 58(10):1311–1316, 2007 17914008

American Psychiatric Association: Diagnostic and Statistical Manual of Mental Disorders, 3rd Edition. Washington, DC, American Psychiatric Association, 1980

American Psychiatric Association: Diagnostic and Statistical Manual of Mental Disorders, 4th Edition. Washington, DC, American Psychiatric Association, 1994

American Psychiatric Association: Diagnostic and Statistical Manual of Mental Disorders, 5th Edition. Arlington, VA, American Psychiatric Association, 2013

Bloom S: The Sanctuary Model, in Treating Complex Traumatic Stress Disorders in Children and Adolescents: Scientific Foundations and Therapeutic Models. Edited by Ford JD, Courtois CA. New York, Guilford, 2013, pp 277–294

Brewin CR, Lanius RA, Novac A, et al: Reformulating PTSD for DSM-V: life after Criterion A. J Trauma Stress 22(5):366–373, 2009 19743480

Briere J: Trauma Symptom Checklist for Children: Professional Manual. Odessa, FL, Psychological Assessment Resources, 1996

Briggs-Gowan MJ, Carter AS, Clark R, et al: Exposure to potentially traumatic events in early childhood: differential links to emergent psychopathology. J Child Psychol Psychiatry 51(10):1132–1140, 2010a 20840502

Briggs-Gowan MJ, Ford JD, Fraleigh L, et al: Prevalence of exposure to potentially traumatic events in a healthy birth cohort of very young children in the northeastern United States. J Trauma Stress 23(6):725–733, 2010b 21171133

Briggs-Gowan MJ, Carter AS, Ford JD: Parsing the effects violence exposure in early childhood: modeling developmental pathways. J Pediatr Psychol 37(1):11–22, 2012 21903730

Brosky BA, Lally SJ: Prevalence of trauma, PTSD, and dissociation in court-referred adolescents. J Interpers Violence 19(7):801–814, 2004 15186537

Byrne DG, Mazanov J: Sources of adolescent stress, smoking and the use of other drugs. Stress Med 15(4):215–227, 1998

Carrion VG, Steiner H: Trauma and dissociation in delinquent adolescents. J Am Acad Child Adolesc Psychiatry 39(3):353–359, 2000 10714056

Cauffman E, Feldman SS, Waterman J, et al: Posttraumatic stress disorder among female juvenile offenders. J Am Acad Child Adolesc Psychiatry 37(11):1209–1216, 1998 9808933

Chilcoat HD, Menard C: Epidemiological investigations: comorbidity of posttraumatic stress disorder and substance use disorder, in Trauma and Substance Abuse: Causes, Consequences, and Treatment of Comorbid Disorders. Edited by Ouimette P, Brown P. Washington, DC, American Psychological Association, 2003, pp 9–28

Clark DB, Lesnick L, Hegedus AM: Traumas and other adverse life events in adolescents with alcohol abuse and dependence. J Am Acad Child Adolesc Psychiatry 36(12):1744–1751, 1997 9401336

Cohen JA, Mannarino AP, Perel JM, et al: A pilot randomized controlled trial of combined trauma-focused CBT and sertraline for childhood PTSD symptoms. J Am Acad Child Adolesc Psychiatry 46(7):811–819, 2007 17581445

Cohen JA, Berliner L, Mannarino A: Trauma focused CBT for children with co-occurring trauma and behavior problems. Child Abuse Negl 34(4):215–224, 2010 20304489

Cohen JA, Mannarino AP, Iyengar S: Community treatment of posttraumatic stress disorder for children exposed to intimate partner violence: a randomized controlled trial. Arch Pediatr Adolesc Med 165(1):16–21, 2011 21199975

Connor DF, Meltzer BM: Pediatric Psychopharmacology. New York, WW Norton, 2006

Connor DF, Ford JD, Arnsten AF, et al: An update on posttraumatic stress disorder in children and adolescents. Clin Pediatr (Phila) Jul 2, 2014 [Epub ahead of print]

Courtois CA, Ford J (eds): Treating Complex Traumatic Stress Disorders: An Evidence-Based Guide. New York, Guilford, 2009

Crimmins SM, Cleary SD, Brownstein HH, et al: Trauma, drugs and violence among juvenile offenders. J Psychoactive Drugs 32(1):43–54, 2000 10801067

Crum RM, La Flair L, Storr CL, et al: Reports of drinking to self-medicate anxiety symptoms: longitudinal assessment for subgroups of individuals with alcohol dependence. Depress Anxiety 30(2):174–183, 2013a 23280888

Crum RM, Mojtabai R, Lazareck S, et al: A prospective assessment of reports of drinking to self-medicate mood symptoms with the incidence and persistence of alcohol dependence. JAMA Psychiatry 70(7):718–726, 2013b 23636710

Dalenberg CJ, Brand BL, Gleaves DH, et al: Evaluation of the evidence for the trauma and fantasy models of dissociation. Psychol Bull 138(3):550–588, 2012 22409505

D'Andrea W, Ford J, Stolbach B, et al: Understanding interpersonal trauma in children: why we need a developmentally appropriate trauma diagnosis. Am J Orthopsychiatry 82(2):187–200, 2012 22506521

Daviss WB, Mooney D, Racusin R, et al: Predicting posttraumatic stress after hospitalization for pediatric injury. J Am Acad Child Adolesc Psychiatry 39(5):576–583, 2000 10802975

Dawes MA, Antelman SM, Vanyukov MM, et al: Developmental sources of variation in liability to adolescent substance use disorders. Drug Alcohol Depend 61(1):3–14, 2000 11064179

de Arellano MA, Lyman DR, Jobe-Shields L, et al: Trauma-focused cognitive-behavioral therapy for children and adolescents: assessing the evidence. Psychiatr Serv 65(5):591–602, 2014 24638076

Dennis M: Global Appraisal of Individual Needs: Administration Guide for the GAIN and Related Measures. Bloomington, IL, Chestnut Health Systems, 1999. Available at: http://gaincc.org/gainss. Accessed April 11, 2015.

DeRosa RR, Rathus JH: Dialectical behavior therapy with adolescents, in Treating Complex Traumatic Stress Disorders in Children and Adolescents. Edited by Ford JD, Courtois, CA. New York, Guilford, 2013, pp 225–247

Finkelhor D, Ormrod RK, Turner HA, et al: Measuring poly-victimization using the Juvenile Victimization Questionnaire. Child Abuse Negl 29(11):1297–1312, 2005 16274741

Finkelhor D, Ormrod RK, Turner HA: Poly-victimization: a neglected component in child victimization. Child Abuse Negl 31(1):7–26, 2007 17224181

Ford JD: Treatment implications of altered neurobiology, affect regulation and information processing following child maltreatment. Psychiatr Ann 35(5):410–419, 2005

Ford JD: Neurobiological and developmental research: clinical implications, in Treating Complex Traumatic Stress Disorders: An Evidence-Based Guide. New York, Guilford, 2009, pp 31–58

Ford JD: Assessing child and adolescent complex traumatic stress reactions. J Child Adolesc Trauma 4(3):217–232, 2011a

Ford JD: Future directions in conceptualizing complex posttraumatic stress syndromes in childhood and adolescence: toward a developmental trauma disorder diagnosis, in Post-traumatic Syndromes in Childhood and Adolescence. Edited by Ardino V. Chichester, UK, Wiley-Blackwell, 2011b, pp 433–448

Ford JD: Posttraumatic stress disorder (PTSD) among youth involved in juvenile justice, in Handbook of Juvenile Forensic Psychology and Psychiatry. Edited by Grigorenko E. New York, Springer, 2012, pp 487–503

Ford JD: Identifying and caring for acutely traumatized children. Consultant for Pediatricians 12(4):182–187, 2013a

Ford JD: Posttraumatic stress disorder (PTSD) and substance abuse treatment, in Encyclopedia of Addictive Behaviors, Vol 3: Interventions for Addiction. Edited by Miller P. New York, Elsevier, 2013b, pp 187–194

Ford JD, Blaustein ME: Systemic self-regulation: a framework for trauma-informed services in residential juvenile justice programs. J Fam Violence 28(7):665–677, 2013

Ford JD, Courtois CA: Complex PTSD, affect dysregulation, and borderline personality disorder. Borderline Personality Disorder and Emotion Dysregulation 1:9, 2014

Ford JD, Hawke J: Trauma affect regulation psychoeducation group and milieu intervention outcomes in juvenile detention facilities. J Aggress Maltreat Trauma 21(4):365–384, 2012

Ford JD, Racusin R, Ellis CG, et al: Child maltreatment, other trauma exposure, and posttraumatic symptomatology among children with oppositional defiant and attention deficit hyperactivity disorders. Child Maltreat 5(3):205–217, 2000 11232267

Ford JD, Courtois CA, Steele K, et al: Treatment of complex posttraumatic self-dysregulation. J Trauma Stress 18(5):437–447, 2005 16281241

Ford JD, Russo EM, Mallon SD: Integrating treatment of posttraumatic stress disorder and substance use disorder. J Couns Dev 85(4):475–489, 2007

Ford JD, Hartman JK, Hawke J, et al: Traumatic victimization, posttraumatic stress disorder, suicidal ideation, and substance abuse risk among juvenile justice-involved youths. J Child Adolesc Trauma 1:75–92, 2008

Ford JD, Connor DF, Hawke J: Complex trauma among psychiatrically impaired children: a cross-sectional, chart-review study. J Clin Psychiatry 70(8):1155–1163, 2009 19573498

Ford JD, Elhai JD, Connor DF, et al: Poly-victimization and risk of posttraumatic, depressive, and substance use disorders and involvement in delinquency in a national sample of adolescents. J Adolesc Health 46(6):545–552, 2010 20472211

Ford JD, Opler LA, Muenzenmaier K, et al: Manual for the Symptoms of Trauma Scale for Children, Research Version (SOTS-C-RV). Farmington, University of Connecticut Health Center, 2011

Ford JD, Chapman JC, Connor DF, et al: Complex trauma and aggression in secure juvenile justice settings. Crim Justice Behav 39(6):694–724, 2012a

Ford JD, Steinberg KL, Hawke J, et al: Randomized trial comparison of emotion regulation and relational psychotherapies for PTSD with girls involved in delinquency. J Clin Child Adolesc Psychol 41(1):27–37, 2012b 22233243

Ford JD, Blaustein M, Habib M, et al: Developmental trauma-focused treatment models, in Treating Complex Traumatic Stress Disorders in Children and Adolescents: Scientific Foundations and Therapeutic Models. Edited by Ford JD, Courtois CA. New York, Guilford, 2013a, pp 261–276

Ford JD, Grasso D, Greene C, et al: Clinical significance of a proposed developmental trauma disorder diagnosis: results of an international survey of clinicians. J Clin Psychiatry 74(8):841–849, 2013b 24021504

Ford JD, Grasso DJ, Hawke J, et al: Poly-victimization among juvenile justice-involved youths. Child Abuse Negl 37(10):788–800, 2013c 23428165

Ford JD, Nader K, Fletcher K: Clinical assessment and diagnosis, in Treating Complex Traumatic Stress Disorders in Children and Adolescents: Scientific Foundations and Therapeutic Models. Edited by Ford JD, Courtois CA. New York, Guilford, 2013d pp 116–139

Ford JD, Spinazzola J, Van der Kolk B, et al: Developmental Trauma Disorder (DTD) field trial, I: evidence of reliability, structure, and validity of the DTD Semistructured Interview (DTD-SI). Paper presented at the annual convention of the International Society for Traumatic Stress Studies, Miami, FL, November 2014

Freyd JJ: Betrayal Trauma. Cambridge, MA, Harvard University Press, 1997

Frisman LK, Ford JD, Lin H, et al: Outcomes of trauma treatment using the TARGET model. Journal of Groups in Addiction and Recovery 3:285–303, 2008

Frueh BC, Elhai JD, Grubaugh A, et al: Assessment and Treatment Planning for PTSD. Hoboken, NJ, Wiley, 2012

Giaconia RM, Reinherz HZ, Hauf AC, et al: Comorbidity of substance use and post-traumatic stress disorders in a community sample of adolescents. Am J Orthopsychiatry 70(2):253–262, 2000 10826037

Gola H, Engler H, Schauer M, et al: Victims of rape show increased cortisol responses to trauma reminders: a study in individuals with war- and torture-related PTSD. Psychoneuroendocrinology 37(2):213–220, 2012 21723669

Grasso DJ, Ford JD, Briggs-Gowan MJ: Early life trauma exposure and stress sensitivity in young children. J Pediatr Psychol 38(1):94–103, 2013 23008502

Grella CE, Joshi V: Treatment processes and outcomes among adolescents with a history of abuse who are in drug treatment. Child Maltreat 8(1):7–18, 2003 12568501

Guffanti G, Galea S, Yan L, et al: Genome-wide association study implicates a novel RNA gene, the lincRNA AC068718.1, as a risk factor for post-traumatic stress disorder in women. Psychoneuroendocrinology 38(12):3029–3038, 2013 24080187

Hall BJ, Bolton PA, Annan J, et al: The effect of cognitive therapy on structural social capital: results from a randomized controlled trial among sexual violence survivors in the Democratic Republic of the Congo. Am J Public Health 104(9):1680–1686, 2014 25033113

Harrington M, Robinson J, Bolton SL, et al: A longitudinal study of risk factors for incident drug use in adults: findings from a representative sample of the U.S. population. Can J Psychiatry 56(11):686–695, 2011 22114923

Hawke JM, Jainchill N, De Leon G: The prevalence of sexual abuse and its impact on onset of drug use among adolescents in therapeutic community drug treatment. J Child Adolesc Subst Abuse 9(3):35–49, 2000

Hawke JM, Jainchill N, De Leon G: Posttreatment victimization and violence among adolescents following residential drug treatment. Child Maltreat 8(1):58–71, 2003 12568505

Hawke J, Ford JD, Kaminer Y, et al: Trauma and PTSD among youths in outpatient treatment for alcohol and other substance use disorders. J Child Adolesc Trauma 2(1):1–14, 2009

Herrenkohl TI, Sousa C, Tajima EA, et al: Intersection of child abuse and children's exposure to domestic violence. Trauma Violence Abuse 9(2):84–99, 2008 18296571

Jaycox LH, Ebener P, Damesek L, et al: Trauma exposure and retention in adolescent substance abuse treatment. J Trauma Stress 17(2):113–121, 2004 15141784

Kaminer Y, Ford JD, Clark D: Assessment and treatment of internalizing disorders, in Clinical Manual of Adolescent Substance Abuse Treatment. Edited by Kaminer Y, Winters K. Washington, DC, American Psychiatric Publishing, 2011, pp 307–347

Kelly JF, Greene MC: Where there's a will there's a way: a longitudinal investigation of the interplay between recovery motivation and self-efficacy in predicting treatment outcome. Psychol Addict Behav 28(3):928–934, 2014 24274437

Kelly PA, Viding E, Wallace GL, et al: Cortical thickness, surface area, and gyrification abnormalities in children exposed to maltreatment: neural markers of vulnerability? Biol Psychiatry 74(11):845–852, 2013 23954109

Kessler RC, Sonnega A, Bromet E, et al: Posttraumatic stress disorder in the National Comorbidity Survey. Arch Gen Psychiatry 52(12):1048–1060, 1995 7492257

Kessler RC, Berglund P, Demler O, et al: Lifetime prevalence and age-of-onset distributions of DSM-IV disorders in the National Comorbidity Survey Replication. Arch Gen Psychiatry 62(6):593–602, 2005 15939837

Kilpatrick DG, Ruggiero KJ, Acierno R, et al: Violence and risk of PTSD, major depression, substance abuse/dependence, and comorbidity: results from the National Survey of Adolescents. J Consult Clin Psychol 71(4):692–700, 2003 12924674

Kilpatrick DG, Resnick HS, Acierno R: Should PTSD Criterion A be retained? J Trauma Stress 22(5):374–383, 2009 19743478

Kühn S, Gallinat J: Gray matter correlates of posttraumatic stress disorder: a quantitative meta-analysis. Biol Psychiatry 73(1):70–74, 2013 22840760

Layne C, Beck C, Rimmasch H, et al: Promoting "resilient" posttraumatic adjustment in childhood and beyond, in Treating Traumatized Children: Risk, Resilience, and Recovery. Edited by Brom D, Pat-Horenczyk R, Ford JD. London, Routledge, 2008, pp 13–47

Lewis-Fernández R, Turner JB, Marshall R, et al: Elevated rates of current PTSD among Hispanic veterans in the NVVRS: true prevalence or methodological artifact? J Trauma Stress 21(2):123–132, 2008 18404629

Manson SM: The wounded spirit: a cultural formulation of post-traumatic stress disorder. Cult Med Psychiatry 20(4):489–498, 1996 8989988

Marrow MT, Knudsen KJ, Olafson E, et al: The value of implementing TARGET within a trauma-informed juvenile justice setting. J Child Adolesc Trauma 5:257–270, 2012

McFarlane AC: Posttraumatic stress disorder: a model of the longitudinal course and the role of risk factors. J Clin Psychiatry 61 (suppl 5):15–20, discussion 21–23, 2000 10761675

McLaughlin KA, Koenen KC, Hill ED, et al: Trauma exposure and post-traumatic stress disorder in a national sample of adolescents. J Am Acad Child Adolesc Psychiatry 52(8):815–830, 2013 23880492

Milan S, Zona K, Acker J, et al: Prospective risk factors for adolescent PTSD: sources of differential exposure and differential vulnerability. J Abnorm Child Psychol 41(2):339–353, 2013 22956298

Mollica RF, Caspi-Yavin Y, Bollini P, et al: The Harvard Trauma Questionnaire: validating a cross-cultural instrument for measuring torture, trauma, and posttraumatic stress disorder in Indochinese refugees. J Nerv Ment Dis 180(2):111–116, 1992 1737972

Myers MG, Brown SA, Mott MA: Coping as a predictor of adolescent substance abuse treatment outcome. J Subst Abuse 5(1):15–29, 1993 8329878

Nader K, Kriegler JA, Blake DD, et al: Clinician-Administered PTSD Scale, Child and Adolescent Version. White River Junction, VT, National Center for PTSD, 1996

Najavits LM: Seeking Safety: A Treatment Manual for PTSD and Substance Abuse. New York, Guilford, 2002

Najavits LM, Hien D: Helping vulnerable populations: a comprehensive review of the treatment outcome literature on substance use disorder and PTSD. J Clin Psychol 69(5):433–479, 2013 23592045

Najavits LM, Gallop RJ, Weiss RD: Seeking safety therapy for adolescent girls with PTSD and substance use disorder: a randomized controlled trial. J Behav Health Serv Res 33(4):453–463, 2006 16858633

Navalta CP, Brown AD, Nisewaner A, et al: Trauma systems therapy, in Treating Complex Traumatic Stress Disorders in Children and Adolescents: Scientific Foundations and Therapeutic Models. Edited by Ford JD, Courtois CA. New York, Guilford, 2013, pp 329–348

Norman SB, Myers US, Wilkins KC, et al: Review of biological mechanisms and pharmacological treatments of comorbid PTSD and substance use disorder. Neuropharmacology 62(2):542–551, 2012 21600225

Parmenter J, Mitchell C, Keen J, et al: Predicting biopsychosocial outcomes for heroin users in primary care treatment: a prospective longitudinal cohort study. Br J Gen Pract 63(612):e499–e505, 2013 23834887

Perkonigg A, Kessler RC, Storz S, et al: Traumatic events and post-traumatic stress disorder in the community: prevalence, risk factors and comorbidity. Acta Psychiatr Scand 101(1):46–59, 2000 10674950

Perkonigg A, Pfister H, Stein MB, et al: Longitudinal course of posttraumatic stress disorder and posttraumatic stress disorder symptoms in a community sample of adolescents and young adults. Am J Psychiatry 162(7):1320–1327, 2005 15994715

Pole N, Gone JP, Kulkarni M: Posttraumatic stress disorder among ethnoracial minorities in the United States. Clinical Psychology: Science and Practice 15(1):35–61, 2008

Ruchkin VV, Schwab-Stone M, Koposov R, et al: Violence exposure, posttraumatic stress, and personality in juvenile delinquents. J Am Acad Child Adolesc Psychiatry 41(3):322–329, 2002 11886027

Seedat S, Lockhat R, Kaminer D, et al: An open trial of citalopram in adolescents with post-traumatic stress disorder. Int Clin Psychopharmacol 16(1):21–25, 2001 11195256

Seedat S, Stein DJ, Ziervogel C, et al: Comparison of response to a selective serotonin reuptake inhibitor in children, adolescents, and adults with posttraumatic stress disorder. J Child Adolesc Psychopharmacol 12(1):37–46, 2002 12014594

Seedat S, Nyamai C, Njenga F, et al: Trauma exposure and post-traumatic stress symptoms in urban African schools: survey in CapeTown and Nairobi. Br J Psychiatry 184(2):169–175, 2004 14754831

Smith P, Perrin S, Dalgleish T, et al: Treatment of posttraumatic stress disorder in children and adolescents. Curr Opin Psychiatry 26(1):66–72, 2013 23201964

Stein RE, Hurlburt MS, Heneghan AM, et al: Chronic conditions among children investigated by child welfare: a national sample. Pediatrics 131(3):455–462, 2013 23420907

Steinberg AM, Brymer MJ, Decker KB, et al: The University of California at Los Angeles Post-traumatic Stress Disorder Reaction Index. Curr Psychiatry Rep 6(2):96–100, 2004 15038911

Stevens SJ, Murphy BS, McKnight K: Traumatic stress and gender differences in relationship to substance abuse, mental health, physical health, and HIV risk behavior in a sample of adolescents enrolled in drug treatment. Child Maltreat 8(1):46–57, 2003 12568504

Sumner JA, Pietrzak RH, Aiello AE, et al: Further support for an association between the memory-related gene WWC1 and posttraumatic stress disorder:
results from the Detroit neighborhood health study. Biol Psychiatry
76(11):e25–e26, 2014 24947539

Teicher MH, Samson JA: Childhood maltreatment and psychopathology: a case
for ecophenotypic variants as clinically and neurobiologically distinct subtypes. Am J Psychiatry 170(10):1114–1133, 2013 23982148

Tolin DF, Foa EB: Sex differences in trauma and posttraumatic stress disorder:
a quantitative review of 25 years of research. Psychol Bull 132(6):959–992,
2006 17073529

van der Kolk BA, Spinazzola J, Blaustein ME, et al: A randomized clinical trial
of eye movement desensitization and reprocessing (EMDR), fluoxetine, and
pill placebo in the treatment of posttraumatic stress disorder: treatment effects and long-term maintenance. J Clin Psychiatry 68(1):37–46, 2007
17284128

Wagner EF, Myers MG, McInnich JL: Stress-coping and temptation-coping as
predictors of adolescent substance use. Addict Behav 24(6):769–779, 1999
10628511

Weathers FW, Blake DD, Schnurr PP et al: The Clinician-Administered PTSD
Scale for DSM-5 (CAPS-5). 2013. Interview available at: www.ptsd.va.gov,
2013. Accessed June 29, 2013.

White S, Acierno R, Ruggiero KJ, et al: Association of CRHR1 variants and posttraumatic stress symptoms in hurricane exposed adults. J Anxiety Disord
27(7):678–683, 2013 24077033

Wittchen HU, Schönfeld S, Thurau C, et al: Prevalence, incidence and determinants of PTSD and other mental disorders: design and methods of the PID-
PTSD+3 study. Int J Methods Psychiatr Res 21(2):98–116, 2012 22605681

Xie P, Kranzler HR, Poling J, et al: Interaction of FKBP5 with childhood adversity on risk for post-traumatic stress disorder. Neuropsychopharmacology
35(8):1684–1692, 2010 20393453

Yehuda R, Daskalakis NP, Lehrner A, et al: Influences of maternal and paternal
PTSD on epigenetic regulation of the glucocorticoid receptor gene in Holo-
caust survivor offspring. Am J Psychiatry 171(8):872–880, 2014 24832930

CHAPTER 10

Suicidal and Nonsuicidal Self-Harm Behaviors and Substance Use Disorders

Christianne Esposito-Smythers, Ph.D.

Alexandra Perloe, M.A.

Kyla Machell, M.A.

Bethany Rallis, Ed.M.

There exists a growing body of literature on the association between adolescent deliberate self-inflicted injury, including suicide attempts (SAs) and nonsuicidal self-injury (NSSI), and substance use disorders (SUDs). This chapter includes a review of the epidemiology, clinical features, etiology, and clinical course of adolescent SAs and NSSI. The theoretical and empirical links between these two self-injurious behaviors and SUDs are then discussed. Current assessment approaches for SAs and NSSI are reviewed, and interventions that incorporate self-injury and SUDs are presented.

SAs and NSSI are distinct yet commonly overlapping behaviors. A *suicide attempt* is defined as a direct, potentially life-threatening self-injurious behavior that is self-inflicted with at least *some intent to die*

This research was supported by grants from the National Institute of Mental Health (R01 MH097703) and the National Institute on Alcohol Abuse and Alcoholism (R01 AA016854), awarded to C. Esposito-Smythers, Ph.D.

(e.g., self-poisoning, severe cutting, hanging, suffocation, jumping from heights, use of firearm). *Nonsuicidal self-injury* is defined as direct and deliberate self-inflicted bodily harm in the *absence of intent to die* (e.g., less severe self-cutting, burning, head banging, self-hitting, scratching to the point of drawing blood) (Nock 2010). In outpatient clinic samples, 33%–37% of adolescents who engage in NSSI report a lifetime SA (Asarnow et al. 2011; Jacobson et al. 2008). Moreover, NSSI prospectively predicts suicidal behavior, even above the impact of prior suicidal behavior (Asarnow et al. 2011). Indeed, a recent review in this area concluded that NSSI is a robust predictor of SAs, with the association greatest among adolescents with more frequent and severe methods of NSSI (Hamza et al. 2012).

Although they co-occur at high rates, SAs and NSSI have many notable differences. Rates of SAs vary by survey method but, nonetheless, are much lower than rates of NSSI. Using data from the National Comorbidity Survey Replication–Adolescent Supplement, the largest nationally representative survey of adolescents to employ structured psychiatric interviews, Nock et al. (2013) found that 4.1% of adolescents made a SA during their lifetime. Rates were found to be higher in a national anonymous survey that employed a self-report instrument; according to the Youth Risk Behavior Surveillance System, 8% of adolescents made a SA in the last year, and 2.7% made an attempt that required medical attention (Kann et al. 2014). Rates are even higher in clinical samples, with 24%–33% of adolescents reporting a prior SA (Asarnow et al. 2011; Jacobson et al. 2008). Large epidemiological studies have not been conducted to assess adolescent NSSI. However, prevalence estimates of adolescent NSSI range from 12% to 46% in community-based samples (Jacobson and Gould 2007; Lloyd-Richardson et al. 2007), and from 39% (Lipschitz et al. 1999) to 68% (Guerry and Prinstein 2010) in clinical samples. Medical lethality and frequency of self-injury also differ for adolescents who engage in SAs and NSSI. SAs tend to involve more lethal methods (e.g., self-poisoning, hanging, more severe cutting in dangerous body areas) relative to NSSI (e.g., less severe cutting, burning, hitting self) (Andover and Gibb 2010). SAs also occur less frequently than NSSI among adolescents who self-injure. For example, Lloyd-Richardson et al. (2007) found the average number of NSSI acts to be 12.87 in a normative community sample. In contrast, Nock et al. (2006) reported an average of only 2.8 lifetime SAs in a sample of patients in a psychiatric hospital.

Because SAs and NSSI are both forms of self-inflicted injury and NSSI predicts SAs, it is not surprising that they share many common correlates, one of which is co-occurrence with SUDs. We begin this chapter with a review of the key features, diagnosis, etiology, and clinical course of treatment for SAs and NSSI among adolescents. Then we discuss the relationship and clinical course of these behaviors with SUDs, including suggested empirical and theoretical links; review current assessment approaches to SAs and NSSI; and present interventions that address self-harm and SUDs. We conclude this chapter with a discussion of potential future directions.

Key Features and Diagnosis of Suicidal and NSSI Behaviors

In DSM-5 (American Psychiatric Association 2013), a SA is listed as a symptom of a major depressive episode, and SAs and NSSI are listed as symptoms of borderline personality disorder. SAs and NSSI are also included in proposed disorders described in the DSM-5 section "Conditions for Further Study." Specifically, proposed criteria for suicidal behavior disorder (Box 10–1) include a SA (not solely suicidal thoughts or plans) in the last 2 years that does not meet criteria for NSSI. The patient cannot have enacted the SA "during a state of delirium or confusion" and cannot have engaged in the SA "solely for a political or religious objective."

Box 10–1. DSM-5 Criteria for Suicidal Behavior Disorder

A. Within the last 24 months, the individual has made a suicide attempt.
   Note: A suicide attempt is a self-initiated sequence of behaviors by an individual who, at the time of initiation, expected that the set of actions would lead to his or her own death. (The "time of initiation" is the time when a behavior took place that involved applying the method.)
B. The act does not meet criteria for nonsuicidal self-injury—that is, it does not involve self-injury directed to the surface of the body undertaken to induce relief from a negative feeling/cognitive state or to achieve a positive mood state.
C. The diagnosis is not applied to suicidal ideation or to preparatory acts.
D. The act was not initiated during a state of delirium or confusion.
E. The act was not undertaken solely for a political or religious objective.

Specify if:
   Current: Not more than 12 months since the last attempt.
   In early remission: 12–24 months since the last attempt.

The DSM-5 proposed criteria for NSSI (Box 10–2) include intentional self-injury to the surface of one's body, in the absence of suicidal intent, for 5 or more days. This behavior is engaged in with the expectation of relief from a negative feeling or cognitive state, to induce a positive mood state, or to resolve interpersonal difficulty. The self-injury must also be associated with either interpersonal difficulties or negative feelings or thoughts, prior preoccupation with NSSI that is difficult to control, and/or frequent thoughts about NSSI even in the absence of action. NSSI can neither be socially sanctioned nor limited to picking scabs or nail biting. NSSI or its consequences must lead to clinically significant distress or impairment. NSSI cannot be better accounted for by other mental disorders nor occur exclusively during other thought or substance-related conditions (psychotic episode, delirium, substance intoxication or withdrawal).

Box 10–2.   DSM-5 Criteria for Nonsuicidal Self-Injury

A. In the last year, the individual has, on 5 or more days, engaged in intentional self-inflicted damage to the surface of his or her body of a sort likely to induce bleeding, bruising, or pain (e.g., cutting, burning, stabbing, hitting, excessive rubbing), with the expectation that the injury will lead to only minor or moderate physical harm (i.e., there is no suicidal intent).

Note: The absence of suicidal intent has either been stated by the individual or can be inferred by the individual's repeated engagement in a behavior that the individual knows, or has learned, is not likely to result in death.

B. The individual engages in the self-injurious behavior with one or more of the following expectations:

1. To obtain relief from a negative feeling or cognitive state.
2. To resolve an interpersonal difficulty.
3. To induce a positive feeling state.

Note: The desired relief or response is experienced during or shortly after the self-injury, and the individual may display patterns of behavior suggesting a dependence on repeatedly engaging in it.

C. The intentional self-injury is associated with at least one of the following:

1. Interpersonal difficulties or negative feelings or thoughts, such as depression, anxiety, tension, anger, generalized distress, or self-criticism, occurring in the period immediately prior to the self-injurious act.
2. Prior to engaging in the act, a period of preoccupation with the intended behavior that is difficult to control.
3. Thinking about self-injury that occurs frequently, even when it is not acted upon.

D. The behavior is not socially sanctioned (e.g., body piercing, tattooing, part of a religious or cultural ritual) and is not restricted to picking a scab or nail biting.

E. The behavior or its consequences cause clinically significant distress or interference in interpersonal, academic, or other important areas of functioning.

F. The behavior does not occur exclusively during psychotic episodes, delirium, substance intoxication, or substance withdrawal. In individuals with a neurodevelopmental disorder, the behavior is not part of a pattern of repetitive stereotypies. The behavior is not better explained by another mental disorder or medical condition (e.g., psychotic disorder, autism spectrum disorder, intellectual disability, Lesch-Nyhan syndrome, stereotypic movement disorder with self-injury, trichotillomania [hair-pulling disorder], excoriation [skin-picking] disorder).

Etiology and Clinical Course of Suicidal and NSSI Behaviors

Rates of SAs rise precipitously from childhood through adolescence. Prevalence of SAs remains quite low through age 12 (<1%), increases in a roughly linear fashion through age 15, and then increases more slowly through age 17 (Nock et al. 2013). Rates of SAs are consistently higher among females than males (Kann et al. 2014; Nock et al. 2013). Racial and ethnic differences are less consistent across national surveys. In the Youth Risk Behavior Surveillance System, Hispanic adolescents reported higher annual rates of SAs than non-Hispanic black and non-Hispanic white adolescents, and non-Hispanic black adolescents reported higher rates than non-Hispanic white adolescents (Kann et al. 2014). In the National Comorbidity Survey Replication–Adolescent Supplement, the only difference found in lifetime rates of SAs was between non-Hispanic black and non-Hispanic white adolescents, with the former exhibiting lower odds of a SA (Nock et al. 2013).

The clinical course of NSSI is similar to that found with SAs. NSSI peaks in adolescence, with an average age at onset between 11 and 15 years (Whitlock 2010), and declines into adulthood (Zanarini et al. 2005). Gender differences in NSSI are not always consistent, although rates generally appear higher in females (e.g., Howe-Martin et al. 2012; Whitlock 2010). The gender discrepancy in NSSI is greater among young adolescents (ages

10–14), with a female-to-male ratio of 8:1, than in later adolescence (ages 15–19), with a ratio of approximately 3:1 (Hawton and Harriss 2008).

With regard to racial and ethnic differences, one study conducted with an ethnically diverse sample of adolescents found that white adolescents reported higher rates of NSSI than did African American or Hispanic adolescents, although the latter two groups did not differ significantly from each other (Muehlenkamp et al. 2010). Other studies suggest that racial and ethnic differences in rates of NSSI vary based on age, gender, and type of NSSI. In a sample of ethnically diverse low-income middle and high school students (Gratz et al. 2012), rates of overall NSSI were higher among African American youth than white youth, particularly among younger African American males; however, rates of *frequent* deliberate self-harm (DSH) did not differ between these two groups. Moreover, when cutting in particular (rather than all types of NSSI) was examined, white females reported higher rates of cutting than did African American females or white males. African American males, however, reported higher rates of cutting than did white males. Race and ethnicity interacted with age, such that white students of high school age, in comparison with same-age African American students, reported higher rates of cutting, but no race differences were present for cutting rates in students of middle school age. Similarly, Lloyd-Richardson et al. (2007) found significantly higher rates of overall NSSI in white adolescents compared to African American adolescents. However, higher rates of moderate/severe NSSI were reported by white youth than African American youth, and higher rates of minor NSSI were reported by African American youth than white youth.

Many reasons may potentially contribute to the sharp rise in SAs and NSSI during adolescence. Increased vulnerability to environmental stress precipitated by the rapid psychological, biological, and social changes that occur during this developmental period may account for increases in SAs (Pelkonen and Marttunen 2003). With growth in cognitive abilities, adolescents may be better able to plan and execute a SA (Grøholt et al. 1998). Developmental changes during adolescence also may contribute to the onset of psychiatric disorders (i.e., mood and substance use disorders) known to increase risk for suicidal behavior (Grøholt et al. 1998; Pelkonen and Marttunen 2003). The same explanations apply equally well to NSSI.

SAs and NSSI share numerous common etiologies, most of which are not specific to these behaviors but predict many forms of maladaptive behavior. Comprehensive reviews in these areas (see Esposito-

Smythers et al. 2014; Whitlock and Selekman 2014) suggest that reliable risk factors include the presence of antecedent (and comorbid) psychiatric disorders (e.g., depressive, anxiety, eating, disruptive behavior, and substance use disorders) and borderline personality traits, heightened emotional states and dysregulation (i.e., negative emotionality, anger, aggression, impulsivity), poor coping and problem-solving skills, childhood physical and sexual abuse, adverse family environments (e.g., high conflict, low cohesion, neglect, poor parental mental health), exposure to SAs and NSSI (e.g., via peers and media), and greater stressful life events. Specific to SAs, prior suicidal behavior is the strongest risk factor for a future SA and suicide completion (Goldston et al. 2009). Familial suicidal behavior (via modeling and/or genetic transmission) is also believed to play an important role (Brent and Melhem 2008).

Cognitive, behavioral, and emotional vulnerabilities may mediate the association between the distal risk factors noted above (e.g., childhood sexual abuse) and later self-injury. Both SAs and NSSI may serve as maladaptive coping tools that yield either temporary or permanent (in the case of completed suicide) avoidance of or solutions to perceived stressors, psychological pain, and physiological arousal. Furthermore, both are often reinforced via desired changes in emotions, physiology, and/or the social environment (e.g., Goldston 2004; Klonsky 2007; Nock 2010; Spirito and Esposito-Smythers 2006).

Relationship and Clinical Course of Suicidal and NSSI Behaviors With SUD

Empirical Support

SUDs have been associated with both SAs and NSSI among adolescents. In a review conducted by Esposito-Smythers and Spirito (2004), rates of alcohol and/or cannabis use disorders among adolescents who attempted suicide ranged from 27% to 50%. The presence of an alcohol use disorder and/or other SUD was associated with a threefold to sixfold increase in SAs. Differences in the age of those in the sample, clinical setting (inpatient vs. outpatient), and assessment method (research diagnostic interview vs. clinical interview) may account for differences across studies (Esposito-Smythers and Spirito 2004).

More recent cross-sectional studies have also found an association between substance use and SAs across community-based and clinical samples. In a nationally representative U.S. sample of 6,438 adolescents,

Nock et al. (2013) found that rates of SUDs (alcohol and illicit drug abuse) were significantly elevated among adolescents with a history of a SA when compared to those without a history of a SA. In a national sample of 3,005 Mexican adolescents, Miller et al. (2011) found that those with alcohol and drug use had a greater likelihood of SAs than adolescents with no substance use, even after controlling for comorbid psychiatric disorders. In a community-based sample of 4,175 adolescents followed over the course of a year, Roberts et al. (2010) found that marijuana use significantly increased the risk of first incidence of a SA (odds ratio [OR]=4.8), even after controlling for the effects of other significant predictors (such as caregiver SAs). In a sample of 1,723 incarcerated youths, Freedenthal et al. (2007) reported that inhalant use, abuse, and dependence were associated with increased risk for a SA, after controlling for the effects of demographic variables, psychiatric symptoms, and trauma history. In a sample of 141 Finnish adolescent patients in a psychiatric hospital diagnosed with conduct disorder, alcohol dependence increased the risk for SAs in females (OR=3.8) and males (OR=9.8) (Ilomäki et al. 2007). Only one published study did not find a relationship between substance use and SAs. In a sample of 289 incarcerated adolescents, a history of alcohol, marijuana, or hard drug use prior to incarceration differentiated youths with versus youths without a history of a SA (Penn et al. 2003).

Some evidence suggests that earlier onset of alcohol and other substance use may increase risk for SAs. In a sample of 31,953 middle and high school students, after controlling for multiple covariates, Swahn and Bossarte (2007) found that preadolescent onset of alcohol use (initiation before age 13) was associated with an increased likelihood of SAs (OR=1.32) relative to adolescent onset (initiation after age 13). Similar results were found in a study conducted with 856 seventh-grade students (Swahn et al. 2008), as well as in a sample of 1,643 adolescents with a history of major depression (Bossarte and Swahn 2011). One study conducted with 503 adolescents with SUDs also found that males who made a SA had a significantly earlier age at onset of alcohol use disorder than did males without this history (Kelly et al. 2004). With regard to other drugs, Wilcox and Anthony (2004) found that early-onset (initiation before age 16) cannabis use and inhalant use were associated with a modest increase in the risk for SAs in a sample of 2,311 adolescents followed into adulthood.

Adolescents with heavier alcohol and drug use may be at particularly high risk for SAs. In a sample of 32,217 middle and high school students, Aseltine et al. (2009) found that heavy episodic drinking was associated with an increased risk for a SA (OR=1.78), after controlling for depressive symptoms. Similarly, Schilling et al. (2009) found that heavy episodic drinking was associated with increased risk for SAs in a sample of 31,953 adolescents, after controlling for demographics, depressive symptoms, and suicidal ideation. Research also suggests that the relationship between substance use and SAs may be stronger for adolescents with more severe substance use (harder drugs, higher lifetime number of substances used) (Wong et al. 2013). More severe substance use may also increase risk for multiple SAs (Pena et al. 2012).

In contrast, many studies also suggest that the relationship between substance use, particularly alcohol use, and SAs is no longer significant after accounting for covariates. In a cross-sectional sample of 2,090 Canadian youths ages 12–13, Afifi et al. (2007) found that alcohol and marijuana use were associated with SAs among males and females in bivariate analyses. However, in adjusted models that controlled for numerous covariates (e.g., multiple health risk behaviors, depressive symptoms, emotional/anxiety symptoms, physical aggression), only marijuana use remained statistically associated with SAs among adolescent males, and no association between alcohol or marijuana use remained for females. Wong et al. (2013) examined the relationship between adolescent substance use and SAs (those that did and did not require medical attention) in a sample of 73,183 high school students. Alcohol and nine other substances had significant bivariate associations with SAs. After controlling for multiple covariates (e.g., sociodemographic variables, interpersonal violence, depressive symptoms, eating disorder symptoms, sexual intercourse), the relationship between alcohol use and SAs that required medical attention was reduced to nonsignificance, although other associations remained. In a longitudinal study that followed 180 adolescents for up to 13 years after psychiatric hospitalization, Goldston et al. (2009) found that SUDs predicted future SAs in bivariate analyses and that this relationship strengthened as adolescents grew older. However, this association was nonsignificant in multivariate analyses. Similar results were found in a large epidemiological sample of 1,420 children and adolescents, ages 9 to 16. SUDs only predicted suicidality (ideation, plans, and/or attempts) in the presence of other mental health disorders, particularly depression, over the course of 3-month follow-up (Foley et al. 2006). These results suggest that SUDs, particularly alcohol, may primarily confer risk for a SA in the presence of other mental health symptoms.

Relatively less research has been conducted to examine the association between NSSI and substance use in adolescent populations. Most studies support an association; however, all but one used a cross-sectional design. In a cross-national community-based sample of 1,862 adolescents, substance use was found to be associated with NSSI (Giletta et al. 2012). In a school-based sample of 211 adolescents, greater substance abuse was reported by youths with than by those without a history of repeated NSSI (≥5 acts) (Howe-Martin et al. 2012). In a study conducted with 4,205 Finnish community adolescents, after adjusting for age and race, Laukkanen et al. (2009) found that the following were associated with an increased risk of past and current NSSI (self-cutting): frequent alcohol consumption, abuse of legal drugs, and cannabis use. In multivariate analyses, frequent alcohol use remained significant for past (but not current) NSSI, whereas drug abuse (legal drugs and cannabis) was associated with current and past NSSI. In a sample of 141 Finnish adolescent patients in a psychiatric hospital diagnosed with conduct disorder, alcohol dependence was associated with an increased risk for NSSI in both females (OR=3.9) and males (OR=5.3) (Ilomäki et al. 2007). In one longitudinal study, a history of alcohol use at baseline predicted NSSI at 1-year follow-up in a sample of 189 depressed adolescent outpatients (Tuisku et al. 2012).

Only a few studies failed to find a consistent association between various types of substance use and NSSI. No association was found between a lifetime history of NSSI and recent alcohol or substance use in a nonclinical sample of 114 Scottish adolescents (Brody and Carson 2012). In a clinical sample of 289 incarcerated adolescents, neither a history of alcohol nor marijuana use prior to incarceration differentiated youths with a history of NSSI from those without such a history (Penn et al. 2003).

A handful of studies that examined DSH did not differentiate between self-harm inflicted with and without suicidal intent. In a sample of 113 Swedish high school students predominantly ages 16–18 years, DSH was positively correlated with alcohol consumption (Andersson et al. 2013). In a sample of 477 Japanese students in junior high school, a significant positive correlation was found between frequency of alcohol use and DSH (self-cutting) in males and females and self-hitting among females (Izutsu et al. 2006). Haavisto et al. (2005) found that alcohol use (getting drunk at least once per week) and a history of any illicit drug use were significantly associated with increased odds of self-harm in a birth cohort of 2,348 Finnish 18-year-old males (alcohol OR=19.0; illicit drug use OR=6.3). In a sample of 2,974 Japanese junior and senior high school students, Matsumoto and Imamura (2008) found significantly more alcohol abuse and experience using illicit drugs among those with versus those without a history of DSH. After controlling for multiple covariates, De Leo and Heller (2004) found that amphetamine use was significantly associated with past-year DSH in a sample of 3,757 Australian high school students (OR=2.5).

Some evidence also indicates that the association between DSH and substance use varies by type of substance used and covariates controlled for in study analyses. In a study that included 4,431 adolescents from Belgium and 4,458 from the Netherlands, multivariate analyses suggested that the use of cannabis, but not of alcohol or hard drugs, was associated with a higher risk of DSH (Portzky et al. 2008). In a school-based sample of 1,699 adolescents in Australia, frequent alcohol use (>3 days in the past week) was associated with DSH in males and females in univariate analyses but was reduced to nonsignificance when adjusted for other variables. Weekly marijuana use was associated with DSH only in females (adjusted and unadjusted analyses) (Patton et al. 1997). Given the discrepancy in study results, particularly when covariates are controlled in analyses, research is needed to better understand the mechanisms that underlie the association between both forms of self-harm behavior and substance use disorders as well as sociodemographics that affect this association.

Theoretical Support

According to a conceptual review paper published by Goldston (2004), there are multiple reasons that suicidal behavior and SUDs may be interrelated. Many of these reasons apply equally well to NSSI. First, all three behaviors may be employed by adolescents as a means to escape and/or achieve relief from perceived insurmountable stress, consistent with the self-medication hypothesis (Khantzian 1997). Second, all three behaviors tend to co-occur with other health risk behavior among many youths, suggesting a common underlying set of traits (e.g., sensation seeking, impulsivity) or unifying syndrome, consistent with problem behavior theory (Donovan and Jessor 1985). Third, adolescents who engage in these three behaviors share many common precipitants and life experiences (e.g., psychiatric disorders, trauma history). Fourth, all three behaviors possess some addictive qualities, for at least a subset of adolescents. Repetitive NSSI, SAs, and substance use may increase in frequency and severity over time for a subset of adolescents despite associated impairment and the life-threatening nature of these behaviors. Although the possibility is not yet well studied, all three conditions may also stem in part from commonalities in altered neurobiological functioning.

Formal theories have also been offered to explain the association between self-harm and SUDs; all of these theories incorporate commonalities suggested by Goldston (2004). Most suggest that substance use typically precedes and increases risk for SAs. According to the cognitive-behavioral theory of suicide (Spirito and Esposito-Smythers 2006), adolescents who attempt suicide tend to have underlying vulnerabilities (e.g., history of trauma, psychiatric disorders) that increase the likelihood that they will experience maladaptive cognitions, behaviors, and emotional responses to stress. When vulnerable adolescents are exposed to a significant stressor (e.g., interpersonal conflict, worsening of psychiatric symptoms), they may cognitively process it in a distorted manner and experience problem-solving difficulties. This response may trigger greater cognitive distortion and emotional dysregulation, as well as eventual maladaptive coping strategies, such as substance use and NSSI. If a stressor persists or an adolescent's substance use (or other maladaptive coping behaviors such as NSSI) generates additional stressors, the adolescent's cognitive and emotional state may worsen, and he or she may contemplate suicide as a means of relief or escape from perceived intolerable and endless emotional pain. In the presence of other environmental risk factors (e.g., access to method, lack of support), the likelihood of making a SA is further heightened.

Hufford (2001) offers a simpler conceptual model for the relationship between alcohol use and SAs, with a focus on proximal and distal associations. When intoxicated, individuals may experience greater psychological distress, aggressiveness (toward self and others), and belief in their ability to attempt suicide (e.g., "alcohol will make me brave enough to attempt suicide"). Intoxication may also inhibit one's ability to use adaptive coping strategies to manage stress. Among adolescents contemplating suicide, this increase in psychological distress, aggression, and positive suicide expectancies may increase the likelihood that an adolescent will act on suicidal thoughts. When examined distally, the consequences of alcohol and substance use may be increased stress (e.g., social, academic, and/or legal problems) and mental health problems, such as depression. As these conditions worsen, a SA may be viewed as a solution to perceived insurmountable problems and emotions. Others (e.g., Goldston 2004) suggest that directionality of this association may vary across individuals (i.e., alcohol leads to a SA, SAs lead to alcohol use, or a spurious relationship exists) and that the association between substance use and suicidal behavior is complex and not fully understood.

With regard to NSSI and SUDs in particular, two theories have been offered that focus on the well-established affect regulation function of these behaviors (Klonsky 2007): the experiential avoidance model

(EAM; Chapman et al. 2006) and the emotional cascade model (ECM; Selby et al. 2008). In the EAM (Chapman et al. 2006), *experiential avoidance* is defined as "the phenomenon that occurs when a person is unwilling to remain in contact with particular private experiences (e.g., bodily sensations, emotions, thoughts, memories, images, behavioral predispositions) and takes steps to alter the form or frequency of these experiences or the contexts that occasion them, even when these forms of avoidance cause behavioral harm" (Hayes et al. 2004, p. 554). *Experiential avoidance* is considered a broader term than *emotional* or *cognitive avoidance* because the former term describes efforts to escape, avoid, or modify a wide range of internal experiences (Howe-Martin et al. 2012). In the EAM, NSSI and SUDs are situated among a broad class of maladaptive experiential avoidance behaviors that commonly co-occur (Chapman et al. 2006).

The EAM describes a cycle that exacerbates a person's reliance on maladaptive experiential avoidance behaviors, such as NSSI and substance use, as a form of emotion regulation (Chapman et al. 2006). First, a person encounters a stimulus that elicits an emotional response (e.g., shame, anger, sadness, frustration). In individuals for whom these emotions are very intense and who lack distress tolerance or other emotion regulation skills, the urge to avoid this seeming emotional torment becomes increasingly strong. Then, the person engages in NSSI and/or substance use and experiences temporary relief as he or she escapes or reduces the intensity of the unwanted emotional arousal. This behavior is negatively reinforcing, and over time, NSSI and substance use become conditioned, near-reflexive responses to unwanted emotional arousal.

According to the ECM (Selby et al. 2008), individuals who ruminate on their negative affect tend to experience an intensification of that affect and eventually engage in dysregulated behavior (e.g., NSSI, substance use) to disrupt and distract from this cascade of emotion (Selby et al. 2008, 2013). Although rumination and catastrophizing may be attempts to regulate emotions, they backfire; instead of calming negative affect, they intensify it. An individual who lacks other emotion regulation skills, and for whom less intense methods of distraction (e.g., a hot or cold shower, watching TV) prove insufficient, may then engage in a distracting behavior that evokes stronger sensations—such as NSSI or substance use—to halt the emotional cascade. Support for the ECM exists for both NSSI and substance use (Selby et al. 2008, 2013). For example, rumination is associated with an increased frequency of these behaviors, even after controlling for broader psychological distress and a deficit of adaptive emotion regulation strategies (Selby et al. 2008). Moreover, more intense rumination predicts greater levels of behavioral dysregulation a month later (Selby et al. 2008).

Addiction models have also been used to explain the etiology of NSSI. Those who engage in NSSI report symptoms consistent with substance dependence, such as tolerance, withdrawal, impairment, and craving. Self-injurers consistently demonstrate an increased pain tolerance and threshold (e.g., Franklin et al. 2012). Although they may perceive the level of physical pain at the same subjective intensity that non-self-injurers do, they are better able to *tolerate* those pain levels (Weinberg and Klonsky 2012). They may also experience the behavior as more rewarding. In a recent laboratory study, individuals with an NSSI history, compared with those with no history, reported significantly greater reductions in negative arousal after a high-intensity electrical shock, although the groups reported comparable subjective levels of self-inflicted pain (Weinberg and Klonsky 2012). Given the association between increased pain tolerance and NSSI, some researchers have conceptualized NSSI as an addictive behavior. Indeed, in a sample of hospitalized adolescents, those who engaged in repeated NSSI described qualities consistent with a dependence or addiction model, such as tolerance (frequency and/or intensity of NSSI had increased to achieve the same effect) and withdrawal (tension level reoccurred if NSSI was discontinued). These adolescents also reported continued NSSI, despite the recognition that it was harmful, and endorsed items describing NSSI as time-consuming and interfering with relationships (Nixon et al. 2002).

Adolescents who engage in self-injury also report "cravings" for NSSI. However, in a study that compared adolescents' cravings for substances and for NSSI (Victor et al. 2012), results suggested that the cravings for NSSI may be more limited and context dependent than cravings for substances. In addition, cravings for NSSI occurred almost entirely in the context of negative emotions, whereas cravings for substances occurred in a variety of contexts. This finding held even when analyses were limited to adolescents who engaged in both substance use and self-injury.

Assessment

In this section, we review important areas to cover when assessing for imminent suicide risk with an adolescent who made a SA (or is at significant risk). We also review some of the most commonly used evidence-based instruments for assessing adolescent suicidal behavior and NSSI across research and clinical settings, including a brief interview, a comprehensive interview, and a self-report instrument. For a comprehensive description of assessment guidelines and tools for youth suicidal behavior and NSSI, see King et al. (2013) and Klonsky and Lewis (2014).

When attempting to determine an adolescent's degree of risk for a future SA, the clinician should begin with an assessment of suicidal ideation and the presence of a suicide plan. If the adolescent has already made an attempt, the clinician should assess the method, intent, precipitant, and reasons for the attempt. Assessing for deterrents to suicide and hopelessness can also be helpful in determining suicide risk. The results of this assessment can be used to inform disposition and treatment planning.

Suicidal ideation precedes almost all suicidal acts. One study found that 88% of adolescents who made a SA reported prior suicidal thoughts (Lewinsohn et al. 1996). However, the degree of suicidal ideation can vary across multiple dimensions. Some adolescents ideate for long periods of time and make detailed suicide plans before attempting, whereas others act impulsively. To adequately assess for severity of suicidal ideation in an interview format, the clinician needs to ask questions to determine the frequency and duration of suicidal thoughts, to address whether suicidal thoughts have been disclosed to another person (particularly an adult), and to elicit the specificity of any suicide plans.

Although numerous instruments have been designed to assess for suicidal thoughts, the most widely used across clinical and research settings is the Suicidal Ideation Questionnaire (Reynolds 1985). It comes in two versions: junior (with 15 items for individuals in grades 7–9) and senior (with 30 items for individuals in grades 10–12). Items are rated on a Likert scale and capture the frequency and severity of suicidal thoughts over the last month. Clinical cutoff scores and critical items are offered to denote adolescents at highest risk.

Method and lethality of SAs are dictated in part by opportunity and availability. The most common methods of attempt are poisoning (overdose of medication) and superficial cutting. Use of other methods may signify greater risk for a repeat attempt and eventual completed suicide (American Academy of Child and Adolescent Psychiatry 2001). Therefore, it is important to inquire about the method of any SAs and access to suicide means (e.g., pills, razors, firearms). The clinician should clearly state that available means should be removed from the home or locked up until the suicidal episode resolves. Lethality of the act is also important to assess. This can be assessed with the Beck Lethality Scale (Beck et al. 1975), which includes separate scales that measure the medical lethality of eight methods of SAs (e.g., shooting, jumping, drug overdose). Each scale is rated from 0 (e.g., fully conscious and alert) to 10 (e.g., death) based on an examination of the adolescent's physical condition, review of medical information, and consultation with any involved mental health professionals.

Although determining method and lethality can help in making a risk assessment, it is important to note that they are not always accurate indicators of suicidal intent. Adolescents do not accurately estimate the degree of lethality associated with suicide methods and acts. Therefore, it is important for the clinician to assess intentionality of the act, including the expected outcome and the degree of planning for the attempt. Adolescents should be asked whether they made a plan, what the details of the plan were, how much time was spent in planning and preparation, whether the plan was disclosed to others, whether they believed the plan would lead to death (and if not, what would happen), whether they really wanted to die (and if not, what they did want), and whether they still feel the same way or believe things will get better with time. The measure of suicidal intent with the most empirical support with adolescents is the Suicide Intent Scale (SIS; Beck et al. 1974); this is a 15-item interview that assesses behavior before and during the most recent SA, including circumstances surrounding the attempt, potential lethality, expectations of rescue, purpose of the attempt, impulsivity, and reaction to the attempt. A self-report version is also available.

The precipitant and reasons for the SA are also important to assess. The most commonly reported precipitants among a sample of adolescents who made a medically serious SA included the end of a relationship (24%) and other interpersonal problems (26%), such as conflict with friends and family members (Beautrais et al. 1997). Although these are seemingly common and transient stressors, they may tip the adolescent "over the edge" in the presence of other stressors and risk factors for suicide, and thus their impact should not be underestimated. Relatedly, the clinician should also determine whether the precipitating stressor has been resolved and the adolescent can avoid similar situations in the future. If not, the adolescent may remain at heightened risk for SAs.

Two additional areas that may help a clinician to determine degree of suicide risk are the perceived presence of deterrents to suicide and the degree of hopelessness. The Brief Reasons for Living Inventory for Adolescents (BRFL-A; Osman et al. 1996) inventory is a 32-item self-report measure that assesses an individual's various reasons for living and attitudes about living versus committing suicide. The BRFL-A includes subscales for family alliance, suicide-related concerns, self-acceptance, peer-acceptance and support, and future optimism. The Hopelessness Scale for Children (Kazdin et al. 1983) is also widely used; it is a 17-item instrument that captures feelings about the future, loss of motivation, and future expectations. Adolescents with no or few reasons for living and greater hopelessness may be at greater risk for a future SA.

A number of well-validated and comprehensive instruments have been used across clinical and research settings to assess for the presence and severity of adolescents' SAs and NSSI. Two commonly used interviews are the Columbia-Suicide Severity Rating Scale (C-SSRS; Posner et al. 2011) and the Self-Injurious Thoughts and Behaviors Interview (SITBI; Nock et al. 2007). The C-SSRS is a very brief interview that assesses suicidal ideation, suicidal behavior (actual, aborted, and interrupted attempts), and preparatory acts or behavior related to a SA. It also inquires about the presence of NSSI. It is available in lifetime, current (last 6 months), and recent (since last visit) versions.

The SITBI is a structured interview that includes five modules assessing the presence, frequency, and characteristics of five types of self-injurious thoughts and behaviors: suicidal ideation, suicidal plans, suicidal gestures, SAs (including aborted and interrupted), and NSSI. Each module begins with a screening question about the lifetime presence of a self-injurious thought or behavior, followed by items that measure age at onset, recent thoughts and behaviors, severity of thoughts and behaviors, probability of future behavior, and precipitants and functions of the behavior. The SITBI is available in long and short forms.

A commonly used self-report measure of SAs and NSSI that has been well validated with adolescents is the Self-Harm Behavior Questionnaire (Gutierrez et al. 2001). This 32-item instrument assesses suicidal ideation, SAs, and suicide gestures, as well as risk-taking behaviors and NSSI. It assesses for the frequency, method, age at onset, need for medical attention, age at most recent episode, disclosure to others, and precipitants.

Intervention

The literature is scant on integrated interventions for adolescent self-harm (SAs and/or NSSI) and SUDs. Only cognitive-behavioral therapy (CBT) has demonstrated some initial promise in the context of randomized clinical trials with adolescents. Specifically, two randomized pilot trials have examined the efficacy of interventions that address both SAs and SUDs; both trials integrated cognitive-behavioral and motivational enhancement techniques. In a study conducted by Esposito-Smythers et al. (2011), an integrated CBT (I-CBT) was compared to enhanced treatment as usual (E-TAU) in the community in a randomized clinical trial with 40 adolescents with co-occurring suicidality (75% with a SA and 25% with significant suicidal ideation) and SUDs (alcohol and/or cannabis use disorder). Participants in the I-CBT condition attended 6 months of weekly sessions (acute treatment), 3 months of biweekly sessions (continuation treatment), and then 3 monthly sessions (maintenance treatment). This protocol included individual, parent training, and family sessions that were provided by two therapists (an adolescent therapist and parent/family therapist). Participants in the I-CBT and E-TAU conditions were also provided with case management and medication management (as needed) with the same board-certified child psychiatrist. Compared with adolescents randomized to E-TAU, those in the I-CBT condition reported fewer SAs, psychiatric hospitalizations, emergency department visits, heavy drinking days, and days of cannabis use over the course of the 18 months. I-CBT and E-TAU showed comparable reductions in suicidal ideation and number of drinking days. This protocol (with a few additional sessions) is currently being tested in a larger randomized clinical trial (grant R01MH097703 from the National Institute of Mental Health) for depressed adolescents psychiatrically evaluated for inpatient or partial hospitalization due to suicide risk who also have made a recent SA, have an SUD, and/or engage in NSSI.

Goldston et al. (2011) tested a CBT relapse prevention (CBT-RP) program for adolescents and young adults (ages 13–20) with co-occurring depression, a SA (or recent plan), and SUD (alcohol and/or cannabis). Rather than being a stand-alone intervention, CBT-RP was designed to augment standard care, with the goal of improving outcomes typically obtained in the community. CBT-RP included a 3-month acute treatment phase (sessions attended weekly) and a 3-month continuation phase (sessions attended weekly to biweekly). One therapist delivered individual, parent, and family sessions. Thirteen adolescents were randomly assigned to CBT-RP+TAU or TAU alone. Although no difference in numbers of SAs was found between groups (only one in each group), the rate of change in suicidal ideation and depressive symptoms (measuring change from baseline to midpoint and then from midpoint to treatment end) was greater in the CBT-RP+TAU condition than in TAU alone. For drinking and marijuana use days, those undergoing TAU, compared with those undergoing CBT-RP+TAU, reported a greater rate of improvement between baseline and midpoint. However, between midpoint and study end, CBT-RP showed a greater rate of improvement in marijuana use days; there were no differences in drinking days. Five of six participants in each group drank 0 or 1 day during the 30 days prior to the study end. Of note, differences in favor of CBT-RP+TAU were achieved despite the fact that those in TAU alone received higher levels of mental health and substance use services (psychiatric hospitalization, intensive substance abuse services, partial day hospital, in-home family services, residential home placement, etc.) (more than 65%) than in the CBT-RP+TAU condition (fewer than 20%).

Although dialectical behavior therapy (DBT) has not yet been explored with adolescents with co-occurring self-harm and SUDs, DBT may hold promise. Linehan and colleagues have examined the effects of DBT on adults with both self-harm behavior (SAs and/or NSSI experienced in the context of borderline personality disorder) and SUDs in randomized clinical trials. When compared to TAU (Linehan et al. 1999) and comprehensive validation therapy plus a 12-step program (Linehan et al. 2002) in pilot trials with substance-dependent women, DBT was associated with greater reductions in substance use and comparable reductions in self-harm. In a larger trial conducted with 101 adults with borderline personality disorder, DBT was associated with higher SUD remission rates, more self-reported days of abstinence from drugs and alcohol, and fewer SAs by 24-month follow-up relative to non–behavioral therapy provided by community-based psychotherapy experts (Harned et al. 2008). Similar to CBT (Taylor et al. 2011), DBT has also shown promise in reducing self-harm (SAs and/or NSSI) in quasi-experimental and open pilot trials with adolescents (e.g., Fischer and Peterson 2014; Fleischhaker et al. 2011).

Summary and Future Directions

As presented in this chapter, a fair amount of research has been done to support an association between adolescent SAs, NSSI, and substance use. However, the nature of this relationship is complex, is poorly understood, and varies across studies. Moreover, the large majority of research in this area is cross-sectional in nature. There is a clear need for longitudinal, prospective studies that examine the development of SAs, NSSI, and SUDs. Longitudinal studies may yield particularly informative data if they assess and analyze potential mediators and moderators of the links between SUDs and self-harm in a longitudinal fashion. To potentially maximize knowledge gained, it would be of particular interest to focus on developmental time points characterized by significant biological, cognitive, and social shifts and reorganization. Developmental transition periods are known to induce significant stress and thus increase risk for maladaptive coping behaviors. Examples include the transition from elementary to middle school, middle school to high school, and high school to college. These naturalistic, ecologically valid time points may represent ideal times not only to study the emergence of SAs, NSSI, and SUDs but also to focus prevention efforts for vulnerable youth, such as those with a history of mental health problems or trauma.

Further testing of integrated cognitive-behavioral protocols for adolescent self-harm (SAs and NSSI), as well as other potentially promising therapies such as DBT, is also sorely needed. By addressing both self-harm and SUDs in one protocol, it is possible to closely monitor both conditions, obtain an understanding of their functional relationship for each individual adolescent, and devise treatment plans accordingly. Repeated practice with a core set of skills to address both conditions over an extended time interval may be necessary to bring about lasting change in self-harm behavior and substance use. Integrated protocols should include skill instruction and repeated practice for adolescents and parents alike to address intra-individual factors as well as interpersonal and contextual factors that maintain these high-risk behaviors. Moreover, the use of a consistent theoretical conceptualization and therapeutic orientation to address both self-harm behaviors and SUDs will result in a simpler treatment plan and thus increase engagement, which may result in greater practice, mastery, and generalization of therapeutic skill.

Although data are scant, there is some evidence that effective intervention for adolescents with co-occurring self-inflicted injury and SUDs may require an active skills-based approach that incorporates individual and family work to simultaneously address both conditions. Much more research is needed to understand the origin, maintenance, and effective treatment of co-occurring suicidal behavior, NSSI, and SUDs.

KEY POINTS

- Suicidal behavior and nonsuicidal self-injury commonly co-occur among adolescents.

- Substance abuse is associated with suicidal behavior and non-suicidal self-injury, although this relationship may be accounted for, in part, by co-occurring mental health symptoms and other common factors.

- Leading theories suggest that substances, suicidal behavior, and nonsuicidal self-injury may all be used to escape negative affect and significant distress, among other reasons.

- Suicidal behavior and nonsuicidal self-injury should be assessed with empirically validated assessment instruments, many of which are free and widely available.

- Cognitive-behavioral and dialectical behavior therapies show the greatest promise to date in reducing substance use and self-harm (suicidal behavior and/or nonsuicidal self-injury) among individuals who present with both conditions.

References

Afifi TO, Cox BJ, Katz LY: The associations between health risk behaviours and suicidal ideation and attempts in a nationally representative sample of young adolescents. Can J Psychiatry 52(10):666–674, 2007 18020114

American Academy of Child and Adolescent Psychiatry: Practice parameter for the assessment and treatment of children and adolescents with suicidal behavior. J Am Acad Child Adolesc Psychiatry 40(7 suppl):24S–51S, 2001 11434483

American Psychiatric Association: Diagnostic and Statistical Manual of Mental Disorders, 5th Edition. Arlington, VA, American Psychiatric Association, 2013

Andersson MJE, Tanna H, Nordin S: Self-image in adolescents with deliberate self-harm behavior. Psych J 2(3):209–216, 2013

Andover MS, Gibb BE: Non-suicidal self-injury, attempted suicide, and suicidal intent among psychiatric inpatients. Psychiatry Res 178(1):101–105, 2010 20444506

Asarnow JR, Porta G, Spirito A, et al: Suicide attempts and nonsuicidal self-injury in the treatment of resistant depression in adolescents: findings from the TORDIA study. J Am Acad Child Adolesc Psychiatry 50(8):772–781, 2011 21784297

Aseltine RH Jr, Schilling EA, James A, et al: Age variability in the association between heavy episodic drinking and adolescent suicide attempts: findings from a large-scale, school-based screening program. J Am Acad Child Adolesc Psychiatry 48(3):262–270, 2009 19182691

Beautrais AL, Joyce PR, Mulder RT: Precipitating factors and life events in serious suicide attempts among youths aged 13 through 24 years. J Am Acad Child Adolesc Psychiatry 36(11):1543–1551, 1997 9394939

Beck AT, Schuyler D, Herman I: Development of suicidal intent scales, in The Prediction of Suicide. Edited by Beck AT, Resnick H, Lettieri D. Bowie, MD, Charles Press, 1974, pp 45–56

Beck AT, Beck R, Kovacs M: Classification of suicidal behaviors, I: quantifying intent and medical lethality. Am J Psychiatry 132(3):285–287, 1975 1115273

Bossarte RM, Swahn MH: The associations between early alcohol use and suicide attempts among adolescents with a history of major depression. Addict Behav 36(5):532–535, 2011 21315518

Brent DA, Melhem N: Familial transmission of suicidal behavior. Psychiatr Clin North Am 31(2):157–177, 2008 18439442

Brody S, Carson CM: Brief report: self-harm is associated with immature defense mechanisms but not substance use in a nonclinical Scottish adolescent sample. J Adolesc 35(3):765–767, 2012 21955549

Chapman AL, Gratz KL, Brown MZ: Solving the puzzle of deliberate self-harm: the experiential avoidance model. Behav Res Ther 44(3):371–394, 2006 16446150

De Leo D, Heller TS: Who are the kids who self-harm? An Australian self-report school survey. Med J Aust 181(3):140–144, 2004 15287831

Donovan JE, Jessor R: Structure of problem behavior in adolescence and young adulthood. J Consult Clin Psychol 53(6):890–904, 1985 4086689

Esposito-Smythers C, Spirito A: Adolescent substance use and suicidal behavior: a review with implications for treatment research. Alcohol Clin Exp Res 28(5 suppl):77S–88S, 2004 15166639

Esposito-Smythers C, Spirito A, Kahler CW, et al: Treatment of co-occurring substance abuse and suicidality among adolescents: a randomized trial. J Consult Clin Psychol 79(6):728–739, 2011 22004303

Esposito-Smythers C, Weismoore J, Zimmermann RP, et al: Suicidal behaviors among children and adolescents, in The Oxford Handbook of Suicide and Self-Injury. Edited by Nock MK. New York, Oxford University Press, 2014 pp 61–81

Fischer S, Peterson C: Dialectical behavior therapy for adolescent binge eating, purging, suicidal behavior, and non-suicidal self-injury: a pilot study. Psychotherapy (Chic) Apr 28, 2014 24773094 [Epub ahead of print]

Fleischhaker C, Böhme R, Sixt B, et al: Dialectical behavioral therapy for adolescents (DBT-A): a clinical trial for patients with suicidal and self-injurious behavior and borderline symptoms with a one-year follow-up. Child Adolesc Psychiatry Ment Health 5(1):3, 2011 21276211

Foley DL, Goldston DB, Costello EJ, et al: Proximal psychiatric risk factors for suicidality in youth: the Great Smoky Mountains Study. Arch Gen Psychiatry 63(9):1017–1024, 2006 16953004

Franklin JC, Aaron RV, Arthur MS, et al: Nonsuicidal self-injury and diminished pain perception: the role of emotion dysregulation. Compr Psychiatry 53(6):691–700, 2012 22208846

Freedenthal S, Vaughn MG, Jenson JM, et al: Inhalant use and suicidality among incarcerated youth. Drug Alcohol Depend 90(1):81–88, 2007 17433572

Giletta M, Scholte RH, Engels RC, et al: Adolescent non-suicidal self-injury: a cross-national study of community samples from Italy, the Netherlands and the United States. Psychiatry Res 197(1–2):66–72, 2012 22436348

Goldston DB: Conceptual issues in understanding the relationship between suicidal behavior and substance use during adolescence. Drug Alcohol Depend 76(suppl):S79–S91, 2004 15555819

Goldston DB, Daniel SS, Erkanli A, et al: Psychiatric diagnoses as contemporaneous risk factors for suicide attempts among adolescents and young adults: developmental changes. J Consult Clin Psychol 77(2):281–290, 2009 19309187

Goldston D, Wells K, Curry J, et al: Relapse prevention for suicidal adolescents with depression and substance abuse. Paper presented at the annual meeting of the American Association of Suicidology, Portland, OR, April 2011

Gratz KL, Latzman RD, Young J, et al: Deliberate self-harm among underserved adolescents: the moderating roles of gender, race, and school-level and association with borderline personality features. Personal Disord 3(1):39–54, 2012 22448860

Grøholt B, Ekeberg O, Wichstrøm L, et al: Suicide among children and younger and older adolescents in Norway: a comparative study. J Am Acad Child Adolesc Psychiatry 37(5):473–481, 1998 9585647

Guerry JD, Prinstein MJ: Longitudinal prediction of adolescent nonsuicidal self-injury: examination of a cognitive vulnerability stress model. J Clin Child Adolesc Psychol 39(1):77–89, 2010 20390800

Gutierrez PM, Osman A, Barrios FX, et al: Development and initial validation of the Self-Harm Behavior Questionnaire. J Pers Assess 77(3):475–490, 2001 11781034

Haavisto A, Sourander A, Multimäki P, et al: Factors associated with ideation and acts of deliberate self-harm among 18-year-old boys: a prospective 10-year follow-up study. Soc Psychiatry Psychiatr Epidemiol 40(11):912–921, 2005 16245189

Hamza CA, Stewart SL, Willoughby T: Examining the link between nonsuicidal self-injury and suicidal behavior: a review of the literature and an integrated model. Clin Psychol Rev 32(6):482–495, 2012 22717336

Harned MS, Chapman AL, Dexter-Mazza ET, et al: Treating co-occurring Axis I disorders in recurrently suicidal women with borderline personality disorder: a 2-year randomized trial of dialectical behavior therapy versus community treatment by experts. J Consult Clin Psychol 76(6):1068–1075, 2008 19045974

Hawton K, Harriss L: The changing gender ratio in occurrence of deliberate self-harm across the lifecycle. Crisis 29(1):4–10, 2008 18389640

Hayes SC, Strosahl K, Wilson KG, et al: Measuring experiential avoidance: a preliminary test of a working model. Psychol Rec 54(4):553–578, 2004

Howe-Martin LS, Murrell AR, Guarnaccia CA: Repetitive nonsuicidal self-injury as experiential avoidance among a community sample of adolescents. J Clin Psychol 68(7):809–829, 2012 22589002

Hufford MR: Alcohol and suicidal behavior. Clin Psychol Rev 21(5):797–811, 2001 11434231

Ilomäki E, Räsänen P, Viilo K, et al: Suicidal behavior among adolescents with conduct disorder—the role of alcohol dependence. Psychiatry Res 150(3):305–311, 2007 17321598

Izutsu T, Shimotsu S, Matsumoto T, et al: Deliberate self-harm and childhood hyperactivity in junior high school students. Eur Child Adolesc Psychiatry 15(3):172–176, 2006 16447027

Jacobson CM, Gould M: The epidemiology and phenomenology of non-suicidal self-injurious behavior among adolescents: a critical review of the literature. Arch Suicide Res 11(2):129–147, 2007 17453692

Jacobson CM, Muehlenkamp JJ, Miller AL, et al: Psychiatric impairment among adolescents engaging in different types of deliberate self-harm. J Clin Child Adolesc Psychol 37(2):363–375, 2008 18470773

Kann L, Kinchen S, Shanklin SL, et al: Youth risk behavior surveillance—United States, 2013. MMWR Surveill Summ 63 (suppl 4):1–168, 2014 24918634

Kazdin AE, French NH, Unis AS, et al: Hopelessness, depression, and suicidal intent among psychiatrically disturbed inpatient children. J Consult Clin Psychol 51(4):504–510, 1983 6619356

Kelly TM, Cornelius JR, Clark DB: Psychiatric disorders and attempted suicide among adolescents with substance use disorders. Drug Alcohol Depend 73(1):87–97, 2004 14687963

Khantzian EJ: The self-medication hypothesis of substance use disorders: a reconsideration and recent applications. Harv Rev Psychiatry 4(5):231–244, 1997 9385000

King CA, Ewell-Foster C, Rogalski KM: Teen Suicide Risk: A Practitioner Guide to Screening, Assessment, and Management. New York, Guilford, 2013

Klonsky ED: The functions of deliberate self-injury: a review of the evidence. Clin Psychol Rev 27(2):226–239, 2007 17014942

Klonsky ED, Lewis SP: Assessment of non-suicidal self-injury, in The Oxford Handbook of Suicide and Self-Injury. Edited by Nock MK. New York, Oxford University Press, 2014, pp 337–354

Laukkanen E, Rissanen ML, Honkalampi K, et al: The prevalence of self-cutting and other self-harm among 13- to 18-year-old Finnish adolescents. Soc Psychiatry Psychiatr Epidemiol 44(1):23–28, 2009 18604615

Lewinsohn PM, Rohde P, Seeley JR: Adolescent suicidal ideation and attempts: prevalence, risk factors, and clinical implications. Clinical Psychology: Science and Practice 3(1):25–46, 1996

Linehan MM, Schmidt H III, Dimeff LA, et al: Dialectical behavior therapy for patients with borderline personality disorder and drug-dependence. Am J Addict 8(4):279–292, 1999 10598211

Linehan MM, Dimeff LA, Reynolds SK, et al: Dialectical behavior therapy versus comprehensive validation therapy plus 12-step for the treatment of opioid dependent women meeting criteria for borderline personality disorder. Drug Alcohol Depend 67(1):13–26, 2002 12062776

Lipschitz DS, Winegar RK, Nicolaou AL, et al: Perceived abuse and neglect as risk factors for suicidal behavior in adolescent inpatients. J Nerv Ment Dis 187(1):32–39, 1999 9952251

Lloyd-Richardson EE, Perrine N, Dierker L, et al: Characteristics and functions of non-suicidal self-injury in a community sample of adolescents. Psychol Med 37(8):1183–1192, 2007 17349105

Matsumoto T, Imamura F: Self-injury in Japanese junior and senior high-school students: prevalence and association with substance use. Psychiatry Clin Neurosci 62(1):123–125, 2008 18289152

Miller M, Borges G, Orozco R, et al: Exposure to alcohol, drugs and tobacco and the risk of subsequent suicidality: findings from the Mexican Adolescent Mental Health Survey. Drug Alcohol Depend 113(2–3):110–117, 2011 20801585

Muehlenkamp JJ, Cowles ML, Gutierrez PM: Validity of the Self-Harm Behavior Questionnaire with diverse adolescents. J Psychopathol Behav Assess 32(2):236–245, 2010

Nixon MK, Cloutier PF, Aggarwal S: Affect regulation and addictive aspects of repetitive self-injury in hospitalized adolescents. J Am Acad Child Adolesc Psychiatry 41(11):1333–1341, 2002 12410076

Nock MK: Self-injury. Annu Rev Clin Psychol 6:339–363, 2010 20192787

Nock MK, Joiner TE Jr, Gordon KH, et al: Non-suicidal self-injury among adolescents: diagnostic correlates and relation to suicide attempts. Psychiatry Res 144(1):65–72, 2006 16887199

Nock MK, Holmberg EB, Photos VI, et al: Self-Injurious Thoughts and Behaviors Interview: development, reliability, and validity in an adolescent sample. Psychol Assess 19(3):309–317, 2007 17845122

Nock MK, Green JG, Hwang I, et al: Prevalence, correlates, and treatment of lifetime suicidal behavior among adolescents: results from the National Comorbidity Survey Replication Adolescent Supplement. JAMA Psychiatry 70(3):300–310, 2013 23303463

Osman A, Kopper BA, Barrios FX, et al: The Brief Reasons for Living Inventory for Adolescents (BRFL-A). J Abnorm Child Psychol 24(4):433–443, 1996 8886940

Patton GC, Harris R, Carlin JB, et al: Adolescent suicidal behaviours: a population-based study of risk. Psychol Med 27(3):715–724, 1997 9153691

Pelkonen M, Marttunen M: Child and adolescent suicide: epidemiology, risk factors, and approaches to prevention. Paediatr Drugs 5(4):243–265, 2003 12662120

Pena JB, Matthieu MM, Zayas LH, et al: Co-occurring risk behaviors among white, black, and Hispanic US high school adolescents with suicide attempts requiring medical attention, 1999–2007: implications for future prevention initiatives. Soc Psychiatry Psychiatr Epidemiol 47(1):29–42, 2012 21153018

Penn JV, Esposito CL, Schaeffer LE, et al: Suicide attempts and self-mutilative behavior in a juvenile correctional facility. J Am Acad Child Adolesc Psychiatry 42(7):762–769, 2003 12819435

Portzky G, De Wilde EJ, van Heeringen K: Deliberate self-harm in young people: differences in prevalence and risk factors between the Netherlands and Belgium. Eur Child Adolesc Psychiatry 17(3):179–186, 2008 17876500

Posner K, Brown GK, Stanley B, et al: The Columbia-Suicide Severity Rating Scale: initial validity and internal consistency findings from three multisite studies with adolescents and adults. Am J Psychiatry 168(12):1266–1277, 2011 22193671

Reynolds WM: Suicidal Ideation Questionnaire. Odessa, FL, Psychological Assessment Resources, 1985

Roberts RE, Roberts CR, Xing Y: One-year incidence of suicide attempts and associated risk and protective factors among adolescents. Arch Suicide Res 14(1):66–78, 2010 20112145

Schilling EA, Aseltine RH Jr, Glanovsky JL, et al: Adolescent alcohol use, suicidal ideation, and suicide attempts. J Adolesc Health 44(4):335–341, 2009 19306791

Selby EA, Anestis MD, Joiner TE: Understanding the relationship between emotional and behavioral dysregulation: emotional cascades. Behav Res Ther 46(5):593–611, 2008 18353278

Selby EA, Franklin J, Carson-Wong A, et al: Emotional cascades and self-injury: investigating instability of rumination and negative emotion. J Clin Psychol 69(12):1213–1227, 2013 23381733

Spirito A, Esposito-Smythers C: Addressing adolescent suicidal behavior: cognitive behavioral strategies, in Child and Adolescent Therapy: Cognitive-Behavioral Procedures, 3rd Edition. Edited by Kendall PC. New York, Guilford, 2006, pp 217–242

Swahn MH, Bossarte RM: Gender, early alcohol use, and suicide ideation and attempts: findings from the 2005 Youth Risk Behavior Survey. J Adolesc Health 41(2):175–181, 2007 17659222

Swahn MH, Bossarte RM, Sullivent EE III: Age of alcohol use initiation, suicidal behavior, and peer and dating violence victimization and perpetration among high-risk, seventh-grade adolescents. Pediatrics 121(2):297–305, 2008 18245421

Taylor LMW, Oldershaw A, Richards C, et al: Development and pilot evaluation of a manualized cognitive-behavioural treatment package for adolescent self-harm. Behav Cogn Psychother 39(5):619–625, 2011 21392417

Tuisku V, Pelkonen M, Kiviruusu O, et al: Alcohol use and psychiatric comorbid disorders predict deliberate self-harm behaviour and other suicidality among depressed adolescent outpatients in 1-year follow-up. Nord J Psychiatry 66(4):268–275, 2012 22087575

Victor SE, Glenn CR, Klonsky ED: Is non-suicidal self-injury an "addiction"? A comparison of craving in substance use and non-suicidal self-injury. Psychiatry Res 197(1–2):73–77, 2012 22401975

Weinberg A, Klonsky ED: The effects of self-injury on acute negative arousal: a laboratory simulation. Motiv Emot 36(2):242–254, 2012

Whitlock J: Self-injurious behavior in adolescents. PLoS Med 7(5):e1000240, 2010 20520850

Whitlock J, Selekman MD: Non-suicidal self-injury across the lifespan, in The Oxford Handbook of Suicide and Self-Injury. Edited by Nock MK. New York, Oxford University Press, 2014 pp. 133–151

Wilcox HC, Anthony JC: The development of suicide ideation and attempts: an epidemiologic study of first graders followed into young adulthood. Drug Alcohol Depend 76(suppl):S53–S67, 2004 15555817

Wong SS, Zhou B, Goebert D, et al: The risk of adolescent suicide across patterns of drug use: a nationally representative study of high school students in the United States from 1999 to 2009. Soc Psychiatry Psychiatr Epidemiol 48(10):1611–1620, 2013 23744443

Zanarini MC, Frankenburg FR, Hennen J, et al: The McLean Study of Adult Development (MSAD): overview and implications of the first six years of prospective follow-up. J Pers Disord 19(5):505–523, 2005 16274279

CHAPTER 11

Schizophrenia and Substance Use Disorders

Kara S. Bagot, M.D.
Robert Milin, M.D., FRCPC

In this chapter, we examine the interaction between schizophrenia/ psychotic disorders and substance use disorders (SUDs), with an emphasis on cannabis use disorder (CUD). The primary focus will be on prodrome and first-episode psychoses because these generally present during adolescence. Exploration of the following is included: epidemiology, features of comorbid disorders, etiology, clinical course, assessment, and interventions.

Epidemiology

Psychosis is a sensory perception in the absence of external stimuli. Psychotic experiences have been attributed to one or more of the following: substance use (intoxication, withdrawal, toxicity); medical conditions (metabolic, endocrine, autoimmune, infectious, neurologic, genetic); acute or chronic poisoning; side effects of medications; loss, grief, or trauma; functional nonpsychotic psychiatric illnesses; and/or a primary psychotic disorder (PPD), including schizophrenia. Psychosis is the third most disabling condition for youth, following depressive disorders and SUDs (World Health Organization 2001).

The lifetime risk of developing schizophrenia is 0.72% (McGrath et al. 2008). Males have an earlier onset of schizophrenia than females (ages 15–25 vs. 19–35 years) and greater incidence of schizophrenia than females (1.4:1) (Sara et al. 2013). *Early-onset schizophrenia* (EOS), defined as onset of schizophrenia prior to age 18, makes up approximately 18% of newly diagnosed cases of schizophrenia. *Childhood-onset schizophrenia* (COS) has an onset prior to age 13 (American Academy of Child and Adolescent Psychiatry 2000), with mean age at onset of 6.9 years and mean age at diagnosis of 9.5 years (Driver et al. 2013). The incidence of COS is estimated to be less than 0.04%, with equal incidence in boys and girls (Driver et al. 2013). Research indicates that less than 1% of those with schizophrenia experience onset prior to age 10 and approximately 5% experience onset prior to age 15 (Pakyurek et al. 2013). The increased prevalence of hallucinatory experiences during adolescence coincides with the time of greatest vulnerability to psychosis and development of addiction, which indicates likely common etiologies of these phenomena.

Clinically high-risk (CHR) or ultra-high-risk populations include those individuals who meet at least one of the following criteria: 1) exhibiting attenuated positive symptoms in the past year, 2) having a brief psychotic episode of less than 1 week's duration, 3) meeting criteria for schizotypal disorder, or 4) having a first-degree relative with a diagnosis of psychotic disorder *and* having at least a 30% decline in functioning (as measured by the Global Assessment of Functioning [GAF] scale) in the past year. The risk of progression to schizophrenia in the CHR population increases with time such that the risk is 22% at 1 year, 29% at 2 years, and 36% after 3 years (Pakyurek et al. 2013). Risk for progression to psychosis continues for up to 10 years following initial recognition of symptoms; poorer baseline functioning, baseline negative symptoms, thought disorders, and longer duration of symptoms are associated with higher risk of conversion (Nelson et al. 2013).

Symptoms of both schizophrenia and SUDs appear in adolescence, especially in males. Prevalence of substance use in adolescents is as high as 25.2% (greater for those over age 15) (Johnston et al. 2013), and approximately 11.4% of adolescents in the general population meet criteria for SUD (Merikangas et al. 2010). Although rates of use of many substances have been on the decline, cannabis use has demonstrated a steady increase, with 6.5% of adolescents using daily (Johnston et al. 2013). Approximately 13% of adolescents ages 12–17 years have used cannabis in the past year, more than 25% of whom meet criteria for CUD (Wu et al. 2014).

SUDs are one of the most common comorbidities among individuals with schizophrenia, affecting up to 50% of this population (Meister et al. 2010). The likelihood of having a comorbid SUD is estimated to be 4.6 times greater in those with schizophrenia than in the general population (Meister et al. 2010). Studies of adolescents with comorbid SUDs and psychosis have reported prevalence rates of approximately 3% for schizophrenia and 7% for schizophreniform disorder (Milin 2008). Prevalence rates of lifetime and current SUDs vary in differing clinical samples, likely because of methodological differences, sample characteristics, and country of origin. In adolescent populations with schizophrenia, the most commonly used substance is cannabis, followed by alcohol, stimulants, hallucinogens, and multiple substances (Meister et al. 2010). In CHR populations, cannabis, alcohol, and tobacco, in that order, are the most commonly abused substances (Addington et al. 2014). Younger age and male gender are consistently found to be associated with schizophrenia and comorbid SUD (Bagot et al. 2015).

Schizophrenia is the most stable diagnosis following first-episode psychosis (FEP), with up to 92% of diagnosed individuals retaining the diagnosis through subsequent assessments (Pope et al. 2013). Studies have found that up to 62% of those experiencing FEP have a lifetime history of SUD (Lambert et al. 2005). Compared with the general population, individuals with FEP are twice as likely to use substances (especially cannabis [used by up to 35% of the individuals] and alcohol); up to half of those who present for treatment abuse substances (Tucker 2009). Increased rates of substance use have also been found among those with prodromal psychotic symptoms (Korkeila et al. 2005).

Diagnosis and Features of Schizophrenia

In the transition from DSM-IV (American Psychiatric Association 1994) to DSM-5 (American Psychiatric Association 2013), not many changes were made to the criteria for the diagnosis of schizophrenia. The criteria have been refined by eliminating the note stating that only one Criterion A symptom is needed if it is either bizarre delusions or auditory hallucinations experienced as running commentary or multiple voices conversing. In DSM-5, two Criterion A symptoms are required, and a person must demonstrate at least one of three positive symptoms for a diagnosis of schizophrenia (Box 11–1). Additionally, given the poor validity and reliability of schizophrenia subtypes, they have been removed from schizophrenia classification in DSM-5.

Box 11–1.   DSM-5 Criteria for Schizophrenia

A. Two (or more) of the following, each present for a significant portion of time during a 1-month period (or less if successfully treated). At least one of these must be (1), (2), or (3):

    1. Delusions.

    2. Hallucinations.

    3. Disorganized speech (e.g., frequent derailment or incoherence).

    4. Grossly disorganized or catatonic behavior.

    5. Negative symptoms (i.e., diminished emotional expression or avolition).

B. For a significant portion of the time since the onset of the disturbance, level of functioning in one or more major areas, such as work, interpersonal relations, or self-care, is markedly below the level achieved prior to the onset (or when the onset is in childhood or adolescence, there is failure to achieve expected level of interpersonal, academic, or occupational functioning).

C. Continuous signs of the disturbance persist for at least 6 months. This 6-month period must include at least 1 month of symptoms (or less if successfully treated) that meet Criterion A (i.e., active-phase symptoms) and may include periods of prodromal or residual symptoms. During these prodromal or residual periods, the signs of the disturbance may be manifested by only negative symptoms or by two or more symptoms listed in Criterion A present in an attenuated form (e.g., odd beliefs, unusual perceptual experiences).

D. Schizoaffective disorder and depressive or bipolar disorder with psychotic features have been ruled out because either 1) no major depressive or manic episodes have occurred concurrently with the active-phase symptoms, or 2) if mood episodes have occurred during active-phase symptoms, they have been present for a minority of the total duration of the active and residual periods of the illness.

E. The disturbance is not attributable to the physiological effects of a substance (e.g., a drug of abuse, a medication) or another medical condition.

F. If there is a history of autism spectrum disorder or a communication disorder of childhood onset, the additional diagnosis of schizophrenia is made only if prominent delusions or hallucinations, in addition to the other required symptoms of schizophrenia, are also present for at least 1 month (or less if successfully treated).

Specify if:

The following course specifiers are only to be used after a 1-year duration of the disorder and if they are not in contradiction to the diagnostic course criteria.

    First episode, currently in acute episode: First manifestation of the disorder meeting the defining diagnostic symptom and time criteria. An *acute episode* is a time period in which the symptom criteria are fulfilled.

First episode, currently in partial remission: *Partial remission* is a period of time during which an improvement after a previous episode is maintained and in which the defining criteria of the disorder are only partially fulfilled.

First episode, currently in full remission: *Full remission* is a period of time after a previous episode during which no disorder-specific symptoms are present.

Multiple episodes, currently in acute episode: Multiple episodes may be determined after a minimum of two episodes (i.e., after a first episode, a remission and a minimum of one relapse).

Multiple episodes, currently in partial remission

Multiple episodes, currently in full remission

Continuous: Symptoms fulfilling the diagnostic symptom criteria of the disorder are remaining for the majority of the illness course, with subthreshold symptom periods being very brief relative to the overall course.

Unspecified

Specify if:

> **With catatonia** (refer to the criteria for catatonia associated with another mental disorder, pp. 119–120, for definition).
>
> > **Coding note:** Use additional code 293.89 (F06.1) catatonia associated with schizophrenia to indicate the presence of the comorbid catatonia.

Specify current severity:

> Severity is rated by a quantitative assessment of the primary symptoms of psychosis, including delusions, hallucinations, disorganized speech, abnormal psychomotor behavior, and negative symptoms. Each of these symptoms may be rated for its current severity (most severe in the last 7 days) on a 5-point scale ranging from 0 (not present) to 4 (present and severe). (See Clinician-Rated Dimensions of Psychosis Symptom Severity in the chapter "Assessment Measures.")
>
> **Note:** Diagnosis of schizophrenia can be made without using this severity specifier.

It remains very difficult to discern clear psychotic episodes in COS because it is normal for children to have rich, fantasy-driven experiences and to engage in imaginative play. Approximately 5% of healthy children experience psychotic symptoms (Driver et al. 2013). Additional factors that may contribute to the diagnostic difficulty are sample bias (more severe, treatment-refractory patients come to clinical attention), a process unique to childhood neurodevelopment, differential neural effects of treatment, or combinations of all aforementioned dynamics. Compared with individuals with EOS, individuals with COS have increased genetic vulnerability; tend to exhibit earlier, more insidious onset; experience greater severity of premorbid impairment (including neurodevelopmental and cytogenetic abnormalities and motor and behavioral dysregulation); and have symptoms that overlap with many other childhood/developmental disorders (e.g., language delay, stereotypies, social withdrawal) (Abidi 2013). In EOS, cognitive symptoms often precede the onset of psychotic symptoms and generally do not fluctuate; instead, they persist regardless of overall illness status (Abidi 2013). As with COS, DSM-5 criteria are applied for diagnosis in adolescents.

Etiology

Neurobiology

There is likely a bidirectional etiological relationship between SUDs and PPDs, inclusive of schizophrenia and related disorders. Increased vulnerability to SUDs among individuals with PPD may reflect the impact neurophysiological changes of psychosis have on neural circuitry involved in reward processing (Chambers et al. 2001). Additionally, a combination of heritability and exposure to environmental risk factors such as substance use may lead to abnormal neurodevelopment, exceeding the threshold needed to manifest psychosis. These relationships are even more salient in the adolescent brain, because puberty marks a critical period for neurodevelopment of brain regions associated with mood and executive function as well as motivation and addiction.

Disruption of the frontostriatal and limbic systems may also result in abnormalities in associative learning and assignment of salience and value to thoughts or events in schizophrenia (Bernacer et al. 2013). These disruptions are important because they may serve as the basis for assigning salience to irrelevant stimuli and erroneously connecting ideas and events, which leads to misperceptions and false beliefs (Bernacer et al. 2013). Additionally, changes in the hippocampal formation and frontal cortex that are seen in individuals with schizophrenia appear to enhance rewarding effects of drugs while reducing inhibitory control over substance-seeking and abuse behaviors. Dysfunction in these brain regions results in alterations in dopaminergic and glutamatergic signaling in the nucleus accumbens, which is associated with motivation (van Nimwegen et al. 2005).

Increasing evidence suggests that illicit substances may act as independent risk factors for psychosis, with the most substantive data available for cannabis, especially in adolescent, young adult, and CHR populations. Adolescence marks the stage at which dopamine sensitization likely begins (Laruelle 2000). Cannabis use triggers repeated activation of the endogenous mesolimbic dopaminergic system, which, in turn, may lead to sensitization of this system and progressive enhancement of acquired susceptibility to psychosis (Laruelle 2000). Delta-9-tetrahydrocannabinol (THC) stimulates the ventral tegmental area, leading to increased dopamine release from the nucleus accumbens and prefrontal cortex, which results in increased dopamine levels in the cerebral cortex. Therefore, exposure to high levels of THC can increase risk for psychosis via neuronal signaling disruption and changes in neurotransmitter expression in the endocannabinoid system (Pope et al. 2003). THC is associated with deficits in learning and recall, as well as both positive and negative psychotic symptoms, and patients with schizophrenia demonstrate greater sensitivity to the effects of THC, and adolescents who use cannabis demonstrate higher rates of schizophrenia (Kumra et al. 2012). Cocaine has also been shown to directly stimulate dopaminergic circuits and may play a role similar to cannabis in generation of psychotic symptoms (van Nimwegen et al. 2005).

Stimulants have also been shown to induce psychotic symptoms. Methamphetamine leads to neurodevelopmental changes that result in a paranoid syndrome similar to what is seen in schizophrenia (van Nimwegen et al. 2005). Additionally, abnormalities in activation of the dorsolateral prefrontal cortex and anterior cingulate cortex that result in cognitive deficits in methamphetamine users may contribute to the development of schizophrenia (Li et al. 2014). Finally, there is some evidence demonstrating increased dopamine levels through inhibitory action of methamphetamine on the dopamine transporter and diminished receptor density in the striatum, nucleus accumbens, and prefrontal cortex (Thirthalli and Benegal 2006). The reduction in this transporter is associated with duration of methamphetamine abuse and severity of positive symptoms.

There may also be a two-hit role in development of comorbidity in that those with schizophrenia alone and those with SUD alone demonstrate similar neurodevelopmental changes. In adolescents with schizophrenia, there is excessive pruning of dopaminergic neurons in the frontal cortex. This hypofrontality increases risk of symptoms seen in schizophrenia, including cognitive dysfunction, alterations in mood, and negative symptoms. It also triggers a reactive hyperdopaminergic mesolimbic state, which increases salience of positive symptoms, inability to switch focus to other salient stimuli, and rigidity. This state mimics that of an addicted brain, in which dopaminergic hypofrontality leads to craving and dysphoria. Adolescents are particularly susceptible to psychotic symptoms because they exhibit low mesolimbic dopamine levels at baseline (van Nimwegen et al. 2005).

There is evidence to suggest that compared to individuals with adult-onset schizophrenia, individuals with COS and EOS, and some with non-schizophrenia psychosis, demonstrate greater progressive losses of cortical gray matter volumes and increases in ventricular volumes, with the rate of loss plateauing during early adulthood (Arango et al. 2008). Decreased gray matter volume has also been found in adolescents with CUD alone (Kumra et al. 2012). This decrease is especially salient in the left superior parietal cortex, a brain region that has been shown to be instrumental in the expression of executive functioning deficits associated with psychosis.

Additionally, smaller gray matter volumes in the left thalamus have been associated with comorbid cannabis use and psychosis, as opposed to either alone, suggesting that exposure to cannabis may increase thalamic dysmorphology and dysfunction beyond that caused by psychosis alone (Kumra et al. 2012). Disruption of the thalamus's role as a relay between the basal ganglia and the cerebral cortex likely results in the cognitive processing deficits at the core of psychosis.

In contrast, studies have also found less overall dysmorphology in those with premorbid cannabis use due to FEP, which has been associated with better premorbid functioning (Cunha et al. 2013). It is likely that among those individuals with comorbid CUD and psychosis, cannabis may act as an environmental risk factor in those who have less of the dysmorphology associated with psychosis.

Genetics

COS and other psychotic disorders appear to be highly heritable. A twin study estimated heritability of 84.5% for COS, with concordance of 88.2% in monozygotic twins and 22.3% in dizygotic twins. Although the incidence of COS is extremely low, at less than 1 per 10,000 children, studies have found common polymorphisms associated with COS, including at the G72/G30 gene locus, the glutamate decarboxylase 1 gene GAD1, dysbindin, and the neuregulin 1 gene NRG1. At-risk individuals with *NRG1* or *GAD1* polymorphisms demonstrate steeper rates of gray and white matter volume loss and frontal gray matter volume loss, respectively, compared with those without these alleles. Additionally, dysbindin and G72/G30 polymorphisms are associated with older age of psychosis onset and better premorbid functioning (Asarnow and Forsyth 2013).

Adolescent cannabis abuse in populations that are biologically vulnerable to psychosis due to a catechol O-methyltransferase gene polymorphism (Val-Met substitution at codon 158) may be associated with a greater risk of development of EOS or other psychotic disorders, especially with cannabis use before age 18, because the Val allele is associated with increased levels of mesolimbic dopamine signaling and lower dopamine levels in the prefrontal cortex (Caspi et al. 2005). Changes in synaptic dopamine activity in the prefrontal cortex occur until adulthood, thus increasing potential sensitivity to environmental influences during adolescence (Lewis 1997).

Course

Schizophrenia generally courses through four phases: prodromal, acute, recovery, and residual (American Academy of Child and Adolescent Psychiatry 2000). The *prodromal phase* is characterized by bizarre behaviors and/or preoccupations, mood dysregulation, changes in motor activity, and social withdrawal/isolation, all of which lead to decrements in functioning. These changes may be sudden or insidious in onset and decline. Additionally, child and adolescent populations have been shown to exhibit more pronounced decrements in premorbid IQ during the prodromal phase (Frangou 2013). The definition of prodromal phase differs for the CHR group, some of whom may have experienced a positive symptom prior to disorder onset but do not meet criteria for full-blown PPD. Additionally, CHR populations have been shown to demonstrate greater cognitive deficits during the prodromal phase, including impairment in attention, working and verbal declarative memory, visuospatial performance, processing speed, and executive functions (Lindgren et al. 2010). At the onset of the first positive symptom, the *acute phase* begins. The first hospitalization occurs during the acute phase, generally more than a year after the onset of positive symptoms. Premorbid substance use is associated with longer duration of untreated psychosis in adolescents, with lifetime cannabis and alcohol use specifically shown to impact treatment delay (Broussard et al. 2013). The *recovery phase* follows, with a preponderance of negative symptoms and continued functional deterioration. The *residual phase* is characterized by less marked functional impairment secondary to negative symptoms and less significant positive symptoms. This phase occurs between acute episodes, but not all adolescents will experience periods of reduced symptom burden (American Academy of Child and Adolescent Psychiatry 2000). Indeed, those with COS are more likely to have more enduring negative symptoms later in the course of illness (Galderisi et al. 2002). Comorbid SUD is associated with poorer overall clinical and functional outcomes, as measured by longer and more frequent hospitalizations, treatment nonadherence, less symptom improvement between acute episodes, poorer insight into illness, poorer quality of life (including increased violence, suicidality, and victimization), and greater health burden (i.e., medical costs) (Pope et al. 2013; Riggs et al. 2008).

There is evidence of different patterns of involvement of brain regions over the course of schizophrenia and with timing of schizophrenia onset. Patients with new-onset schizophrenia do not demonstrate decrements in amygdala and temporal lobe volumes, as do patients with chronic schizophrenia (Vita et al. 2006). However, patients with FEP demonstrate ventricular enlargement and decreased brain volume and hippocampal size (Vita et al. 2006). Compared with patients with adult-onset schizophrenia, patients with EOS tend to exhibit less progressive loss of gray matter (Arango et al. 2008).

Relationship and Course With Specific SUDs

Cannabis Use

Past-year prevalence of cannabis use in adolescents ages 12–17 is estimated to be 13.4%, with more than 25% of these individuals meeting criteria for CUD (Wu et al. 2014). Evidence shows that cannabis use can precipitate transient psychotic and affective experiences and prodromal symptoms, including hallucinations, paranoia, depression, and anxiety (Andréasson et al. 1987; Stefanis et al. 2004). Initiation of cannabis use prior to age 16 appears to have a stronger effect on development of psychotic illness (McGrath et al. 2010; Moore et al. 2007). Research shows that compared with individuals who initiate use in late adolescence, children who initiate cannabis use prior to age 12 are three times more likely to have the highest 10% of scores on "psychotic experiences," and those with initiation of use between ages 12 and 15 are somewhat more likely to experience severe psychotic symptoms (Schubart et al. 2011). This association remains even after dichotomizing users into high-frequency and low-frequency users (Leeson et al. 2012). The association between early cannabis use and later psychosis appears to be more robust for CHR adolescents, who demonstrate a greater rate of conversion to functional psychosis within 1 year of prodrome compared with their non-cannabis-using counterparts (Kristensen and Cadenhead 2007). Baseline cannabis use has been shown to predict emergence of psychotic disorders in adolescents at high risk for psychosis at 4-year follow-up, especially in those with parietal lobe dysmorphology associated with cognitive deficits and delusions (Henquet et al. 2005; Kumra et al. 2012). Additionally, in those with greater genetic vulnerability plus early cannabis use, the literature demonstrates a 50% risk of developing schizophrenia when both parents are affected and an 80% risk in the second monozygotic twin if one is affected by schizophrenia (Arango et al. 2008). High-potency cannabis, with greater concentrations of THC and decreased cannabidiol content, has been found to have a robust association with later psychosis. This is likely due to the impact of THC on brain regions associated with psychosis, via CB1 receptors, and the absence of the antipsychotic effects of, and mediation of the psychogenic effects of THC by, cannabidiol (DiForti et al. 2015).

Cannabis use appears to be highly associated with symptoms that meet diagnostic criteria for schizophrenia. Studies show that cannabis use increases the probability of later psychosis twofold to sixfold, with dose-dependent increases in risk based on potency, frequency, duration, and amount of use (DiForti et al. 2015). These risk possibilities hold true for sibling pairs as well (Andréasson et al. 1987; Henquet et al. 2005; McGrath et al. 2010; Moore et al. 2007). Age at cannabis use onset of 15 years or younger has been associated with more severe hallucinations, paranoia, negative symptoms, grandiosity, and thought disorders, with greater frequency and/or duration of use increasing effect sizes of these relationships (Schubart et al. 2011; Stefanis et al. 2004). However, some studies suggest that CHR adolescents demonstrate fewer negative symptoms (Auther et al. 2012; Baeza et al. 2009). With regard to social and academic functioning, adolescents whose cannabis use predates psychosis onset tend to exhibit better social functioning and less social anhedonia than nonusers, even among CHR populations (Auther et al. 2012; Compton et al. 2011). There is diverging evidence on the impact of premorbid cannabis use on cognition, likely because of differing sample characteristics and measures of neurocognition examined in published studies. For example, one study found that CHR adolescents who met criteria for CUD demonstrated higher IQs (Auther et al. 2012), whereas another study found that cannabis users who used less frequently had higher IQs (Leeson et al. 2012). Studies do not identify any differences between cannabis users and nonusers at FEP in working memory, learning, attention, and executive functioning, but they do show that cannabis users have better ability to plan (de la Serna et al. 2010). However, the data are consistent that cannabis users function more poorly academically than nonusers, as a function of frequency of use and age at onset of use (Compton et al. 2011; Schimmelmann et al. 2012).

Lifetime CUD is associated with onset of psychosis, or prodromal symptoms, approximately 3 years earlier than those without premorbid CUD; acute presentation (daily users); earlier age at first psychiatric hospitalization; and a higher risk of relapse, with evidence of a dose-response effect (Compton et al. 2011; Galvez-Buccollini et al. 2012; Moore et al. 2007). Indeed, there is a greater association of hospital admission for psychosis with cannabis use than with use of other substances (Sara et al. 2013). Persistent cannabis users with comorbid psychotic illness have poorer medication adherence, increased rate and duration of hospital admissions for psychiatric illness, and greater illness severity (Schimmelmann et al. 2012). Of those adolescents with baseline cannabis use, over half decrease or stop use with treatment for FEP (Schimmelmann et al. 2012). Age at cannabis use onset has been shown to predict persistent cannabis use, with mean age of initiation of 14.5 years for persistent users and 17 years for those who achieve abstinence (Leeson et al. 2012). Cannabis users who achieve abstinence have been shown to have fewer and less severe positive and negative symptoms and to function better overall than persistent users, those who initiate cannabis use after psychosis, and those who never used cannabis (Baeza et al. 2009).

Stimulant Use

Limited data are available on the effects of adolescent stimulant abuse on emergence of psychotic disorders. Thus, we look to the adult literature, as presented in the following paragraphs, to evaluate possible relationships between stimulant use and schizophrenia.

The literature demonstrates a 10 times greater prevalence of cannabis and stimulant use disorders in individuals with FEP than in the general population, with more than 20% of those with comorbid psychosis abusing stimulants (Sara et al. 2013). Amphetamine-based stimulants have been shown to induce psychotic symptoms in those with psychosis, likely via enhanced dopamine activity (Sara et al. 2013). Many cases of comorbid stimulant use and psychotic disorders appear to be drug-induced psychosis or consistent with brief psychosis as opposed to schizophrenia. However, one study found a correlation between methamphetamine use and symptoms of schizophrenia, both positive (delusions and hallucinations) and negative (Srisurapanont et al. 2003). Another study demonstrated a sevenfold increased risk of schizophrenia with methamphetamine use in those with first-degree relatives with schizophrenia (Li et al. 2014); Li et al. concluded that methamphetamine use may contribute to development of schizophrenia and leads to neural changes consistent with cognitive deficits in schizophrenia. Similarly, another study demonstrated a five times greater risk of development of schizophrenia in individuals with relatives who had methamphetamine-induced psychosis. Risk increased as a function of relatives' duration of amphetamine use and severity of psychosis (Chen et al. 2005). Those with genetic vulnerability to schizophrenia may use earlier and more frequently or in greater quantities, leading to more severe psychosis.

Case reports of Japanese young adults demonstrate possible sensitization to psychosis with initiation of regular methamphetamine use, leading to delusions, paranoia, and ideas of reference. However, these youths retained their ability to function. With continued use, the individuals may experience further progression of psychosis, with development of unremitting symptoms that significantly impair functioning, including delusions with greatly diminished reality testing and insight, as well as hallucinations. Although latency between initiation of use and emergence of psychotic symptoms appears to vary greatly, the mean latency in this young adult Japanese cohort was 5 years. Ujike and Sato (2004) also found that risk of development of psychosis increased with duration of methamphetamine use beyond 6 months. Methamphetamine users who have been hospitalized for psychosis have also been shown to have a higher risk of subsequent diagnosis of schizophrenia compared with hospitalized non–substance users; the risk for methamphetamine users was similar to that for cannabis users (Callaghan et al. 2012).

Alcohol Use

Alcohol use has been shown to be prevalent among individuals with psychosis, especially among the CHR population (Addington et al. 2014; Barrowclough et al. 2014). Alcohol use disorder has been shown to negatively impact the course of psychosis but has not been shown to contribute to the potential risk of developing a psychotic disorder (Barrowclough et al. 2014). There is no evidence to suggest a temporal relationship between development of alcohol use disorder and onset of psychotic symptoms (Compton et al. 2009), although one study demonstrates that low levels of alcohol use predict conversion to psychosis in CHR youths (Buchy et al. 2014). Those youths with psychosis and concomitant alcohol abuse demonstrate poorer outcomes, including increased hospital admissions. The literature on the impact of alcohol use on psychosis remains inconclusive, with studies reporting mixed results regarding negative and positive symptoms. With regard to psychiatric symptomatology, Barrowclough et al. (2014) suggested that the most deleterious effect of alcohol on those with comorbid psychosis is its impact on depression. Finally, pre-psychosis alcohol use in adolescence may contribute to later dependence in those who develop schizophrenia (Jeanblanc et al. 2014).

Conclusions

The literature to date appears to validate the association between cannabis use and development of psychosis. The early preliminary data also demonstrate a relationship between stimulant use and psychotic symptoms; however, the strength and extent of this association has yet to be determined. For all other substances of abuse, there is insufficient evidence of resultant effect on psychosis (except alcohol use, which has no predictive value but does have a negative impact on outcome). Although the reported effects on psychotic outcomes vary by substance, there is converging evidence that substance-induced and substance-preceded psychotic episodes are not benign. Indeed, it has been shown that continued use of substances during treatment for FEP is associated with poorer treatment outcomes in relation to symptom severity and utilization of the health system (Wisdom et al. 2011).

Assessment

Identifying schizophrenia in child and adolescent populations may be difficult given the varying neurodevelopmental stages at presentation. Therefore, in individuals suspected of having psychotic symptoms, it is important to evaluate the following: 1) persistence and duration of symptoms, 2) course, 3) functional impairment (e.g., social, academic), 4) identifiable causal factors (i.e., SUD, medical illness), and 5) reality testing and insight. Symptoms that are infrequent and cause a low level of distress are often associated with retention of *insight*—thoughts that the patient can identify as coming from his or her own mind—and do not significantly impair functioning. Additionally, evaluation of youths' ability to adapt to and successfully navigate the developmental changes inherent to the period of adolescence may inform the diagnostic assessment. Late childhood and adolescence are marked by neurodevelopmental changes in cognition; therefore, adolescents should demonstrate progressive enhancement of executive functioning, memory, attention, and overall intellectual ability.

It is important to differentiate FEP in an individual with a PPD and concurrent SUD from etiology that is substance induced (i.e., substance-induced psychotic disorder [SIPD]), because treatment and outcomes may differ. Patients with SIPD have been shown to be more likely to meet criteria for substance dependence, experience visual hallucinations, and have less severe psychotic symptoms (Fraser et al. 2012). Youths with SIPD are also more likely to have a history of legal involvement, history of trauma, and higher levels and rates of SUDs (including cannabis, stimulants, and polysubstance). Features of cannabis-induced psychosis specifically include affect dysregulation, bizarre thought content and behaviors, grandiosity, hallucinations, euphoria, increased psychomotor activity, delusions, paranoia, and aggressive tendencies (Kulhalli et al. 2007). SIPD may not be benign, because youths may transition to having a PPD. As a result, medical follow-up over time is essential to determine psychosis outcome. Notably, youths with a PPD and concurrent SUD are more likely to have an immediate family history of psychosis, less insight, and lower levels of hostility and anxiety than youths with SIPD (Fraser et al. 2012).

Diagnostic clarity is further compromised in adolescents with comorbid SUD, because periods of sustained abstinence are required to make a diagnosis of schizophrenia. Indeed, the impact of ongoing substance use, and even cessation, may be great and may induce psychotic symptoms unconnected to a functional psychotic disorder. However, it has been suggested that psychotic symptoms that persist into a period of abstinence (duration based on known properties of a substance of abuse) without clinical improvement should be treated as a functional psychotic disorder (Milin and Walker 2011). Accuracy in diagnosis is essential for recommending appropriate treatment and reaching an optimal outcome. Comorbid SUD has been associated with longer duration of untreated psychosis and results in poorer long-term prognosis (Milin and Walker 2011). Clinical and sociodemographic differences between youths with SIPD and youths with a PPD may be used to aid clinical diagnosis during assessment.

Opportunistic interviews and screening during primary care visits are essential, because youths may not readily disclose substance use or psychotic symptoms and therefore may not come to the attention of mental health providers until later in the disease progression. Screening procedures should be coupled with developmentally informed brief interventions to address SUDs.

Treatment Interventions

Owing to the paucity of studies of youth PPD/FEP and comorbid SUDs, interventions for youth are often based on extrapolations from adult FEP data. Early intervention is recommended to reduce long-term disability and improve outcomes.

Interdisciplinary Treatment

For those with FEP and/or EOS, specialized early intervention services are recommended, consisting of educational support, behavioral and social skills interventions, cognitive rehabilitation, medication management, substance use programs, and psychosocial services. Importantly, integrated treatment with communication between providers is crucial to prevent gaps and inconsistencies in treatment, as well as to address the complex needs of patients with comorbidity. Psychoeducation and engaging youths and their families in all aspects of treatment are also essential to prevent noncompliance, which is common among youth populations with comorbidities. Family-focused therapy has been shown to decrease interfamily conflict through improved communication, stress management, and problem-solving skills, leading to decreased psychotic symptomatology and better social functioning (O'Brien et al. 2006). Indeed, family-focused therapy may act prophylactically on positive psychotic symptoms in CHR adolescents but, compared with family psychoeducation (which focuses on symptom prevention), family-focused therapy may have less of an effect on social and role functioning in late adolescence (Miklowitz et al. 2014).

Cognitive therapy has shown utility in helping youths traverse and address developmental challenges inherent to childhood-onset illness, including social dysfunction and neurocognitive and intellectual deficits (Abidi 2013). It appears that combining cognitive-behavioral therapy (CBT) with motivational interviewing may help to reduce substance use, decrease positive symptoms, and increase functioning for up to 18 months following treatment, with longer interventions demonstrating the greatest promise, especially among heavy users (Baker et al. 2010; Haddock et al. 2003). Brief interventions have been shown to be less effective than 10 sessions of CBT or motivational interviewing or a combination of the two (Baker et al. 2010).

In CHR youths, social cognitive remediation has been shown to be beneficial for reducing impairments in their ability to accurately perceive, interpret, and understand others in the world and what occurs in the world (Statucka and Walder 2013). In turn, these social cognitive improvements—specifically, gains in affect recognition—have been shown to lead to a better functional outcome. Improvements are apparent across modalities, including computer-based, visual materials, written vignettes, and group and individual therapy (Statucka and Walder 2013). Cognitive remediation has also been shown to improve executive and adaptive functioning in adolescents with EOS who are stabile with pharmacotherapy, to reduce caregiver burden on parents of youths with EOS, and to maintain acute gains (Puig et al. 2014). Although cognitive remediation has demonstrated efficacy in EOS and CHR youths, there are no studies demonstrating its efficacy in treating youths with either FEP or EOS with concurrent SUD.

In patients with FEP and concurrent SUDs, research demonstrates that when substance use is addressed with psychoeducation (individual, group, and family) and relapse prevention in concert with treatment for psychosis, the number of patients who actively abuse substances may decrease over the course of the first 3–18 months of treatment. CBT has been found to be as effective as psychoeducation in treating those with FEP and comorbid CUD. In a small study comparing brief individualized motivational interviewing coupled with coping and problem-solving strategies for substance use versus standard inpatient care, no difference was found between groups in postdischarge substance use. This finding indicates that brief interventions in an acute setting may not be as effective at reducing substance use as treatments of longer duration with closer follow-up in outpatient settings. Indeed, it has been proposed that interventions targeted for substance use are most effective 3–6 months following initiation of treatment for psychosis (Wisdom et al. 2011). Additionally, it is likely that the commonalities, such as the use of pharmacotherapy, interventions delivered in stages, and ongoing long-term outreach by clinicians, for psychosis treatment and substance use interventions lead to reductions in substance use. In adolescents with CUD and comorbid mental illness, preliminary evidence supports the efficacy of recovery-oriented early intervention services within public sector psychiatry (Werder 2012).

Given the association between duration of prodromal symptoms and risk of progression to psychosis in the CHR population, increased vigilance in identifying subthreshold psychotic symptoms in primary care settings, along with prompt psychiatric referral, is essential for improving outcome. Psychosocial interventions specific to realms of functioning that are often diminished in CHR populations, including neurocognitive, social cognitive, academic, employment, and familial, are crucial because these interventions may prevent or slow transition to a full-blown psychotic disorder (Nelson et al. 2013).

Pharmacotherapy

Pharmacotherapy remains the mainstay of treatment for psychotic disorders. First-generation antipsychotics (FGAs) target dopamine receptors globally, whereas second-generation antipsychotics (SGAs) indirectly target dopamine and other receptors (i.e., histaminic and adrenergic receptors). The global blockade by FGAs increases the risk of extrapyramidal side effects, including akathisia, parkinsonism, and dystonias. Children appear to be more sensitive to the extrapyramidal side effects of FGAs, with some research demonstrating permanence of these side effects in this population (Abidi 2013). The multireceptor blockade by SGAs can result in metabolic dysfunction (e.g., dyslipidemia, weight gain, hypercholesterolemia, glucose intolerance), cardiac abnormalities, sedation, and anticholinergic effects, as well as extrapyramidal side effects. FGAs such as olanzapine and risperidone are associated with significant weight gain in youths ages 8–19 years, and olanzapine is associated with lipid and liver dysfunction (Findling et al. 2010).

In patients with both psychotic and substance use disorders, there has been some evidence of worsening substance use in those treated with FGAs (Riggs et al. 2008). Some studies demonstrate greater efficacy of SGAs in the treatment of schizophrenia with comorbid SUD. However, ongoing cannabis use may negatively impact the trajectory of positive symptoms and symptoms of disorganization (i.e., thought disorders, bizarre behavior) of patients receiving risperidone and olanzapine during treatment of FEP. Additionally, compared with nonusers, patients with ongoing cannabis use have experienced greater partial response or nonresponse to SGAs (Pelayo-Terán et al. 2014). Nevertheless, there has been promising evidence for olanzapine (compared with risperidone) in reducing cannabis craving, likely due to olanzapine's low occupancy and high dissociation rates at the dopamine type 2 receptor (Machielsen et al. 2012). The greatest preliminary evidence, however, in adult populations, is for clozapine, with improvements in psychosis coupled with decrements in substance use (as found in case reports and retrospective studies for alcohol, cannabis, cocaine, and nicotine) as well as cannabis craving (Brunette et al. 2006; Green et al. 2008; Zhornitsky et al. 2010). There are also case reports of clozapine's efficacy in youth with comorbid cannabis use and treatment-refractory psychosis (Rahmani et al. 2014).

Clozapine's inhibitory effect on several receptors, including dopamine type 2 (weak) and α_2-noradrenergic receptors, may dampen the reward circuitry that underlies SUDs (Riggs et al. 2008); however, because patients taking clozapine require increased monitoring with regular laboratory work because of the potential for agranulocytosis and leukopenia, this medication is not considered first-line treatment. Despite the promising efficacy of clozapine in adults with schizophrenia and comorbid SUD, and limited evidence in adolescents, the only antipsychotics approved by the U.S. Food and Drug Administration for youths ages 13–17 are haloperidol, chlorpromazine, olanzapine, risperidone, quetiapine, and aripiprazole, with aripiprazole and olanzapine demonstrating efficacy for prodromal symptoms (Abidi 2013; Woods et al. 2003, 2007). The effect of SGAs on multiple receptors likely addresses symptoms seen in child and adolescent populations, including early cognitive dysfunction, aggression, and impulsivity. Compared with adults, children and adolescents are not as likely to maintain consistent treatment over the course of a year, and symptom response tends to plateau at about 8 weeks of treatment during the acute phase (Findling et al. 2010). Long-acting injectable risperidone has been shown to be efficacious in FEP and early phases of psychotic illness, even in young populations (Parellada 2007). Because both adolescents and patients with comorbid SUD have high rates of medication noncompliance and high relapse rates, depot medications may be of greater utility.

Preliminary evidence from a Japanese study suggests that perospirone, a newer SGA that is not available in the United States, may be effective in improving positive symptoms and delaying onset of psychosis in CHR populations (Tsujino et al. 2013). Given the properties of this multireceptor agonist/antagonist, perospirone may have the potential to positively impact positive and negative psychotic symptoms, cognitive deficits, and anxiety.

Close monitoring for unfavorable effects is warranted because the risk of adverse side effects from antipsychotic medications is higher in youth. Monotherapy and use of the lowest effective dose are recommended to decrease the risk of side effects. The literature demonstrates 90% efficacy of antipsychotic medications in youths who are compliant with treatment, with 40%–60% achieving the residual phase within the first year (Abidi 2013). More than 66% of those who remain compliant with pharmacotherapy will have positive symptoms remit and functionality improve. Approximately 50% of these youths are able to resume age-appropriate educational and social activities. Pharmacotherapy should be maintained for 2 years, with return to normal functioning prior to considering discontinuation. Only about 20% of youths will be able to successfully discontinue antipsychotics without recurrence of symptoms (Abidi 2013). In those with FEP or EOS and comorbid SUD (especially those with CUD), relapse rates are higher despite multidisciplinary treatment, even in the context of medication adherence (Malla et al. 2008).

Summary and Future Directions

Symptoms of schizophrenia and SUD typically emerge during adolescence and often have overlapping clinical presentations and confounding etiology. Different substances of abuse act on differing neurophysiological and chemical pathways, resulting in varying patterns of use and resultant clinical impact. Methodological challenges that remain in determining the etiology of psychosis in the context of SUDs have to do with significant polysubstance misuse, which hinders clinicians' ability to separate individual effects. However, cannabis has the most evidence of neurodevelopmental and clinical impact to date (Bagot et al. 2015).

Additionally, scant information is available on specific strategies to successfully address symptoms in youths with psychosis and comorbid substance use. However, there does seem to be a consensus that pharmacotherapy in combination with early psychosocial intervention decreases symptoms and increases functioning. Further research is needed on the efficacy of specific pharmacological and psychological interventions (as well as length and content of intervention and duration of effects) in the unique population of adolescents with comorbid cannabis use and primary psychotic illness.

KEY POINTS

- Substance use disorder (SUD) is one of the most common co-morbidities in individuals with psychotic disorders and portends negative outcomes.

- Symptoms of both schizophrenia and SUDs emerge in adolescence and may have similar presentations, especially in regard to cannabis use disorder (CUD).

- There is likely a bidirectional etiological relationship between SUDs and psychotic disorders that is further impacted by environmental and genetic risk factors.

- The evidence appears to validate an association between CUD and psychosis, with early preliminary evidence of a significant association between stimulant use disorders and psychosis as well.

- A combination of pharmacotherapy and psychosocial intervention appears to be the most efficacious in adolescents with comorbid SUD and psychosis.

References

Abidi S: Psychosis in children and youth: focus on early-onset schizophrenia. Pediatr Rev 34(7):296–305, quiz 305–306, 2013 23818084

Addington J, Case N, Saleem MM, et al: Substance use in clinical high risk for psychosis: a review of the literature. Early Interv Psychiatry 8(2):104–112, 2014 24224849

American Academy of Child and Adolescent Psychiatry: AACAP official action: summary of the practice parameters for the assessment and treatment of children and adolescents with schizophrenia. J Am Acad Child Adolesc Psychiatry 39(12):1580–1582, 2000 11128338

American Psychiatric Association: Diagnostic and Statistical Manual of Mental Disorders, 4th Edition. Washington, DC, American Psychiatric Association, 1994

American Psychiatric Association: Diagnostic and Statistical Manual of Mental Disorders, 5th Edition. Arlington, VA, American Psychiatric Association, 2013

Andréasson S, Allebeck P, Engström A, et al: Cannabis and schizophrenia: a longitudinal study of Swedish conscripts. Lancet 2(8574):1483–1486, 1987 2892048

Arango C, Moreno C, Martínez S, et al: Longitudinal brain changes in early onset psychosis. Schizophr Bull 34(2):341–353, 2008 18234701

Asarnow RF, Forsyth JK: Genetics of childhood-onset schizophrenia. Child Adolesc Psychiatr Clin N Am 22(4):675–687, 2013 24012080

Auther AM, McLaughlin D, Carrión RE, et al: Prospective study of cannabis use in adolescents at clinical high risk for psychosis: impact on conversion to psychosis and functional outcome. Psychol Med 42(12):2485–2497, 2012 22716931

Baeza I, Graell M, Moreno D, et al: Cannabis use in children and adolescents with first episode psychosis: influence on psychopathology and short-term outcome (CAFEPS study). Schizophr Res 113(2–3):129–137, 2009 19427172

Bagot KS, Milin R, Kaminer Y: Adolescent initiation of cannabis use and early onset psychosis. Subst Abus March 16, 2015 [Epub ahead of print]

Baker AL, Hides L, Lubman DI: Treatment of cannabis use among people with psychotic or depressive disorders: a systematic review. J Clin Psychiatry 71(3):247–254, 2010 20331929

Barrowclough C, Eisner E, Bucci S, et al: The impact of alcohol on clinical outcomes in established psychosis: a longitudinal study. Addiction 109(8):1297–1305, 2014 24773575

Bernacer J, Corlett PR, Ramachandra P, et al: Methamphetamine-induced disruption of frontostriatal reward learning signals: relation to psychotic symptoms. Am J Psychiatry 170(11):1326–1334, 2013 23732871

Broussard B, Kelley ME, Wan CR, et al: Demographic, socio-environmental, and substance-related predictors of duration of untreated psychosis (DUP). Schizophr Res 148(1–3):93–98, 2013 23746486

Brunette MF, Drake RE, Xie H, et al: Clozapine use and relapses of substance use disorder among patients with co-occurring schizophrenia and substance use disorders. Schizophr Bull 32(4):637–643, 2006 16782758

Buchy L, Perkins D, Woods SW, et al: Impact of substance use on conversion to psychosis in youth at clinical high risk of psychosis. Schizophr Res 156(2–3):277–280, 2014 24837058

Callaghan RC, Cunningham JK, Allebeck P, et al: Methamphetamine use and schizophrenia: a population-based cohort study in California. Am J Psychiatry 169(4):389–396, 2012 22193527

Caspi A, Moffitt TE, Cannon M, et al: Moderation of the effect of adolescent-onset cannabis use on adult psychosis by a functional polymorphism in the catechol-O-methyltransferase gene: longitudinal evidence of a gene X environment interaction. Biol Psychiatry 57(10):1117–1127, 2005 15866551

Chambers RA, Krystal JH, Self DW: A neurobiological basis for substance abuse comorbidity in schizophrenia. Biol Psychiatry 50(2):71–83, 2001 11526998

Chen CK, Lin SK, Sham PC, et al: Morbid risk for psychiatric disorder among the relatives of methamphetamine users with and without psychosis. Am J Med Genet B Neuropsychiatr Genet 136B(1):87–91, 2005 15892150

Compton MT, Kelley ME, Ramsay CE, et al: Association of pre-onset cannabis, alcohol, and tobacco use with age at onset of prodrome and age at onset of psychosis in first-episode patients. Am J Psychiatry 166(11):1251–1257, 2009 19797432

Compton MT, Broussard B, Ramsay CE, et al: Pre-illness cannabis use and the early course of nonaffective psychotic disorders: associations with premorbid functioning, the prodrome, and mode of onset of psychosis. Schizophr Res 126(1–3):71–76, 2011 21036542

Cunha PJ, Rosa PG, Ayres Ade M, et al: Cannabis use, cognition and brain structure in first-episode psychosis. Schizophr Res 147(2–3):209–215, 2013 23672820

de la Serna E, Mayoral M, Baeza I, et al: Cognitive functioning in children and adolescents in their first episode of psychosis: differences between previous cannabis users and nonusers. J Nerv Ment Dis 198(2):159–162, 2010 20145493

DiForti M, Marconi A, Carra E, et al: Proportion of patients in south London with first-episode psychosis attributable to use of high potency cannabis: a case-control study. Lancet Psychiatry 2(3):233–238, 2015

Driver DI, Gogtay N, Rapoport JL: Childhood onset schizophrenia and early onset schizophrenia spectrum disorders. Child Adolesc Psychiatr Clin N Am 22(4):539–555, 2013 24012072

Findling RL, Johnson JL, McClellan J, et al: Double-blind maintenance safety and effectiveness findings from the Treatment of Early Onset Schizophrenia Spectrum (TEOSS) study. J Am Acad Child Adolesc Psychiatry 49(6):583–594, quiz 632, 2010 20494268

Frangou S: Neurocognition in early onset schizophrenia. Child Adolesc Psychiatr Clin N Am 22(4):715–726, 2013 24012082

Fraser S, Hides L, Philips L, et al: Differentiating first episode substance induced and primary psychotic disorders with concurrent substance use in young people. Schizophr Res 136(1–3):110–115, 2012 22321667

Galderisi S, Maj M, Mucci A, et al: Historical, psychopathological, neurological, and neuropsychological aspects of deficit schizophrenia: a multicenter study. Am J Psychiatry 159(6):983–990, 2002 12042187

Galvez-Buccollini JA, Proal AC, Tomaselli V, et al: Association between age at onset of psychosis and age at onset of cannabis use in non-affective psychosis. Schizophr Res 139(1–3):157–160, 2012 22727454

Green AI, Noordsy DL, Brunette MF, et al: Substance abuse and schizophrenia: pharmacotherapeutic intervention. J Subst Abuse Treat 34(1):61–71, 2008 17574793

Haddock G, Barrowclough C, Tarrier N, et al: Cognitive-behavioural therapy and motivational intervention for schizophrenia and substance misuse: 18-month outcomes of a randomised controlled trial. Br J Psychiatry 183:418–426, 2003 14594917

Henquet C, Krabbendam L, Spauwen J, et al: Prospective cohort study of cannabis use, predisposition for psychosis, and psychotic symptoms in young people. BMJ 330(7481):11, 2005 15574485

Jeanblanc J, Balguerie K, Coune F, et al: Light alcohol intake during adolescence induces alcohol addiction in a neurodevelopmental model of schizophrenia. Addict Biol Apr 13, 2014 24725220 [Epub ahead of print]

Johnston LD, O'Malley PM, Bachman JG, et al: Monitoring the Future: National Survey Results on Drug Use, 1975–2013, Vol I: Secondary School Students. Ann Arbor, MI, Institute for Social Research, 2013

Korkeila JA, Svirskis T, Heinimaa M, et al: Substance abuse and related diagnoses in early psychosis. Compr Psychiatry 46(6):447–452, 2005 16275212

Kristensen K, Cadenhead KS: Cannabis abuse and risk for psychosis in a prodromal sample. Psychiatry Res 151(1–2):151–154, 2007 17383738

Kulhalli V, Isaac M, Murthy P: Cannabis-related psychosis: presentation and effect of abstinence. Indian J Psychiatry 49(4):256–261, 2007 20680137

Kumra S, Robinson P, Tambyraja R, et al: Parietal lobe volume deficits in adolescents with schizophrenia and adolescents with cannabis use disorders. J Am Acad Child Adolesc Psychiatry 51(2):171–180, 2012 22265363

Lambert M, Conus P, Lubman DI, et al: The impact of substance use disorders on clinical outcome in 643 patients with first-episode psychosis. Acta Psychiatr Scand 112(2):141–148, 2005 15992396

Laruelle M: The role of endogenous sensitization in the pathophysiology of schizophrenia: implications from recent brain imaging studies. Brain Res Brain Res Rev 31(2–3):371–384, 2000 10719165

Leeson VC, Harrison I, Ron MA, et al: The effect of cannabis use and cognitive reserve on age at onset and psychosis outcomes in first-episode schizophrenia. Schizophr Bull 38(4):873–880, 2012 21389110

Lewis DA: Development of the prefrontal cortex during adolescence: insights into vulnerable neural circuits in schizophrenia. Neuropsychopharmacology 16(6):385–398, 1997 9165494

Li H, Lu Q, Xiao E, et al: Methamphetamine enhances the development of schizophrenia in first-degree relatives of patients with schizophrenia. Can J Psychiatry 59(2):107–113, 2014 24881129

Lindgren M, Manninen M, Laajasalo T, et al: The relationship between psychotic-like symptoms and neurocognitive performance in a general adolescent psychiatric sample. Schizophr Res 123(1):77–85, 2010 20729039

Machielsen M, Beduin AS, Dekker N, et al: Differences in craving for cannabis between schizophrenia patients using risperidone, olanzapine or clozapine. J Psychopharmacol 26(1):189–195, 2012 21768161

Malla A, Norman R, Bechard-Evans L, et al: Factors influencing relapse during a 2-year follow-up of first-episode psychosis in a specialized early intervention service. Psychol Med 38(11):1585–1593, 2008 18205969

McGrath J, Saha S, Chant D, et al: Schizophrenia: a concise overview of incidence, prevalence, and mortality. Epidemiol Rev 30:67–76, 2008 18480098

McGrath J, Welham J, Scott J, et al: Association between cannabis use and psychosis-related outcomes using sibling pair analysis in a cohort of young adults. Arch Gen Psychiatry 67(5):440–447, 2010 20194820

Meister K, Burlon M, Rietschel L, et al: Dual diagnosis psychosis and substance use disorders in adolescents—part 1 [in German]. Fortschr Neurol Psychiatr 78(2):81–89, 2010 20146152

Merikangas KR, He JP, Burstein M, et al: Lifetime prevalence of mental disorders in U.S. adolescents: results from the National Comorbidity Survey Replication—Adolescent Supplement (NCS-A). J Am Acad Child Adolesc Psychiatry 49(10):980–989, 2010 20855043

Miklowitz DJ, O'Brien MP, Schlosser DA, et al: Family focused treatment for adolescents and young adults at high risk for psychosis: results of a randomized trial. J Am Acad Child Adolesc Psychiatry 53(8):848–858, 2014 25062592

Milin R: Comorbidity of Schizophrenia and Substance Use Disorders in Adolescents and Young Adults. New York, Routledge, 2008

Milin R, Walker S: Life Cycle: Adolescent Substance Abuse. Philadelphia, PA, Lippincott Williams & Wilkins, 2011

Moore TH, Zammit S, Lingford-Hughes A, et al: Cannabis use and risk of psychotic or affective mental health outcomes: a systematic review. Lancet 370(9584):319–328, 2007 17662880

Nelson B, Yuen HP, Wood SJ, et al: Long-term follow-up of a group at ultra high risk ("prodromal") for psychosis: the PACE 400 study. JAMA Psychiatry 70(8):793–802, 2013 23739772

O'Brien MP, Gordon JL, Bearden CE, et al: Positive family environment predicts improvement in symptoms and social functioning among adolescents at imminent risk for onset of psychosis. Schizophr Res 81(2–3):269–275, 2006 16309893

Pakyurek M, Yarnal R, Carter C: Treatment of psychosis in children and adolescents: a review. Adolesc Med State Art Rev 24(2):420–432, ix, 2013 24298756

Parellada E: Long-acting injectable risperidone in the treatment of schizophrenia in special patient populations. Psychopharmacol Bull 40(2):82–100, 2007 17514188

Pelayo-Terán JM, Diaz FJ, Pérez-Iglesias R, et al: Trajectories of symptom dimensions in short-term response to antipsychotic treatment in patients with a first episode of non-affective psychosis. Psychol Med 44(1):37–50, 2014 23461899

Pope HG Jr, Gruber AJ, Hudson JI, et al: Early onset cannabis use and cognitive deficits: what is the nature of the association? Drug Alcohol Depend 69(3):303–310, 2003 12633916

Pope MA, Joober R, Malla AK: Diagnostic stability of first-episode psychotic disorders and persistence of comorbid psychiatric disorders over 1 year. Can J Psychiatry 58(10):588–594, 2013 24165106

Puig O, Penadés R, Baeza I, et al: Cognitive remediation therapy in adolescents with early onset schizophrenia: a randomized controlled trial. J Am Acad Child Adolesc Psychiatry 53(8):859–868, 2014 25062593

Rahmani M, Paul S, Nguyen ML: Treatment of refractory substance-induced psychosis in adolescent males with a genetic predisposition to mental illness. Int J Adolesc Med Health 26(2):297–301, 2014 24762642

Riggs P, Levin F, Green AI, et al: Comorbid psychiatric and substance abuse disorders: recent treatment research. Subst Abus 29(3):51–63, 2008 19042206

Sara G, Burgess P, Malhi GS, et al: Differences in associations between cannabis and stimulant disorders in first admission psychosis. Schizophr Res 147(2–3):216–222, 2013 23684162

Schimmelmann BG, Conus P, Cotton S, et al: Prevalence and impact of cannabis use disorders in adolescents with early onset first episode psychosis. Eur Psychiatry 27(6):463–469, 2012 21616646

Schubart CD, van Gastel WA, Breetvelt EJ, et al: Cannabis use at a young age is associated with psychotic experiences. Psychol Med 41(6):1301–1310, 2011 20925969

Srisurapanont M, Ali R, Marsden J, et al: Psychotic symptoms in methamphetamine psychotic in-patients. Int J Neuropsychopharmacol 6(4):347–352, 2003 14604449

Statucka M, Walder DJ: Efficacy of social cognition remediation programs targeting facial affect recognition deficits in schizophrenia: a review and consideration of high-risk samples and sex differences. Psychiatry Res 206(2–3):125–139, 2013 23375627

Stefanis NC, Delespaul P, Henquet C, et al: Early adolescent cannabis exposure and positive and negative dimensions of psychosis. Addiction 99(10):1333–1341, 2004 15369572

Thirthalli J, Benegal V: Psychosis among substance users. Curr Opin Psychiatry 19(3):239–245, 2006 16612208

Tsujino N, Nemoto T, Morita K, et al: Long-term efficacy and tolerability of perospirone for young help-seeking people at clinical high risk: a preliminary open trial. Clin Psychopharmacol Neurosci 11(3):132–136, 2013 24465249

Tucker P: Substance misuse and early psychosis. Australas Psychiatry 17(4):291–294, 2009 19301164

Ujike H, Sato M: Clinical features of sensitization to methamphetamine observed in patients with methamphetamine dependence and psychosis. Ann NY Acad Sci 1025:279–287, 2004 15542728

van Nimwegen L, de Haan L, van Beveren N, et al: Adolescence, schizophrenia and drug abuse: a window of vulnerability. Acta Psychiatr Scand Suppl (427):35–42, 2005 15877720

Vita A, De Peri L, Silenzi C, et al: Brain morphology in first-episode schizophrenia: a meta-analysis of quantitative magnetic resonance imaging studies. Schizophr Res 82(1):75–88, 2006 16377156

Werder K: Addressing marijuana use as an early intervention in youth with serious mental illness. Presented at the 8th International Conference on Early Psychosis: From Neurobiology to Public Policy, San Francisco, CA, October 2012

Wisdom JP, Manuel JI, Drake RE: Substance use disorder among people with first-episode psychosis: a systematic review of course and treatment. Psychiatr Serv 62(9):1007–1012, 2011 21885577

Woods SW, Breier A, Zipursky RB, et al: Randomized trial of olanzapine versus placebo in the symptomatic acute treatment of the schizophrenic prodrome. Biol Psychiatry 54(4):453–464, 2003 12915290

Woods SW, Tully EM, Walsh BC, et al: Aripiprazole in the treatment of the psychosis prodrome: an open-label pilot study. Br J Psychiatry Suppl 51:s96–s101, 2007 18055946

World Health Organization: Mental Health: New Understanding, New Hope. The World Health Report. Geneva, Switzerland, World Health Organization, 2001

Wu LT, Brady KT, Mannelli P, et al: Cannabis use disorders are comparatively prevalent among nonwhite racial/ethnic groups and adolescents: a national study. J Psychiatr Res 50:26–35, 2014 24342767

Zhornitsky S, Rizkallah E, Pampoulova T, et al: Antipsychotic agents for the treatment of substance use disorders in patients with and without comorbid psychosis. J Clin Psychopharmacol 30(4):417–424, 2010 20631559

CHAPTER 12

Eating Disorders and Substance Use Disorders

Jessica H. Baker, Ph.D.
Lauren M. Metzger, LCSWA
Cynthia M. Bulik, Ph.D.

Eating disorders and substance use disorders (SUDs) pose a significant threat to the health of adolescents. When evaluating adolescents with either type of disorder, a clinician should complete a thorough evaluation for the other because of the significant comorbidity between the two and the associated risks that arise when both disorders are present. In addition, when evaluating adolescents with both disorders, one must consider not only common substances abused by adolescents, such as alcohol and illicit drugs, but also substances that are associated with eating disorders. Laxatives, diuretics, diet pills, emetics, unregulated supplements, and anabolic steroids are all potentially abused by individuals with eating disorders and carry significant health risks that may be amplified in those who also abuse alcohol or other drugs. Despite the serious associated risks, empirically based treatments for comorbid eating disorders and SUDs are lacking.

Diagnosis and Epidemiology of Eating Disorders

Anorexia Nervosa

In DSM-5 (American Psychiatric Association 2013), anorexia nervosa (AN) is characterized by a significantly low body weight that is below what is minimally normal or expected, fear of gaining weight, undue influence of body weight on self-evaluation, denial of seriousness of low body weight, and distorted perception of body image (Box 12–1). This definition of AN differs in two significant ways from that in DSM-IV (American Psychiatric Association 1994). First, the weight criterion for a diagnosis was "broadened" from less than 85% of ideal body weight to a weight that is less than minimally normal or expected, allowing for more clinical judgment in making a diagnosis. Second, DSM-5 dropped amenorrhea as a diagnostic criterion for AN. Amenorrhea was removed for several reasons, including that it was not relevant when diagnosing male patients or when diagnosing female patients who had not yet reached menarche or who were taking birth control and that empirical research has shown few, if any, clinical differences (e.g., symptom severity, treatment required) between females with and without amenorrhea (Attia and Roberto 2009). DSM-5 also requires that current severity be indicated when making an AN diagnosis, using severity specifiers that are based on body mass index (BMI): mild (BMI≥17), moderate (BMI=16–16.99), severe (BMI=15–15.99), or extreme (BMI<15). Clinical judgment can be used to increase the level of severity if deemed necessary based on factors such as clinical symptoms reported, need for supervision, or degree of functional impairment. *Functional impairment* can be defined as decreased ability to perform activities of daily living and social, occupational, or academic obligations. In DSM-5, two subtypes of AN remain: restricting and binge-eating/purging subtypes. Restricting AN reflects symptomatology characterized by maintaining low body weight and weight loss predominantly through dieting, fasting, and/or excessive exercise. AN binge-eating/purging subtype is characterized by recurrent episodes of binge-eating and/or purging behaviors in conjunction with low body weight.

Box 12–1.   DSM-5 Criteria for Anorexia Nervosa

A. Restriction of energy intake relative to requirements, leading to a significantly low body weight in the context of age, sex, developmental trajectory, and physical health. *Significantly low weight* is defined as a weight that is less than minimally normal or, for children and adolescents, less than that minimally expected.

B. Intense fear of gaining weight or of becoming fat, or persistent behavior that interferes with weight gain, even though at a significantly low weight.

C. Disturbance in the way in which one's body weight or shape is experienced, undue influence of body weight or shape on self-evaluation, or persistent lack of recognition of the seriousness of the current low body weight.

Coding note: The ICD-9-CM code for anorexia nervosa is **307.1,** which is assigned regardless of the subtype. The ICD-10-CM code depends on the subtype (see below).

Specify whether:

(F50.01) Restricting type: During the last 3 months, the individual has not engaged in recurrent episodes of binge eating or purging behavior (i.e., self-induced vomiting or the misuse of laxatives, diuretics, or enemas). This subtype describes presentations in which weight loss is accomplished primarily through dieting, fasting, and/or excessive exercise.

(F50.02) Binge-eating/purging type: During the last 3 months, the individual has engaged in recurrent episodes of binge eating or purging behavior (i.e., self-induced vomiting or the misuse of laxatives, diuretics, or enemas).

Specify if:

In partial remission: After full criteria for anorexia nervosa were previously met, Criterion A (low body weight) has not been met for a sustained period, but either Criterion B (intense fear of gaining weight or becoming fat or behavior that interferes with weight gain) or Criterion C (disturbances in self-perception of weight and shape) is still met.

In full remission: After full criteria for anorexia nervosa were previously met, none of the criteria have been met for a sustained period of time.

Specify current severity:

The minimum level of severity is based, for adults, on current body mass index (BMI) (see below) or, for children and adolescents, on BMI percentile. The ranges below are derived from World Health Organization categories for thinness in adults; for children and adolescents, corresponding BMI percentiles should be used. The level of severity may be increased to reflect clinical symptoms, the degree of functional disability, and the need for supervision.

Mild: BMI $\geq$ 17 kg/m^2

Moderate: BMI 16–16.99 kg/m^2

Severe: BMI 15–15.99 kg/m^2

Extreme: BMI < 15 kg/m^2

DSM-IV AN has a lifetime prevalence of approximately 0.9% for females and 0.3% for males (Hudson et al. 2007). For adolescent populations, the National Adolescent Comorbidity Survey Replication–Adolescent Supplement reported a prevalence of 0.3% for AN, with subthreshold or atypical presentations being more common (Swanson et al. 2011). The observed median age at AN onset was 12.3 years. Adolescents with AN are often depressed and experience functional impairment with friends and family compared with the functioning of their healthy peers (Stice et al. 2013). Because of the broader DSM-5 criteria, more adolescents may be diagnosed with AN who would not have previously met full criteria according to DSM-IV.

Bulimia Nervosa

Bulimia nervosa (BN) is characterized by recurrent episodes of binge eating followed by inappropriate compensatory behaviors that are meant to prevent weight gain (Box 12–2). A binge episode involves 1) eating a large quantity of food in a discrete period of time and 2) feeling a loss of control over eating. DSM-IV specified that these behaviors had to occur, on average, twice per week for 3 months and not exclusively during the course of AN. However, DSM-5 only requires this combination of behaviors to occur at least once per week for 3 months. In BN, as in AN, body weight and shape are among the most important factors that influence self-evaluation. For BN, degree of severity is based on the average number of inappropriate compensatory behavior episodes per week (and may be increased based on other symptoms and level of functional disability): mild (1–3 episodes), moderate (4–7 episodes), severe (8–13 episodes), or extreme (14 or more episodes). DSM-5 no longer includes subtypes of BN as outlined in DSM-IV.

Box 12–2. DSM-5 Criteria for Bulimia Nervosa

A. Recurrent episodes of binge eating. An episode of binge eating is characterized by both of the following:

  1. Eating, in a discrete period of time (e.g., within any 2-hour period), an amount of food that is definitely larger than what most individuals would eat in a similar period of time under similar circumstances.
  2. A sense of lack of control over eating during the episode (e.g., a feeling that one cannot stop eating or control what or how much one is eating).

B. Recurrent inappropriate compensatory behaviors in order to prevent weight gain, such as self-induced vomiting; misuse of laxatives, diuretics, or other medications; fasting; or excessive exercise.

C. The binge eating and inappropriate compensatory behaviors both occur, on average, at least once a week for 3 months.

D. Self-evaluation is unduly influenced by body shape and weight.

E. The disturbance does not occur exclusively during episodes of anorexia nervosa.

Specify if:

In partial remission: After full criteria for bulimia nervosa were previously met, some, but not all, of the criteria have been met for a sustained period of time.

In full remission: After full criteria for bulimia nervosa were previously met, none of the criteria have been met for a sustained period of time.

Specify current severity:

The minimum level of severity is based on the frequency of inappropriate compensatory behaviors (see below). The level of severity may be increased to reflect other symptoms and the degree of functional disability.

Mild: An average of 1–3 episodes of inappropriate compensatory behaviors per week.

Moderate: An average of 4–7 episodes of inappropriate compensatory behaviors per week.

Severe: An average of 8–13 episodes of inappropriate compensatory behaviors per week.

Extreme: An average of 14 or more episodes of inappropriate compensatory behaviors per week.

Reprinted from the *Diagnostic and Statistical Manual of Mental Disorders*, 5th Edition. Arlington, VA, American Psychiatric Association, 2013. Used with permission. Copyright © 2013 American Psychiatric Association.

Swanson et al. (2011) report a mean prevalence for DSM-IV BN of 1.3% for adolescent girls and 0.5% for adolescent boys across the United States. With the required frequency of binge-eating and purging behaviors decreased to once a week in DSM-5, it is also probable that an increased number of youths will be diagnosed with BN.

Binge-Eating Disorder

Previously included in DSM-IV in the eating disorder not otherwise specified category, binge-eating disorder (BED) is now recognized as a distinct eating disorder in DSM-5 (Box 12–3). It is marked by recurrent episodes of binge eating that are not associated with regular inappropriate compensatory behaviors. For a diagnosis of BED, at least three of the following criteria must be met during a binge episode: eating more rapidly than normal, eating until uncomfortably full, eating large quantities of food when not physically hungry, eating alone because of embarrassment, and feeling disgusted, depressed, or guilty after the binge.

Binge eating must occur, on average, once per week for 3 months. The frequency of weekly binge-eating episodes and degree of functional impairment determine the appropriate severity specifier: mild (1–3 episodes), moderate (4–7 episodes), severe (8–13 episodes), or extreme (14 or more episodes).

Box 12–3. DSM-5 Criteria for Binge-Eating Disorder

A. Recurrent episodes of binge eating. An episode of binge eating is characterized by both of the following:
   1. Eating, in a discrete period of time (e.g., within any 2-hour period), an amount of food that is definitely larger than what most people would eat in a similar period of time under similar circumstances.
   2. A sense of lack of control over eating during the episode (e.g., a feeling that one cannot stop eating or control what or how much one is eating).
B. The binge-eating episodes are associated with three (or more) of the following:
   1. Eating much more rapidly than normal.
   2. Eating until feeling uncomfortably full.
   3. Eating large amounts of food when not feeling physically hungry.
   4. Eating alone because of feeling embarrassed by how much one is eating.
   5. Feeling disgusted with oneself, depressed, or very guilty afterward.
C. Marked distress regarding binge eating is present.
D. The binge eating occurs, on average, at least once a week for 3 months.
E. The binge eating is not associated with the recurrent use of inappropriate compensatory behavior as in bulimia nervosa and does not occur exclusively during the course of bulimia nervosa or anorexia nervosa.
Specify if:
   In partial remission: After full criteria for binge-eating disorder were previously met, binge eating occurs at an average frequency of less than one episode per week for a sustained period of time.
   In full remission: After full criteria for binge-eating disorder were previously met, none of the criteria have been met for a sustained period of time.
Specify current severity:
The minimum level of severity is based on the frequency of episodes of binge eating (see below). The level of severity may be increased to reflect other symptoms and the degree of functional disability.
   Mild: 1–3 binge-eating episodes per week.
   Moderate: 4–7 binge-eating episodes per week.

Severe: 8–13 binge-eating episodes per week.
Extreme: 14 or more binge-eating episodes per week.

BED is more common among adults than among children and adolescents, and it still ranks as the most widespread eating disorder. According to DSM-IV, prevalence for adolescents is about 1.6% (Swanson et al. 2011), whereas according to DSM-5, BED prevalence is somewhat higher, ranging between 1.6% and 3.0% (Smink et al. 2014; Stice et al. 2013). Furthermore, there is evidence that loss-of-control eating during childhood significantly predicts threshold and subthreshold BED in adolescence (Hilbert and Brauhardt 2014; Tanofsky-Kraff et al. 2011). *Loss-of-control eating* encompasses all episodes in which there is a subjective sense that one cannot stop eating or that one feels a loss of control over eating, regardless of the amount of food actually consumed. This terminology and definition can be useful for children and adolescents given their differing energy needs and ability to quantify accurately what they are eating.

Other Specified Feeding or Eating Disorders

Constellations of symptoms that do not meet the full criteria for AN, BN, or BED are grouped in a new DSM-5 category: other specified feeding or eating disorder. Presentations of other specified feeding or eating disorder include atypical AN (significant weight loss, but weight is still in normal to above normal range), subsyndromal BN and BED (low frequency of behaviors or limited duration), purging disorder (purging behaviors not associated with binge-eating episodes), and night eating syndrome (recurrent, distressing episodes of waking in the night to eat or excessive eating after evening meals).

The DSM-IV catchall diagnosis of eating disorder not otherwise specified was the diagnosis received by a majority of individuals when presenting for eating disorder treatment. Although changes in DSM-5 were aimed to reduce the number of individuals receiving unspecified diagnoses, it is unclear yet whether other specified feeding or eating disorder will similarly become an umbrella diagnosis.

Obesity

Obesity is not classified as a psychiatric disorder. Adults (age 20 and older) are considered obese if they have a BMI greater than or equal to

30 (Centers for Disease Control and Prevention 2012). To be considered obese, children and adolescents must have a BMI at or above the 95th percentile for individuals of the same age and sex. The prevalence of obesity in childhood and adolescence is estimated at 16.9% (Ogden et al. 2012). It is also not uncommon for obese adolescents to engage in disordered eating behaviors. Binge eating in particular may be relatively common in this population and can often be associated with depression and low self-esteem (Ackard et al. 2003; Pasold et al. 2014).

Etiology of Eating Disorders

The etiology of eating disorders is not entirely clear; however, some risk factors for their development have been identified. In a comprehensive review of the literature, Jacobi et al. (2004) identified several risk factors, including gender, dieting, and general psychological disturbance/negative emotionality. Because of the large sex-related difference in the prevalence of eating disorders (especially AN and BN), being female may be one of the most potent risk factors for their development. However, this risk is nonspecific because rates of other psychological disturbances are also elevated in females. Dieting is also considered an important precursor to eating disorders. Cross-sectional studies consistently find that voluntary dieting behaviors precede the onset of an eating disorder, with approximately 70% of women with BN reporting dieting before the onset of binge eating (Pederson Mussell et al. 1997).

   Longitudinal studies provide evidence that various forms of psychopathology predate eating disorder symptoms (Jacobi et al. 2004). Most of the theories have been discussed in light of the high comorbidity observed between eating disorders and anxiety disorders and between eating disorders and affective disorders. For example, in a study by Bulik et al. (1997), women with anxiety disorder and an eating disorder—90% with AN and 94% with BN—indicated that the anxiety disorder predated the eating disorder. However, a limited number of studies have examined the chronology of eating disorder onset and other comorbid conditions in adolescents. Negative emotionality has also been identified as a nonspecific risk factor for eating disorders in adolescents (Leon et al. 1999). Other personality characteristics (e.g., novelty seeking, impulsivity) are also associated with eating disorders (for review see Cassin and von Ranson 2005), but few studies have examined a causal link.

Familial and genetic factors also play an important role in eating disorder vulnerability. Individuals who have a family member with an eating disorder are up to 11 times more likely to develop an eating disorder themselves, and twin studies indicate that approximately 40%–60% of the risk for AN, BN, and BED is accounted for by genetic factors (Trace et al. 2013). Few studies have parsed genetic factors by age at onset, but preliminary evidence suggests that genetic factors may be more important in the risk for developing eating disorders during middle adolescence through adulthood than at younger ages (Klump et al. 2007). Molecular genetic studies of eating disorders have not yet provided definitive answers about the specific genetic factors involved in eating disorder risk, in part because of low statistical power secondary to small sample sizes. However, large genome-wide association studies are currently aimed at identifying the genes involved in the etiology of eating disorders (Trace et al. 2013).

Clinical Course of Eating Disorders

Eating disorders are associated with considerable psychiatric and physical health risks. AN, BN, and BED are commonly comorbid with depression, anxiety, and SUDs (Baker et al. 2010; Kaye et al. 2004; Perez et al. 2004). AN also has the highest mortality rate of any psychiatric disorder (Chesney et al. 2014). Comorbid AN and alcohol use disorder are particularly important because there is substantial mortality in women with this comorbid presentation (Keel et al. 2003). In addition, eating disorders are associated with substantial medical complications. BN is commonly associated with electrolyte imbalances and oral, gastrointestinal, renal, and endocrine complications, whereas AN is associated with complications that include renal problems, chronic pain, irritable bowel syndrome, osteoporosis, and cardiac arrhythmias (Mehler and Krantz 2003; Mehler et al. 2004). The consequences of BED and obesity are similar and include increased risk for coronary heart disease, diabetes, metabolic syndrome, and hypertension (Bulik et al. 2002; Hudson et al. 2010).

Course of Eating Disorders and Relationship With SUDs

Adult Populations

To date, a majority of studies of comorbid eating disorders and SUDs have focused on adult populations, whereas adolescent research has often focused on broad or subthreshold definitions, related symptomatology, or treatment-seeking samples. Specifically, adult women with an eating disorder or SUD are four times more likely to develop the other disorder compared with the general population (Gadalla and Piran 2007b). A nationally representative population-based study observed that individuals with BN reported a lifetime history of 33.7% for alcohol use disorder, 22.7% for an illicit drug use disorder, and 36.8% for any SUD (Hudson et al. 2007).

A meta-analysis of studies examining the comorbidity between eating disorders and alcohol use disorders in individuals ages 10–65 years confirms a moderate association between eating disorders and SUDs. In clinical samples, a mean effect size of 0.53 was observed for BN/bulimic behaviors and of 0.06 for AN. In community samples, a mean effect size for BN/bulimic behaviors was 0.56, for AN it was 0.24, and for BED it was 0.40 (Gadalla and Piran 2007a). SUDs are also comorbid with adult BED. Approximately 24%–46% of adults with BED have a lifetime comorbidity of an SUD (Grilo et al. 2009; Javaras et al. 2008; Kessler et al. 2013). Specifically, reports observe that about 17%–20% of individuals have an alcohol use disorder and 11%–14% have an illicit drug use disorder.

Although the association between SUD and eating disorders in adults is stronger with BN and BED than with AN, SUDs do occur more frequently in women with AN than in the general population, especially in those women with the binge-eating/purging subtype of AN (Bulik et al. 2004a; Root et al. 2010). The prevalence of SUDs in adults with AN binge-eating/purging subtype appears comparable to that in adults with normal-weight BN (Bulik et al. 2004a).

Of interest, the National Epidemiologic Survey on Alcohol and Related Conditions determined that obese men and women are at decreased risk for incident alcohol abuse and drug dependence compared with their normal-weight peers (Pickering et al. 2011). At the 3-year follow-up, 8.7% of normal-weight men met an alcohol abuse diagnosis versus 3.1% of obese men, with similar results for women (3.9% vs. 2.0%). Rates of drug dependence in obese men and women were low, estimated at 0.8% for men and 0.3% for women. The mechanism for this effect is not entirely clear.

Adolescent Populations

As in adults, there is significant comorbidity between eating disorder and SUD symptomatology in youth. One large, nationally representative epidemiological study (Swanson et al. 2011), reporting combined data from male and female adolescents, observed that 9% of adolescents with AN had a lifetime history of an alcohol use disorder and 13% had an illicit drug use disorder. Among those with BN, 14% had a lifetime history of an alcohol use disorder and 20% had a lifetime history of an illicit drug use disorder, and among those with BED, 14% had a lifetime history of an alcohol use disorder and 23% had a lifetime history of an illicit drug use disorder.

In a community sample of girls ages 11–15 years, 4.64% of the sample met broad diagnostic criteria for an eating disorder, and among those with an eating disorder, 37.8% also met broad criteria for an SUD—a percentage that is significantly higher than that for girls without an eating disorder (Stice et al. 2001). In a sample of adolescent girls presenting for evaluation at an eating disorder treatment program, 5.9% met full criteria for substance abuse, with alcohol and cannabis being the most commonly abused substances (Mann et al. 2014).

Eating disorders and related symptomatology are also frequently observed in adolescents with SUDs. Of adolescent girls ages 13–17 with an SUD, 2.6% had an eating disorder (Wu et al. 2011). Arias et al. (2009) also observed that 26.4% of adolescents ages 13–18 (combined girls and boys) in treatment for an alcohol use disorder had at least one eating disorder symptom: 8.6% were underweight, 3.4% reported recurrent binge eating, and 2.9% reported purging. The number of eating disorder symptoms endorsed was associated with increased alcohol consumption, increased social and psychological problems linked to alcohol use, and an increased number of alcohol-related physical symptoms reported.

Finally, substance use is increased in adolescents with eating disorders. In the large-scale Growing Up Today Study, latent class analyses revealed latent classes resembling BN, BED, and purging disorder in girls. Classes resembling BN had the highest probability of current binge drinking, and those resembling BN and purging disorder were more likely to report current drug use (compared with classes identified as asymptomatic, exhibiting weight/shape concerns, reporting overeating, or resembling BED) (Swanson et al. 2014). BN, BED, and purging disorder classes were also predictive of later binge drinking and drug use. Similarly, a school-based sample of 4,746 adolescents (mean age 14.9 years) with threshold, subthreshold, and no eating disorder diagnosis (AN, BN, and BED) showed that substance use increased with the severity of the eating disorder classification (Ackard et al. 2011).

Analogous findings are observed in treatment-seeking samples. For example, in a sample of youths ages 12–18 with eating disorders (90% female), the lifetime prevalence of any substance use was reported to be 24.6% in adolescents with AN, 48.7% in adolescents with BN, and 28.6% in adolescents with DSM-IV eating disorder not otherwise specified (Mann et al. 2014). The most commonly used substance is alcohol, followed by cannabis, tobacco, and cocaine. Youths with BN were also more likely to use tobacco than were youths with AN, and more frequent binge-purge episodes were significantly associated with alcohol, tobacco, and cannabis use.

Empirical studies examining the comorbidity between BED and SUDs during adolescence are in their infancy; however, there is a clear relationship between binge eating and substance use (Ross and Ivis 1999; Sonneville et al. 2013). Similarly, although the relationship between obesity and substance use during adolescence has been examined, data on prevalence of the comorbidity remain somewhat sparse in comparison with data on AN and BN with comorbid substance use. Longitudinal data from two cohort studies—Identifying the Determinants of Eating and Activity and Etiology of Childhood Obesity—indicated that alcohol use around age 14 predicted decreased BMI z score at 2-year follow-up but that cigarette smoking predicted an increase in body fat at the same follow-up (Pasch et al. 2012). These findings were not bidirectional, in that body composition at age 14 did not predict subsequent substance use. Obese girls also appear to engage in more smoking, drinking, and marijuana use compared with normal-weight girls, yet this same pattern was not observed for boys (Farhat et al. 2010).

Huang et al. (2013) analyzed data from the 1979 National Longitudinal Survey of Youth and explored trajectories for adolescents based on cigarette smoking, alcohol use, marijuana use, and weight. Adolescents who were at heightened risk for alcohol use were more likely to be in the low-risk trajectory for obesity compared with adolescents who were in the low alcohol use trajectory. Cigarette smoking and marijuana use trajectories revealed the opposite when paired with the weight trajectory. High-risk use of both substances was positively associated with obesity.

Although less research has compared the comorbidity between eating disorder and SUD diagnoses in youths than in adults, the patterns of results are similar. Specifically, findings support higher rates of substance use and abuse in girls with eating disorder symptoms and vice versa; higher rates of substance use and abuse in girls with BN or bulimic symptoms than in those with AN; and an inverse association between obesity and alcohol use and abuse.

Race, Ethnicity, and Gender

A limitation in the literature on eating disorder and SUD comorbidity is the lack of data on the role of race/ethnicity and gender in risk, outcome, and clinical presentation, especially in adolescent samples. Granillo et al. (2005) explored the association between eating disorder symptoms and substance use in Latina adolescents and found significant positive correlations. Specifically, correlations were observed for dietary restraint, bulimic symptomatology, being a current smoker, ever drinking alcohol, heavy alcohol consumption, and other drug use. A combination of acculturation and poor body image was also associated with greatest risk for substance use in Latino adolescents (Nieri et al. 2005). Finally, in a treatment-seeking sample of adolescents, racial and ethnic minorities were at the greatest risk for alcohol and illicit drug use (Mann et al. 2014). However, some studies also found no racial/ethnic differences in the association between eating and substance use symptoms in adolescent and college-age samples (Granner et al. 2001, 2002).

Substantially less is known about comorbidity of eating disorders and substance abuse in adolescent males specifically, in part because studies often combine samples of boys and girls. However, a difference often observed between boys and girls is the motivation behind weight-change behaviors and reasons for body dissatisfaction. For example, boys often report a desire to be more muscular rather than a desire to be thin, with estimates suggesting that between 20% and 30% of adolescent boys desire a larger, more muscular body (Ricciardelli and McCabe 2004). Additionally, boys are more often dissatisfied with their bodies when they are underweight or overweight, and in combination with wanting to be more muscular, this can increase risk for abuse of weight gain supplements (e.g., protein powders) or steroid use during adolescence. In adult men, the extreme body image dissatisfaction that may lead to eating disorder symptoms or the misuse of supplements has been termed *reverse anorexia* or *muscle dysmorphia* (Pope et al. 1993).

With regard to muscle dissatisfaction, supplement use, and substance use in adolescent boys, Growing Up Today Study researchers found that approximately 2% of boys reported high concerns with muscularity and the use of supplements, growth hormone derivatives, or steroids to achieve desired body type (Field et al. 2014). Furthermore, boys reporting both high concerns about muscularity and thinness were more likely to use drugs, whereas boys with high concerns about muscularity who used supplements to enhance physical appearance were more likely to engage in frequent binge drinking. Finally, similar to observations about girls, cigarette use, binge drinking, and illicit drug use are significantly associated with eating disorder symptomatology in boys (Parkes et al. 2008; Pisetsky et al. 2008).

Chronology of Onset

Also of clinical interest is the relative age at onset of eating disorders and SUDs. Exploring patterns of onset among adults with AN and BN, we and our colleagues found that, in general, individuals reported that onset of the eating disorder preceded that of the SUD. Only one-third reported the onset of the SUD preceding that of the eating disorder (Baker et al. 2013; Bulik et al. 2004a).

Adult women who initially present with an eating disorder are also at prolonged risk for an alcohol use disorder. Over the course of 9 years, Franko et al. (2005) observed that 10% of patients with AN or BN developed an alcohol use disorder. Symptoms of AN and BN in early adolescence may also predict later substance use problems (Field et al. 2012; Measelle et al. 2006); however, findings have not been consistent. The strong drive for thinness often observed in eating disorders may increase risk for later substance misuse in an attempt to lose weight.

In comparisons of individuals with AN, BN, or BED with and without SUDs, those with the comorbid pattern, in general, tend to report higher rates of impulsivity, novelty seeking, depression, and anxiety (Baker et al. 2013; Bulik et al. 2004a; Peterson et al. 2005). Specifically, adult women with BN and an alcohol use disorder display a pattern of greater impulsiveness across a broad array of domains. Referred to as a "multi-impulsive" group, these women with BN often engage in other impulsive behaviors, such as excessive alcohol consumption, frequent illicit drug use, stealing, self-harm, borderline personality features, and sexual promiscuity (Fichter et al. 1994; Lacey and Evans 1986). This pattern of behaviors is observed in approximately 40% of treatment-seeking individuals with BN (Lacey 1993). Extra care and safety planning measures may need to be taken with this multi-impulsive group because these individuals are at higher risk for self-harming and parasuicidal behaviors. Similarities have been observed in an adolescent sample, but more research is needed to determine whether these same patterns are observed in adolescents (Thompson-Brenner et al. 2008).

Hypotheses of Comorbidity

Several hypotheses have been developed to explain the comorbidity between eating disorders and SUDs. Wolfe and Maisto (2000) discussed these hypotheses and reviewed the empirical evidence for each. First, it has been proposed that an addictive personality style is the predisposing factor for both BN and SUDs. Individuals may have certain personality traits (e.g., impulsivity) that predispose them to becoming "addicted" (Wolfe and Maisto 2000) to both food and substances. However, investigations comparing personality characteristics of women with eating disorders to women with SUDs have found both similarities and differences.

Second, some individuals may be more susceptible to social and cultural pressures for the thin ideal and for experimenting with substances that are common in adolescence, resulting in an increased risk for both eating disorders and substance abuse. However, this does not explain why most adolescents can engage in dieting and recreational drug use without developing either disorder.

Third, individuals with eating disorders may use substances to regulate affect. This hypothesis arises from the fact that women with eating disorders have disproportionately high rates of anxiety and depressive disorders. However, it is also possible that individuals with eating disorders use substances to dampen bulimic urges or as a way to deal with the self-disgust that follows binge eating.

Fourth, with the removal of food, alcohol and drugs may increase in reinforcement value, because food is no longer an available reinforcer. Although animal studies find that food deprivation increases self-administration of commonly abused licit and illicit drugs (Carr 2002), how these findings translate to humans is still unclear.

Finally, given the frequent comorbidity observed between eating disorders and SUDs, one critical question is whether the two disorders are etiologically related. This issue has been tackled to some extent by family and twin studies involving adult samples. Initial family studies observed an increased likelihood of an SUD in first-degree relatives of adult probands (i.e., individuals with the disorder of interest) with BN. However, when controlling for proband SUD, findings indicated that the two disorders are transmitted independently (Lilenfeld et al. 1997). In other words, the increased risk of an SUD in family members of individuals with BN is accounted for by the SUD in the proband.

Unlike family studies, twin studies are able to decompose the correlation between two disorders into genetic and environmental components. In contrast to family studies, twin studies indicate a shared familial association in adults. The first report by Kendler et al. (1995) applied a twin model to the lifetime history of six psychiatric disorders, including BN and alcoholism. A majority of the genetic vulnerability to alcoholism was independent from the other disorders; however, there was a small amount of genetic overlap with BN.

Examining the genetic overlap between BN and several SUDs, including an alcohol use disorder, regular smoking (defined as ever engaging in an average of at least seven episodes of smoking per month), and an illicit drug use disorder, further corroborates a genetic overlap between eating disorders and SUDs. Results found a small to moderate overlap in the genetic factors contributing to BN and all SUDs examined

(Baker et al. 2007, 2010). Genetic overlap has also been observed between bulimic behaviors and alcohol use disorder symptomatology in adolescents at age 17 (Slane et al. 2014); however, this same overlap was not observed in young adulthood. Clearly, more research is needed in this area to further clarify the inconsistencies in findings across family and twin studies and to address whether the same findings are observed in adolescent samples.

Abuse of Other Substances Related to Eating Disorders

Not only do individuals with eating disorders engage in use and abuse of "typical" substances of abuse (e.g., alcohol), but substances ingested for the purpose of weight loss, purging, appetite suppression, and weight gain supplementation can also be abused. Clinicians must be vigilant in assessment for the use and abuse of prescription and over-the-counter medications such as supplements, laxatives, diuretics, and emetics. In addition, individuals may smoke and use excessive amounts of caffeine as ways to control appetite and promote weight loss. More information can be found in the literature about the types of substances abused for these purposes, along with how they are detected, their toxicity levels, and signs of tolerance and withdrawal (Bulik et al. 2004b; Hildebrandt et al. 2011).

When screening younger patients, the clinician needs to be careful not to introduce new ideas for weight loss or purging by questioning about the use of specific substances or behaviors. The best strategy for assessment is to use open-ended approaches that address what substances the patient has tried in an effort to lose or gain weight, control appetite, purge, or modify muscle. In sum, individuals with eating disorders often go to dangerous lengths to control weight and shape, and a thorough assessment is necessary to document the patient's full gamut of eating disorder behaviors.

Assessment of Comorbid Eating Disorders and SUDs

Owing to the significant co-occurrence of eating disorders and SUDs, clinicians should routinely screen for eating disorders in patients who present with substance use problems and vice versa. Given the possible prolonged risk of developing the comorbid disorder, this screening should occur not only at initial assessment but also throughout the duration of treatment.

Routine screening for eating disorders is not complex and does not have to involve time-consuming, comprehensive clinical interviews—

which primary care physicians and clinicians may not have time for. Similar to the rapid screening approach developed for alcoholism (CAGE—questions about cutting down, annoyance with criticism, feelings of guilt, and eye-openers; Ewing 1984), Morgan et al. (1999) developed the SCOFF questionnaire in England for eating disorder screening, and this questionnaire has been modified for use in the United States (Perry et al. 2002). The SCOFF consists of five questions and has been shown to be reliable and valid. Importantly, however, positive screens must be followed up with a comprehensive eating disorder assessment.

Self-report measures of eating disorder attitudes and behaviors that can be used to screen for eating disorder symptomatology include the Eating Disorder Inventory (EDI; Garner 1991), Eating Attitudes Test (EAT; Garner and Garfinkel 1979), and Eating Disorders Examination Questionnaire (EDE-Q; Fairburn and Beglin 1994). Comprehensive clinical interviews to assess eating disorder symptomatology and diagnosis include the Eating Disorders Examination (EDE; Fairburn and Cooper 1993), Module H of the Structured Clinical Interview for DSM-IV (Module H SCID) (First et al. 1997), the Yale-Brown-Cornell Eating Disorder Scale (YBC-EDS; Sunday et al. 1995), and the Structured Interview for Anorexic and Bulimic Disorders (SIAB; Fichter et al. 1998).

Treatment for Eating Disorders and SUDs in Adolescents

Treatment research on comorbid eating disorders and SUDs remains limited. There is a growing field of treatment research for eating disorders in adolescents; however, many of these studies still focus on behavioral interventions for adolescents with AN. Few clinical trials have directed efforts exclusively toward adolescents with BN or BED. Pharmacologically, only a limited number of placebo-controlled trials have been conducted with adolescents, and results are mixed at best. Thus, little is known about tailoring pharmacological treatments for adolescents with AN, BN, or BED.

Treatment of Anorexia Nervosa

A complete medical evaluation, nutritional counseling, and supervised refeeding should be the first steps in the treatment of AN. Outpatient multidisciplinary teams composed of psychiatrists, therapists, dietitians, and family practitioners can manage mild to moderate cases of AN. For individuals who have medical complications or fall below 75%

of their ideal body weight, hospitalization is usually considered. Several professional organizations, including the American Psychiatric Association (Yager et al. 2010) and the Academy for Eating Disorders (2012), have developed guidelines for the treatment of AN.

A systematic review of cognitive-behavioral therapy (CBT) in the treatment of AN (covering a range of ages) concluded that although improvements were shown in outcome areas such as BMI, eating disorder symptoms, and general psychopathology, CBT was not reliably superior to other forms of treatment such as dietary counseling, interpersonal therapy (IPT), or behavioral family therapy (Galsworthy-Francis and Allan 2014). However, findings were not broken down by age. Family-based treatment (FBT) has been the widest studied behavioral intervention for AN and is efficacious for treating adolescent AN. One meta-analysis suggested that although there were no outcome differences between FBT and individual therapy at end of treatment, FBT demonstrated maintained improvements at 6 and 12 months posttreatment (Couturier et al. 2013).

Treatment of Bulimia Nervosa

Although family-based approaches may be the treatment of choice for AN, family-based approaches for BN have been less widely studied. However, these approaches do show promise. A randomized controlled comparison of FBT and supportive psychotherapy concluded that adolescents receiving FBT were significantly more likely to be binge/purge abstinent at posttreatment and 6-month follow-up (le Grange et al. 2007). In comparison with FBT, a variation of CBT was also more effective at reducing binge eating in adolescents with BN; however, this difference was not evident at 12 months posttreatment (Schmidt et al. 2007). In contrast, individual CBT and group CBT are empirically supported forms of treatment for BN in adults and are effective in reducing the core behavioral and psychological symptoms. In addition, when compared to IPT, CBT achieves more rapid reduction of symptoms (Wilson et al. 2002). Limitations still apply for applications with adolescents because few studies stratify treatment outcome by age of patient.

Fluoxetine remains the only medication for BN approved by the U.S. Food and Drug Administration; the recommended dosage is 60 mg/day. In adult patients with BN, administration of fluoxetine for 6–18 weeks was shown to reduce psychological symptoms and binge-eating and purging behaviors but only for a short period of time (Fluoxetine Bulimia Nervosa Collaborative Study Group 1992). The optimal duration of treatment and strategy for maintenance of treatment gains, as well as the efficacy and appropriateness of fluoxetine for BN treatment in adolescents, are still unclear. Caution should be taken when prescribing fluoxetine to adolescents, because of the potential risks associated with selective serotonin reuptake inhibitor antidepressants, including bone thinning, an increase in suicidal thoughts, and serotonin syndrome, which causes flu-like symptoms and can be fatal. Adolescents taking psychiatric medications should have symptoms monitored by their physician on a regular basis.

Treatment of Binge-Eating Disorder

Treatment for BED tends to focus on reduction of either binge eating or weight. CBT is often the psychotherapy of choice for reducing binge-eating behaviors, similar to treatment of BN, whereas behavioral weight loss approaches have been found to be successful at targeting outcomes around weight but not binge eating (Grilo et al. 2011). Unfortunately, the treatment research for adolescents with BED is only beginning to emerge, likely because this disorder is more often diagnosed in adulthood.

However, there has been some promising treatment research on loss-of-control eating in adolescents. A pilot study comparing IPT and standard-of-care health education to prevent weight gain in a sample of girls with and without loss-of-control eating found that IPT was more effective than the health education in reducing loss-of-control episodes (Tanofsky-Kraff et al. 2010). Mazzeo et al. (2013) are developing a culturally sensitive manualized treatment protocol for loss-of-control eating called Linking Individuals Being Emotionally Real (LIBER8); this intervention incorporates components of dialectical behavior therapy and CBT. CBT and enhanced CBT have also been suggested as weight-management methods in children and adolescents who are obese and engage in disordered eating behaviors (Wilfley et al. 2011).

Treatment: Looking Ahead

In addition to the need for an increased understanding of the optimal treatment approaches for adolescents with eating disorders, information is urgently needed about optimal treatment approaches for adolescents who have a comorbid SUD. In theory, there are three options for the treatment of comorbid eating disorders and SUDs: 1) a treatment program or provider specializing in dual diagnosis can treat both disorders simultaneously, 2) treatment for substance abuse or dependence can be followed by specialized eating disorder treatment, and 3) specialized eating disorder treatment can be followed by specialized substance disorder treatment. Unfortunately, there is no empirical evidence to suggest which treatment approach is optimal or most appropriate for which patients. Therefore, clinical judgment and treatment availability are often the primary factors in deciding the sequencing of treatment. Regardless of whether the disorders are treated simultaneously or independently, a vital piece of any treatment is assisting the patient to recognize the relationship between the eating disorder and the SUD. Commitment to recovery from both disorders will be needed, especially considering that relapse from one disorder may cause relapse or increased symptoms of the other disorder. Prevention plans must be well established and are essential in addressing the differences and similarities in relapse risk for each disorder.

One option for treating both disorders simultaneously is dialectical behavior therapy, which has been used with success in the treatment of patients with eating disorders and comorbid SUD (Courbasson et al. 2012). Another viable option is CBT, which has been successful in the treatment of eating and substance disorders independently; however, CBT treatment protocols need to be adapted for the co-occurrence of these disorders because the use of treatment protocols developed for one disorder will miss key behavioral and psychological features of the other disorder. To date, we are aware of no controlled studies examining the efficacy of integrated CBT treatment protocols for the co-occurrence of eating disorders and SUDs. It has also been suggested that treatment should focus on the common maintaining mechanisms of both disorders, including ambivalence about change, deficits in interpersonal functioning, exposure to triggers and response prevention, and impulsivity (Sysko and Hildebrandt 2009).

Motivational interviewing (MI) may be another viable option in the treatment of co-occurring eating disorders and SUDs, because some evidence suggests that MI is efficacious in increasing motivation for change in both disorders independently (see Chapter 3 "Screening, Assessment, and Treatment Options for Youths With a Substance Use Disorder"). MI was originally developed to aid in the treatment of SUDs, but it has gained popularity as an adjunct approach in treating other conditions such as eating disorders. It focuses on helping a patient to resolve ambivalence around treatment and unhealthy behaviors by evoking intrinsic motivation for change while recognizing the patient's autonomy. When paired with CBT in the treatment of eating disorders, MI may support recovery by strengthening the therapeutic alliance and ensuring that interventions are adapted to the patient's readiness for change. Clinicians working with patients who have a dual eating and substance disorder diagnosis may benefit from learning and incorporating MI skills into treatment to increase patient motivation to change and engagement in treatment (see discussion of MI in Chapter 3 "Screening, Assessment, and Treatment Options for Youths With a Substance Use Disorder").

Finally, the use of pharmacological agents early in treatment is discouraged in patients with comorbid disorders, especially if the patient is low weight, because pharmacological agents may exacerbate symptoms of the SUD. Similarly, practitioners treating SUDs should not encourage or recommend diet and exercise plans that have not been approved by a dietitian who specializes in eating disorders and is working with the patient. Unfortunately, many patients who have co-occurring eating disorder and substance use problems seek treatment from multiple providers and treatment programs because few treatment programs are equipped to address the problems simultaneously.

Summary and Future Directions

Comorbid eating disorders and SUDs are a common clinical occurrence during adulthood, and similar comorbidities are observed during adolescence. Although this comorbid pattern is well established and widely recognized, it remains understudied. From an etiological and treatment perspective, continued research should address the nature of the comorbid process, the mechanisms underlying vulnerability to both conditions, and combined prevention and treatment approaches, with a specific focus on adolescent populations.

KEY POINTS

- There is significant comorbidity of eating disorders and substance use disorder symptomatology in youth.

- Assessment of potentially abusable substances in adolescents should include use of laxatives, diuretics, diet pills, emetics, unregulated supplements, and anabolic steroids.

- Treatment options include one or more of the following: dietary counseling, motivational interviewing, interpersonal therapy, cognitive-behavioral therapy, and dialectical behavior therapy.

References

Academy for Eating Disorders: Critical Points for Early Recognition and Medical Risk Management in the Care of Individuals with Eating Disorders. Deerfield, IL, Academy for Eating Disorders, 2012. Available at: http://aedweb.org/web/downloads/Guide-English.pdf. Accessed June 2, 2014.

Ackard DM, Neumark-Sztainer D, Story M, et al: Overeating among adolescents: prevalence and associations with weight-related characteristics and psychological health. Pediatrics 111(1):67–74, 2003 12509556

Ackard DM, Fulkerson JA, Neumark-Sztainer D: Psychological and behavioral risk profiles as they relate to eating disorder diagnoses and symptomatology among a school-based sample of youth. Int J Eat Disord 44(5):440–446, 2011 20872753

American Psychiatric Association: Diagnostic and Statistical Manual of Mental Disorders, 4th Edition. Washington, DC, American Psychiatric Press, 1994

American Psychiatric Association: Diagnostic and Statistical Manual of Mental Disorders, 5th Edition. Arlington, VA, American Psychiatric Press, 2013

Arias JE, Hawke JM, Arias AJ, et al: Eating disorder symptoms and alcohol use among adolescents in substance abuse treatment. Subst Abus 3:81–91, 2009 24357933

Attia E, Roberto CA: Should amenorrhea be a diagnostic criterion for anorexia nervosa? Int J Eat Disord 42(7):581–589, 2009 19621464

Baker JH, Mazzeo SE, Kendler KS: Association between broadly defined bulimia nervosa and drug use disorders: common genetic and environmental influences. Int J Eat Disord 40(8):673–678, 2007 17868121

Baker JH, Mitchell KS, Neale MC, et al: Eating disorder symptomatology and substance use disorders: prevalence and shared risk in a population based twin sample. Int J Eat Disord 43(7):648–658, 2010 20734312

Baker JH, Thornton LM, Strober M, et al: Temporal sequence of comorbid alcohol use disorder and anorexia nervosa. Addict Behav 38(3):1704–1709, 2013 23254222

Bulik CM, Sullivan PF, Fear JL, et al: Eating disorders and antecedent anxiety disorders: a controlled study. Acta Psychiatr Scand 96(2):101–107, 1997 9272193

Bulik CM, Sullivan PF, Kendler KS: Medical and psychiatric morbidity in obese women with and without binge eating. Int J Eat Disord 32(1):72–78, 2002 12183948

Bulik CM, Klump KL, Thornton L, et al: Alcohol use disorder comorbidity in eating disorders: a multicenter study. J Clin Psychiatry 65(7):1000–1006, 2004a 15291691

Bulik C, Slof S, Sullivan P: Eating disorders and substance use disorders, in Dual Diagnosis: Substance Abuse and Comorbid Medical and Psychiatric Conditions, 2nd Edition. Edited by Rounsaville B, Kranzler H. New York, Marcel Dekker, 2004b, pp 317–348

Carr KD: Augmentation of drug reward by chronic food restriction: behavioral evidence and underlying mechanisms. Physiol Behav 76(3):353–364, 2002 12117572

Cassin SE, von Ranson KM: Personality and eating disorders: a decade in review. Clin Psychol Rev 25(7):895–916, 2005 16099563

Centers for Disease Control and Prevention: Basics about childhood obesity, in Overweight and Obesity. Atlanta, GA, Centers for Disease Control and Prevention, 2012. Available at: http://www.cdc.gov/obesity/childhood/basics.html. Accessed June 2, 2014.

Chesney E, Goodwin GM, Fazel S: Risks of all-cause and suicide mortality in mental disorders: a meta-review. World Psychiatry 13(2):153–160, 2014 24890068

Courbasson C, Nishikawa Y, Dixon L: Outcome of dialectical behaviour therapy for concurrent eating and substance use disorders. Clin Psychol Psychother 19(5):434–449, 2012 21416557

Couturier J, Kimber M, Szatmari P: Efficacy of family based treatment for adolescents with eating disorders: a systematic review and meta-analysis. Int J Eat Disord 46(1):3–11, 2013 22821753

Ewing JA: Detecting alcoholism. The CAGE questionnaire. JAMA 252(14):1905–1907, 1984 6471323

Fairburn C, Beglin SJ: Assessment of eating disorders: interview or self-report questionnaire? Int J Eat Disord 16(4):363–370, 1994 7866415

Fairburn C, Cooper Z: The Eating Disorders Examination, 12th Edition, in Binge-Eating: Nature, Assessment and Treatment. Edited by Fairburn C, Wilson G. New York, Guilford, 1993, pp 317–360

Farhat T, Iannotti RJ, Simons-Morton BG: Overweight, obesity, youth, and health-risk behaviors. Am J Prev Med 38(3):258–267, 2010 20171527

Fichter MM, Quadflieg N, Rief W: Course of multi-impulsive bulimia. Psychol Med 24(3):591–604, 1994 7991741

Fichter MM, Herpertz S, Quadflieg N, et al: Structured Interview for Anorexic and Bulimic Disorders for DSM-IV and ICD-10: updated (third) revision. Int J Eat Disord 24(3):227–249, 1998 9741034

Field AE, Sonneville KR, Micali N, et al: Prospective association of common eating disorders and adverse outcomes. Pediatrics 130(2):e289–e295, 2012 22802602

Field AE, Sonneville KR, Crosby RD, et al: Prospective associations of concerns about physique and the development of obesity, binge drinking, and drug use among adolescent boys and young adult men. JAMA Pediatr 168(1):34–39, 2014 24190655

First M, Spitzer R, Gibbon M, et al: Structured Clinical Interview for DSM-IV Axis I Disorders, Research Version, Patient Edition. New York, Biometrics Research, New York State Psychiatric Institute, 1997

Fluoxetine Bulimia Nervosa Collaborative Study Group: Fluoxetine in the treatment of bulimia nervosa: a multicenter, placebo-controlled, double-blind trial. Arch Gen Psychiatry 49(2):139–147, 1992 1550466

Franko DL, Dorer DJ, Keel PK, et al: How do eating disorders and alcohol use disorder influence each other? Int J Eat Disord 38(3):200–207, 2005 16216020

Gadalla T, Piran N: Co-occurrence of eating disorders and alcohol use disorders in women: a meta analysis. Arch Womens Ment Health 10(4):133–140, 2007a 17533558

Gadalla T, Piran N: Eating disorders and substance abuse in Canadian men and women: a national study. Eat Disord 15(3):189–203, 2007b 17520452

Galsworthy-Francis L, Allan S: Cognitive behavioural therapy for anorexia nervosa: a systematic review. Clin Psychol Rev 34(1):54–72, 2014 24394285

Garner D: Eating Disorder Inventory-2: Professional Manual. Odessa, FL, Psychological Assessment Resources, 1991

Garner DM, Garfinkel PE: The Eating Attitudes Test: an index of the symptoms of anorexia nervosa. Psychol Med 9(2):273–279, 1979 472072

Granillo T, Jones-Rodriguez G, Carvajal SC: Prevalence of eating disorders in Latina adolescents: associations with substance use and other correlates. J Adolesc Health 36(3):214–220, 2005 15737777

Granner ML, Abood DA, Black DR: Racial differences in eating disorder attitudes, cigarette, and alcohol use. Am J Health Behav 25(2):83–99, 2001 11297045

Granner ML, Black DR, Abood DA: Levels of cigarette and alcohol use related to eating-disorder attitudes. Am J Health Behav 26(1):43–52, 2002 11795605

Grilo CM, White MA, Masheb RM: DSM-IV psychiatric disorder comorbidity and its correlates in binge eating disorder. Int J Eat Disord 42(3):228–234, 2009 18951458

Grilo CM, Masheb RM, Wilson GT, et al: Cognitive-behavioral therapy, behavioral weight loss, and sequential treatment for obese patients with binge-eating disorder: a randomized controlled trial. J Consult Clin Psychol 79(5):675–685, 2011 21859185

Hilbert A, Brauhardt A: Childhood loss of control eating over five-year follow-up. Int J Eat Disord 47(7):758–761, 2014 24899359

Hildebrandt T, Lai JK, Langenbucher JW, et al: The diagnostic dilemma of pathological appearance and performance enhancing drug use. Drug Alcohol Depend 114(1):1–11, 2011 21115306

Huang DYC, Lanza HI, Anglin MD: Association between adolescent substance use and obesity in young adulthood: a group-based dual trajectory analysis. Addict Behav 38(11):2653–2660, 2013 23899428

Hudson JI, Hiripi E, Pope HG Jr, et al: The prevalence and correlates of eating disorders in the National Comorbidity Survey Replication. Biol Psychiatry 61(3):348–358, 2007 16815322

Hudson JI, Lalonde JK, Coit CE, et al: Longitudinal study of the diagnosis of components of the metabolic syndrome in individuals with binge-eating disorder. Am J Clin Nutr 91(6):1568–1573, 2010 20427731

Jacobi C, Hayward C, de Zwaan M, et al: Coming to terms with risk factors for eating disorders: application of risk terminology and suggestions for a general taxonomy. Psychol Bull 130(1):19–65, 2004 14717649

Javaras KN, Pope HG, Lalonde JK, et al: Co-occurrence of binge eating disorder with psychiatric and medical disorders. J Clin Psychiatry 69(2):266–273, 2008 18348600

Kaye WH, Bulik CM, Thornton L, et al: Comorbidity of anxiety disorders with anorexia and bulimia nervosa. Am J Psychiatry 161(12):2215–2221, 2004 15569892

Keel PK, Dorer DJ, Eddy KT, et al: Predictors of mortality in eating disorders. Arch Gen Psychiatry 60(2):179–183, 2003 12578435

Kendler KS, Walters EE, Neale MC, et al: The structure of the genetic and environmental risk factors for six major psychiatric disorders in women: phobia, generalized anxiety disorder, panic disorder, bulimia, major depression, and alcoholism. Arch Gen Psychiatry 52(5):374–383, 1995 7726718

Kessler RC, Berglund PA, Chiu WT, et al: The prevalence and correlates of binge eating disorder in the World Health Organization World Mental Health Surveys. Biol Psychiatry 73(9):904–914, 2013 23290497

Klump KL, Burt SA, McGue M, et al: Changes in genetic and environmental influences on disordered eating across adolescence: a longitudinal twin study. Arch Gen Psychiatry 64(12):1409–1415, 2007 18056549

Lacey JH: Self-damaging and addictive behaviour in bulimia nervosa: a catchment area study. Br J Psychiatry 163:190–194, 1993 8075910

Lacey JH, Evans CD: The impulsivist: a multi-impulsive personality disorder. Br J Addict 81(5):641–649, 1986 3539167

le Grange D, Crosby RD, Rathouz PJ, et al: A randomized controlled comparison of family based treatment and supportive psychotherapy for adolescent bulimia nervosa. Arch Gen Psychiatry 64(9):1049–1056, 2007 17768270

Leon G, Fulkerson J, Perry C, et al: Three to four-year prospective evaluation of risk factors for disordered eating and assessment of psychopathology in adolescent girls and boys. J Youth Adolesc 28(2):181–196, 1999

Lilenfeld LR, Kaye WH, Greeno CG, et al: Psychiatric disorders in women with bulimia nervosa and their first-degree relatives: effects of comorbid substance dependence. Int J Eat Disord 22(3):253–264, 1997 9285262

Mann AP, Accurso EC, Stiles-Shields C, et al: Factors associated with substance use in adolescents with eating disorders. J Adolesc Health 55(2):182–187, 2014 24656448

Mazzeo SE, Kelly NR, Stern M, et al: LIBER8 design and methods: an integrative intervention for loss of control eating among African American and white adolescent girls. Contemp Clin Trials 34(1):174–185, 2013 23142669

Measelle JR, Stice E, Hogansen JM: Developmental trajectories of co-occurring depressive, eating, antisocial, and substance abuse problems in female adolescents. J Abnorm Psychol 115(3):524–538, 2006 16866592

Mehler PS, Krantz M: Anorexia nervosa medical issues. J Womens Health (Larchmt) 12(4):331–340, 2003 12804340

Mehler PS, Crews C, Weiner K: Bulimia: medical complications. J Womens Health (Larchmt) 13(6):668–675, 2004 15333281

Morgan JF, Reid F, Lacey JH: The SCOFF questionnaire: assessment of a new screening tool for eating disorders. BMJ 319(7223):1467–1468, 1999 10582927

Nieri T, Kulis S, Keith VM, et al: Body image, acculturation, and substance abuse among boys and girls in the Southwest. Am J Drug Alcohol Abuse 31(4):617–639, 2005 16320438

Ogden CL, Carroll MD, Kit BK, et al: Prevalence of obesity and trends in body mass index among U.S. children and adolescents, 1999–2010. JAMA 307(5):483–490, 2012 22253364

Parkes SA, Saewyc EM, Cox DN, et al: Relationship between body image and stimulant use among Canadian adolescents. J Adolesc Health 43(6):616–618, 2008 19027652

Pasch KE, Velazquez CE, Cance JD, et al: Youth substance use and body composition: does risk in one area predict risk in the other? J Youth Adolesc 41(1):14–26, 2012 21853355

Pasold TL, McCracken A, Ward-Begnoche WL: Binge eating in obese adolescents: emotional and behavioral characteristics and impact on health-related quality of life. Clin Child Psychol Psychiatry 19(2):299–312, 2014 23749140

Pederson Mussell M, Mitchell JE, Fenna CJ, et al: A comparison of onset of binge eating versus dieting in the development of bulimia nervosa. Int J Eat Disord 21(4):353–360, 1997 9138047

Perez M, Joiner TE Jr, Lewinsohn PM: Is major depressive disorder or dysthymia more strongly associated with bulimia nervosa? Int J Eat Disord 36(1):55–61, 2004 15185272

Perry L, Morgan J, Reid F, et al: Screening for symptoms of eating disorders: reliability of the SCOFF screening tool with written compared to oral delivery. Int J Eat Disord 32(4):466–472, 2002 12386911

Peterson CB, Miller KB, Crow SJ, et al: Subtypes of binge eating disorder based on psychiatric history. Int J Eat Disord 38(3):273–276, 2005 16142786

Pickering RP, Goldstein RB, Hasin DS, et al: Temporal relationships between overweight and obesity and DSM-IV substance use, mood, and anxiety disorders: results from a prospective study, the National Epidemiologic Survey on Alcohol and Related Conditions. J Clin Psychiatry 72(11):1494–1502, 2011 21457678

Pisetsky EM, Chao YM, Dierker LC, et al: Disordered eating and substance use in high-school students: results from the Youth Risk Behavior Surveillance System. Int J Eat Disord 41(5):464–470, 2008 18348283

Pope HG Jr, Katz DL, Hudson JI: Anorexia nervosa and "reverse anorexia" among 108 male bodybuilders. Compr Psychiatry 34(6):406–409, 1993 8131385

Ricciardelli LA, McCabe MP: A biopsychosocial model of disordered eating and the pursuit of muscularity in adolescent boys. Psychol Bull 130(2):179–205, 2004 14979769

Root TL, Pinheiro AP, Thornton L, et al: Substance use disorders in women with anorexia nervosa. Int J Eat Disord 43(1):14–21, 2010 19260043

Ross HE, Ivis F: Binge eating and substance use among male and female adolescents. Int J Eat Disord 26(3):245–260, 1999 10441240

Schmidt U, Lee S, Beecham J, et al: A randomized controlled trial of family therapy and cognitive behavior therapy guided self-care for adolescents with bulimia nervosa and related disorders. Am J Psychiatry 164(4):591–598, 2007 17403972

Slane JD, Klump KL, McGue M, et al: Genetic and environmental factors underlying comorbid bulimic behaviours and alcohol use disorders: a moderating role for the dysregulated personality cluster? Eur Eat Disord Rev 22(3):159–169, 2014 24616026

Smink FR, van Hoeken D, Oldehinkel AJ, et al: Prevalence and severity of DSM-5 eating disorders in a community cohort of adolescents. Int J Eat Disord 47(6):610–619, 2014 24903034

Sonneville KR, Horton NJ, Micali N, et al: Longitudinal associations between binge eating and overeating and adverse outcomes among adolescents and young adults: does loss of control matter? JAMA Pediatr 167(2):149–155, 2013 23229786

Stice E, Presnell K, Bearman SK: Relation of early menarche to depression, eating disorders, substance abuse, and comorbid psychopathology among adolescent girls. Dev Psychol 37(5):608–619, 2001 11552757

Stice E, Marti CN, Rohde P: Prevalence, incidence, impairment, and course of the proposed DSM-5 eating disorder diagnoses in an 8-year prospective community study of young women. J Abnorm Psychol 122(2):445–457, 2013 23148784

Sunday SR, Halmi KA, Einhorn A: The Yale-Brown-Cornell Eating Disorder Scale: a new scale to assess eating disorder symptomatology. Int J Eat Disord 18(3):237–245, 1995 8556019

Swanson SA, Crow SJ, Le Grange D, et al: Prevalence and correlates of eating disorders in adolescents: results from the National Comorbidity Survey Replication Adolescent Supplement. Arch Gen Psychiatry 68(7):714–723, 2011 21383252

Swanson SA, Horton NJ, Crosby RD, et al: A latent class analysis to empirically describe eating disorders through developmental stages. Int J Eat Disord 47(7):762–772, 2014 24909947

Sysko R, Hildebrandt T: Cognitive-behavioural therapy for individuals with bulimia nervosa and a co-occurring substance use disorder. Eur Eat Disord Rev 17(2):89–100, 2009 19130465

Tanofsky-Kraff M, Wilfley DE, Young JF, et al: A pilot study of interpersonal psychotherapy for preventing excess weight gain in adolescent girls at-risk for obesity. Int J Eat Disord 43(8):701–706, 2010 19882739

Tanofsky-Kraff M, Shomaker LB, Olsen C, et al: A prospective study of pediatric loss of control eating and psychological outcomes. J Abnorm Psychol 120(1):108–118, 2011 21114355

Thompson-Brenner H, Eddy KT, Satir DA, et al: Personality subtypes in adolescents with eating disorders: validation of a classification approach. J Child Psychol Psychiatry 49(2):170–180, 2008 18093115

Trace SE, Baker JH, Peñas-Lledó E, et al: The genetics of eating disorders. Annu Rev Clin Psychol 9:589–620, 2013 23537489

Wilfley DE, Kolko RP, Kass AE: Cognitive-behavioral therapy for weight management and eating disorders in children and adolescents. Child Adolesc Psychiatr Clin N Am 20(2):271–285, 2011 21440855

Wilson GT, Fairburn CC, Agras WS, et al: Cognitive-behavioral therapy for bulimia nervosa: time course and mechanisms of change. J Consult Clin Psychol 70(2):267–274, 2002 11952185

Wolfe WL, Maisto SA: The relationship between eating disorders and substance use: moving beyond co-prevalence research. Clin Psychol Rev 20(5):617–631, 2000 10860169

Wu LT, Gersing K, Burchett B, et al: Substance use disorders and comorbid Axis I and II psychiatric disorders among young psychiatric patients: findings from a large electronic health records database. J Psychiatr Res 45(11):1453–1462, 2011 21742345

Yager J, Devlin MJ, Halmi KA, et al: Practice Guideline for the Treatment of Patients With Eating Disorders, 3rd Edition. Arlington, VA, American Psychiatric Association, 2010. Available at: http://psychiatryonline.org/pb/assets/raw/sitewide/practice_guidelines/guidelines/eatingdisorders.pdf. Accessed June 30, 2014.

CHAPTER 13

Youth Gambling Problems

Jeffrey L. Derevensky, Ph.D.

The landscape of gambling continues to evolve, with greater availability and easier accessibility and more diverse gambling opportunities for both youths and adults. An increasing number of jurisdictions are expanding options for a wide variety of gambling possibilities, including lotteries, bingo venues, and casinos. Additionally, sports-wagering opportunities, Internet gambling sites, electronic gambling machines, and mobile gambling apps are proliferating. Globally, gambling represents one of the fastest-changing and fastest-growing industries in the world. In the United States, only two states had casinos in 1988. In 2014, 39 states had casino gambling of some kind, and more governors and legislatures are contemplating developing "destination" casino resorts. Even in those states that already have casino operations, legislators view the significant tax revenues as far outweighing any social costs and are opting for expanding gambling (either land based, online, or both). Internationally, the proliferation of casinos and other forms of gambling continues. Macau, a small island between Hong Kong and China, is the new mecca of the gambling world, with revenues significantly outpacing those in Las Vegas. Other jurisdictions in the United States, Europe,

Special thanks to Lynette Gilbeau for her many valuable suggestions.

307

Asia, Australasia, Canada, and South America are clamoring to build new gambling venues. The largest U.S. gambling corporations have greatly expanded their operations internationally to capitalize on the growing demand. Gambling opportunities have become so widespread that it is difficult to find jurisdictions in which some form of gambling is not government controlled, regulated, organized, or owned. In those jurisdictions where legalized gambling is banned, underground and illicit gambling exists, with Internet and mobile gambling readily accessible. Gambling throughout the world has become a socially acceptable pastime and a growing form of entertainment in spite of the recognized social and personal costs associated with excessive problematic gambling.

Although governments, mental health workers, and public policy experts remain concerned about gambling, there have been studies that have pointed out positive advantages for individuals when they are engaged in social recreational gambling. Such studies have reported that gambling in moderation is associated with enhanced memory, problem-solving skills, mathematical proficiency, and concentration for the elderly (Shaffer and Korn 2002). Individuals engage in gambling as a social experience to reduce stress (Everard et al. 2000; Hope and Havir 2002; Vander Bilt et al. 2004) and for enhancement of self-esteem (Loroz 2004; Volberg et al. 1997). There is little doubt that gambling has moved from being considered "sin and vice" to a socially acceptable form of entertainment in most parts of the world.

Traditionally viewed as an adult activity, gambling has captured the imagination of young people because of its social acceptability, its support and endorsement by governments, and the glitz and glamour of casinos. Its popularity among youths has increased in part because numerous movies and television shows have depicted gambling's glamour and excitement (e.g., *Rounders, Blade Runner, Casino Royale, 21, Vegas*), and the televised world championship poker tournaments have shown young people winning millions of dollars (many of the recent World Series of Poker tournament winners have been in their 20s). Although most jurisdictions have legislative statutes prohibiting children and adolescents from engaging in government-sponsored and/or regulated forms of gambling (e.g., lottery, casinos, horse racing, machine gambling, Internet wagering), there remains little doubt that many young people continue to be actively engaged in forms of gambling that are both regulated and nonregulated (e.g., card games and sports wagering among peers).

Studies completed throughout North America, Europe, Australia, New Zealand, Asia, South America, and South Africa all point to the popularity of gambling by adolescents. Survey findings and reviews of prevalence studies examining youth gambling behavior have consistently revealed that adolescents (ages 12–17 years) have managed to participate, to some degree, in practically all forms of social, government-sanctioned, and nonregulated gambling available in their homes and communities. Youths are commonly involved in playing cards (poker, while it appears to have lost some of its glamor, is still popular), dice, and board games with family and friends; sports wagering with peers; betting with peers on games of personal skill (e.g., pool, bowling, basketball); playing arcade or video games for money; purchasing lottery tickets; wagering at horse and dog tracks; gambling in bingo halls and card rooms; playing slot machines and table games in casinos; gambling on video lottery/poker terminals; wagering on the Internet; and placing bets with a bookmaker (Derevensky 2012; Derevensky and Gupta 2004a, 2007; Griffiths and Parke 2010; Griffiths and Wood 2007; Volberg et al. 2010; Wardle et al. 2011).

Adolescents' wagering behaviors have often been found to be dependent on a number of factors, including the local availability and accessibility of games, the geographic proximity of gaming locations, the youth's gender and type of game (gambling is more popular among males than females; males prefer sports wagering, whereas girls report engaging in lottery purchases more often), and the individual's age (older adolescents are more likely to engage in video lottery/poker terminal and casino playing because these venues are more easily accessed). Interaction between adolescents and type of gambling is also influenced by gender and cultural/ethnic background (see Ellenbogen et al. 2007; Gupta and Derevensky 1998a, 2004; St-Pierre et al. 2011; Volberg et al. 2010; Wardle et al. 2011).

The gambling behavior of adolescents, similar to that of adults, can best be viewed along a continuum, ranging from nongambling to social/occasional/recreational gambling to problem/pathological/disordered gambling. In DSM-5 (American Psychiatric Association 2013), the most serious form of gambling problems is now referred to as *gambling disorder.* Although the diagnostic criteria in DSM-5 have dropped from 10 to 9 items (Box 13–1), three severity specifiers for gambling disorder are now included: mild (4–5 criteria met), moderate (6–7 criteria met), and severe (8–9 criteria met). (Others use the term *problem gambling* for individuals not reaching the diagnostic threshold [Parhami et al. 2014].) Within the adolescent gambling literature, the terms *social/occasional gambling* and *nonproblematic/recreational gambling* are typically used to denote occasional, infrequent use with few or minimal gambling-related associated problems; *at-risk gambling* often refers to some gambling-related problems that do not reach the diagnostic criteria for pathological/disordered gambling on a gambling severity screen; and *disordered, problem, pathological,* and *compulsive gambling* describe behaviors that are indicative of and associated with excessive gambling-related problems.

Box 13–1. DSM-5 Criteria for Gambling Disorder

A. Persistent and recurrent problematic gambling behavior leading to clinically significant impairment or distress, as indicated by the individual exhibiting four (or more) of the following in a 12-month period:

   1. Needs to gamble with increasing amounts of money in order to achieve the desired excitement.
   2. Is restless or irritable when attempting to cut down or stop gambling.
   3. Has made repeated unsuccessful efforts to control, cut back, or stop gambling.
   4. Is often preoccupied with gambling (e.g., having persistent thoughts of reliving past gambling experiences, handicapping or planning the next venture, thinking of ways to get money with which to gamble).
   5. Often gambles when feeling distressed (e.g., helpless, guilty, anxious, depressed).
   6. After losing money gambling, often returns another day to get even ("chasing" one's losses).
   7. Lies to conceal the extent of involvement with gambling.
   8. Has jeopardized or lost a significant relationship, job, or educational or career opportunity because of gambling.
   9. Relies on others to provide money to relieve desperate financial situations caused by gambling.

B. The gambling behavior is not better explained by a manic episode.

Specify if:

   Episodic: Meeting diagnostic criteria at more than one time point, with symptoms subsiding between periods of gambling disorder for at least several months.

   Persistent: Experiencing continuous symptoms, to meet diagnostic criteria for multiple years.

Specify if:

   In early remission: After full criteria for gambling disorder were previously met, none of the criteria for gambling disorder have been met for at least 3 months but for less than 12 months.

   In sustained remission: After full criteria for gambling disorder were previously met, none of the criteria for gambling disorder have been met during a period of 12 months or longer.

Specify current severity:
Mild: 4–5 criteria met.
Moderate: 6–7 criteria met.
Severe: 8–9 criteria met.

Reprinted from the *Diagnostic and Statistical Manual of Mental Disorders,* 5th Edition. Arlington, VA, American Psychiatric Association, 2013. Used with permission. Copyright © 2013 American Psychiatric Association.

The most popular forms of gambling that emerge repeatedly among adolescents include card playing, lottery purchases (scratch tickets are significantly more popular than lottery draws such as Powerball), dice and board games with family and friends, games of personal skill with peers, sports betting (primarily with peers but also through lottery outlets and/or with a bookmaker; Nevada is currently accepting sports wagering via online sites, and several U.S. states are challenging the prohibitions concerning sports wagering), and bingo (Derevensky 2012), with a growing number of youths engaged in these games via the Internet (Derevensky and Gupta 2007; Griffiths and Parke 2010; McBride and Derevensky 2009a, 2009b, 2012; Shead et al. 2010).

Adolescent Problem Gambling

Meta-analyses have been remarkably consistent in suggesting that adolescents as a group constitute a high-risk population for gambling problems, with males more likely than females to gamble, experience gambling-related problems, and reach criteria for pathological/disordered gambling (Abbott et al. 2004; Derevensky 2012; Volberg et al. 2010; Wardle et al. 2011; Welte et al. 2007). After examining the international research data, Volberg et al. (2010) concluded that although there were significant methodological differences across prevalence studies, the best estimates indicate that between 60% and 80% of adolescents report having engaged in some form of gambling for money during the past year (depending on age and/or accessibility, for legalized gambling, ages vary across jurisdictions and are often dependent on the type of gambling); most of these youths are best described as social, recreational, and occasional gamblers. Nevertheless, ample evidence suggests that 2%–8% of adolescents have a very serious gambling problem and another 10%–15% are at risk of developing a gambling problem (Abbott et al. 2004; Derevensky and Gupta 2000; Productivity Commission 2010; Shaffer and Hall 1996; Volberg et al. 2010). Despite the methodological difficulties and differences involved

when comparing data sets (see Derevensky et al. 2003 for further explanations of the variability concerning adolescent problem gambling rates),
there seems to be ample evidence that adolescent problem gambling rates
exceed those of adults and that among adults (age 18 and older), those
ages 18–25 have the highest prevalence rates of gambling problems.

Nomenclature, instrumentation, and methodological issues exist in
the measurement of adolescent pathological gambling and need to be
directly addressed (see Stinchfield 2010 and Volberg et al. 2010 for a discussion of methodological issues concerning instrumentation). Nevertheless, there remains an overwhelming consensus that gambling and
wagering among youths is a relatively common and popular activity
and that a small, identifiable population experiences serious gambling-
related problems (Derevensky 2012; Ipsos MORI 2009; Shead et al. 2010;
Wardle et al. 2011).

Similar to adults with gambling problems, adolescents with gambling problems have been reported to experience a wide range of social,
economic, personal, academic, mental health, familial, and legal problems. These adolescents have also been shown to have a disproportionately high level of delinquent and criminal behavior, disruption of
familial relationships, poor academic and work performance, and difficult peer relationships. Furthermore, adolescent pathological gamblers have been reported to have high rates of suicidal ideation and
suicide attempts and diverse mental health and behavioral problems
(Blaszczynski and Nower 2002; Derevensky and Gupta 2004a; Derevensky et al. 2007; Dickson et al. 2008; Felsher et al. 2010; Griffiths et al. 2009;
Shead et al. 2010; Temcheff et al. 2014a).

In an early study, Derevensky and Gupta (2000), using the DSM-IV–
Juvenile (DSM-IV-J) gambling severity screen for adolescents, found
that among adolescents identified as pathological gamblers, 91% reported having a preoccupation with gambling; 85% indicated chasing
losses; 70% lied to family members, peers, and friends about their gambling; 61% used their lunch money and/or allowance for gambling; 61%
became tense and restless when trying to reduce their gambling; 57% reported spending increasing amounts of money on gambling; 52% reported that gambling was a way of escaping problems; 27% reported
missing school (more than five times) to gamble during the past year;
24% had stolen money from a family member to gamble without his or
her knowledge; 24% sought help for serious financial concerns resulting
from their gambling; 21% indicated gambling-related familial problems; and 12% reported having stolen money from outside the family to
gamble. In adolescents, as in adults, the hallmark symptoms of a prob-

lem gambler are a preoccupation with the activity and chasing one's losses in an attempt to recoup gambling funds lost. This preoccupation can take a number of different forms (e.g., watching gambling-related shows, playing online social casino games for virtual currency, reading books or watching movies with gambling-related themes, paying extraordinary attention to sporting events, watching online poker tournaments), but these behaviors eventually result in the individual increasing his or her gambling (both frequency and amount wagered) and ultimately his or her losses. The gambling industry has an adage: "The more you gamble, the more you lose."

A growing body of literature suggests that pathological/disordered gamblers are not a homogeneous group and that some types or forms of gambling, impacted by structural or situational factors, may be more problematic and symptomatic of problem gamblers (e.g., slot machines and electronic gambling machines have been called the "crack cocaine" of gambling because they were designed to lead to repetitive play [addiction]; Schüll 2012). It is important to note that the predominant reason youths gamble in the first place is for the enjoyment, excitement, and entertainment associated with gambling. Making money is not the primary reason initially given for gambling, but it often propels the problem gambler to keep gambling in an effort to recoup losses. Similarly, because the thrill of gambling can plateau, individuals often increase both the frequency and the amounts of money wagered to keep gambling exciting and to maintain or enhance the adrenaline rush derived.

Although most individuals, including adolescents and young adults, gamble for the enjoyment, entertainment, and excitement, other factors also come into play. Some individuals gamble for the competition; others view gambling as a potential profession; others use gambling as a way of fulfilling needs, including coping with adversity or escaping from daily stressors (related to school, family, or work); and still others use gambling as a form of socialization, as an escape from boredom or mental and physical health issues (e.g., to reduce anxiety and depression), to relieve loneliness, or to pass time. Most adolescents report that they gamble for multiple reasons.

Although there are many biopsychosocial detriments associated with problem gambling, an understanding of the structural and situational characteristics is similarly important. By examining the structural characteristics (those characteristics that facilitate the acquisition, development, and/or maintenance of gambling behavior, irrespective of individual factors), one can develop a better understanding of the allure of gambling. As Schüll (2012) pointed out, some forms of gambling—in particular, gambling machines (also referred to as slots, video lottery terminals, electronic gambling machines, or pokies)—have the propensity to induce addictive behaviors. Parke and Griffiths (2007) argued that ever since the first slot machine was introduced to the general public in 1895, the gaming industry has employed a multitude of design features (which have changed significantly over time) to entice individuals to try their luck and to maintain their gambling. Similar structural characteristics are found in other forms of gambling. Additional structural characteristics that affect gambling include stake size; event frequency; probability of winning; jackpot size; skill or perceived skill; near-miss opportunities; light, color, and sound effects; payouts given as credits versus money; and the use of clocks on machines. Griffiths (1993) argued that the structural characteristics of a particular type of gambling may act as a reinforcer for continued gambling (based on a Skinnerian behavioral model), may satisfy an individual's psychological and physical needs, and may actually promote or facilitate excessive gambling.

In addition to structural characteristics that impact gambling, situational factors similarly play an important role. Such situational factors include ease of accessibility, geographical distances that must be traveled to gamble, cultural differences, parental attitudes, and age requirements (which can differ depending on the type of gambling, with lottery purchases often having lower minimum age requirements than casino playing).

Correlates and Risk Factors Associated With Problem Gambling

Problem gambling, like many other mental health disorders, has been shown to have multiple associated risk factors (Shead et al. 2010). It is generally accepted that adolescents with gambling problems or disorders are not a homogeneous group; they differ in their motivations to gamble and in the associated correlates and the weightings of the risk factors contributing to their gambling. Indeed, there is no single constellation of risk factors that alone can predict with certainty that an individual will develop a gambling disorder. Also, many of the identified risk factors are similarly associated with other mental health and/or addictive disorders, which helps to explain why disordered gambling is now being viewed as a behavioral addiction (American Psychiatric Association 2013).

Considerable research during the last 25 years has focused on identifying the risk factors associated with excessive gambling problems and has identified possible protective factors as a way of minimizing the problems through early intervention (Derevensky 2012; Derevensky and Gupta 2004a; Shead et al. 2010). Although there are multiple constellations of risk factors that in conjunction with a lack of specific protective factors likely place certain individuals at high risk for a specific problem, there is a growing recognition that the etiology underlying gambling problems is not universal, that the constellation of risk factors may be different for various individuals, and that a number of distinct pathways may exist that lead to pathological gambling (Gupta et al. 2013; Nower and Blaszczynski 2004). Notably, these pathways also have implications for the treatment of gambling disorders.

Recent strides toward an understanding of the onset and developmental course of gambling problems suggest the importance of adopting a biopsychosocial-environmental framework. Research on behavioral patterns, correlates, and risk factors associated with adolescent gambling and problem gambling has led to varied findings: Gambling remains more popular among males than females, and more adolescent males than females exhibit pathological gambling behaviors (Derevensky 2012; Derevensky and Gupta 2004a; Volberg et al. 2010; Wardle et al. 2011). Disordered gambling among adolescent males has been found to be from two to four times as prevalent as among females (Derevensky and Gupta 2004a; Stinchfield and Winters 1998; Volberg et al. 2010). Males have also been found to make higher gross wagers (Derevensky et al. 1996), gamble earlier, gamble on more diverse activities, gamble more frequently, spend more time and money, and experience more gambling-related problems than females. Parents have been found to be more likely to encourage their son's gambling; males are more likely to gamble with their siblings, with parents not being particularly concerned about their children's gambling behaviors independent of their gender (Campbell et al. 2011).

Among adolescents, there is often a rapid movement from social gambler to problem/disordered gambler (Derevensky and Gupta 1999; Gupta and Derevensky 1998a; Volberg et al. 2010). Adolescent problem gamblers report initiating gambling at approximately age 10–11 years, which is earlier than the initiation age of peers who report gambling but have few gambling-related problems (Derevensky and Gupta 2001; Gupta and Derevensky 1997, 1998b; Vitaro et al. 2004; Volberg et al. 2010). Also, many youth problem gamblers report having had very early gambling experiences and an early "big win" (Griffiths 1995;

Gupta and Derevensky 1997; Productivity Commission 1999; Wynne et al. 1996).

The initial gambling experiences of pathological/disordered gamblers often occur with family members in their own homes (Gupta and Derevensky 1997), with older siblings being an early influence. As children mature, their gambling patterns change, with the peer group becoming more dominant and gambling activities changing with interest and accessibility. Adolescents with gambling problems are also more likely to report having parents who are perceived as gambling excessively, are involved in other addictive behaviors, and/or have been involved in illegal activities (Griffiths 1995; Raylu and Oei 2002; Wood and Griffiths 1998).

The peer group plays an important role in endorsing or promoting gambling. Having a friend with a gambling problem appears to be a risk factor, with upward of 40% of disordered gamblers reporting having friends with gambling (Dickson et al. 2008) or substance use (Barnes et al. 1999) problems. The normalization of gambling is supported by adolescents' positive attitudes toward gambling as a highly socially acceptable behavior and pastime (Derevensky 2012).

Although adolescents often fail to comprehend the consequences of their gambling behaviors, many are cognizant of the problems associated with excessive gambling, do not perceive themselves as having a gambling problem (Hardoon et al. 2003), and view the risks associated with disordered gambling as long-term consequences and not of immediate concern (Gillespie et al. 2005).

Cultural differences among adolescents have had an impact on gambling behavior, and prevalence rates have been shown to vary from one country to another (Volberg et al. 2010). These variations may reflect different data collection methodologies or situational factors (e.g., availability, accessibility, age restrictions). Stinchfield (2000), in a large-scale study of Minnesota adolescents, reported that 30% of American Indian adolescents gambled weekly, followed by 22% of Mexican American and African American youth, and 4%–5% of Asian and Caucasian youth. In a more recent study, Arndt and Palmer (2013) reported significant racial/ethnic differences among students who gambled. White (26.0%) and Asian (25.8%) adolescents had the least lifetime exposure, and Latino (30.1%), African American (32.6%), and American Indian (34.1%) adolescents had the highest exposure. In a study in Quebec, Canada, Ellenbogen et al. (2007) reported significant cultural differences in adolescent gambling behaviors among Francophones (French-speaking families), Anglophones (English-speaking families), and allophones (families whose mother tongue was neither English nor French), with allophone adolescents exhibiting the highest rates of problem gambling.

A number of personality traits have been shown to differentiate adolescent problem gamblers from their peers. Problem gamblers have been found to score more highly on measures of excitability and extroversion, tend to have difficulty conforming to societal norms, and experience difficulties with self-discipline (Gupta et al. 2006; Ste-Marie et al. 2006). These problem gamblers also experience higher levels of state and trait anxiety (Gupta and Derevensky 1998b; Ste-Marie et al. 2002), are greater risk takers (Abbott et al. 2004; Nower et al. 2004a; Zuckerman 1994), and are more self-blaming and guilt prone (Gupta and Derevensky 2000). Adolescent problem gamblers exhibit higher scores on measures of disinhibition, boredom susceptibility, impulsivity, and other self-regulatory behaviors (e.g., self-indulgence) (Gupta et al. 2013; Nower et al. 2004a, 2004b; Shead et al. 2010). Adolescents with gambling problems also have been shown to score lower on measures of self-esteem (Gupta and Derevensky 1998b, 2004).

A multiplicity of school-related problems, including increased truancy, delinquent antisocial behaviors, conduct disorders, and poor academic performance, have been shown to be associated with increased gambling problems (Derevensky 2012; Gupta and Derevensky 1998a). Problem gamblers are more likely to have repeated a grade in school and to report a greater frequency of attention-deficit/hyperactivity disorder and conduct-related problems.

Adolescents with gambling disorders have been found to exhibit multiple mental health problems, including high levels of anxiety and depressive symptomatology (Felsher et al. 2010; Gupta and Derevensky 1998b; Gupta et al. 2006), which is consistent with the Pathways Model of problem gambling (Gupta et al. 2013; Nower and Blaszczynski 2004). Additionally, youths with severe gambling problems remain at greater risk for suicidal behaviors (Nower et al. 2004b).

Gambling and Comorbid Substance Use

A growing body of evidence from studies of adults supports phenomenological, clinical, epidemiological, and biological links between problem/disordered gambling and substance use (tobacco, alcohol, and drugs) (Grant and Chamberlain 2013; Grant and Potenza 2005; Maccallum and Blaszczynski 2002; McGrath and Barrett 2009; Petry et al. 2005; Potenza et al. 2004; Raylu and Oei 2002; Wareham and Potenza 2010). Initial analyses using the 2001–2002 U.S. National Epidemiologic Sur-

vey on Alcohol and Related Conditions suggested that 73.2% of patho-
logical/disordered gamblers had an alcohol use disorder, 60.4% had
nicotine dependency, and 38.1% had a drug use disorder (Petry et al.
2005). Parhami et al. (2014), in a longitudinal study using this same data
set, reported that 3 years after the initial interviews, gamblers in general
were at increased risk for a substance use disorder. Problem gamblers
in particular were similarly found to report high rates of multiple comorbid disorders, and this relationship increased with the severity of
the individual's gambling problem. Other studies, however, have suggested a more limited relationship.

Among adolescent problem gamblers, the relationship is less clear.
In a study of 97 substance-abusing adolescents attending an outpatient
treatment center, Kaminer et al. (2002) did not find a significant relationship between substance abuse and pathological gambling. Following
these findings, Kaminer and Haberek (2004) similarly failed to find a
significant relationship between substance-abusing teens and pathological gambling. Nevertheless, there is a growing body of evidence suggesting strong associations between excessive alcohol and other drug
use and pathological gambling among adolescents (Cook et al. 2010;
Derevensky and Gupta 2004a; Gupta and Derevensky 1998a, 1998b;
Lynch et al. 2004; Petry and Tawfik 2001). (It is important to note, however, that researchers have not determined the directions of causality
and the multiple factors influencing the development of gambling problems and substance use [Barnes et al. 1999].) The fact that all of these behaviors may be interrelated is perhaps suggestive that problem
gambling occurs within a problem-behavior syndrome or framework
(Barnes et al. 2011; Derevensky 2012; Jessor 1998; Petry and Tawfik
2001). It also may be that individuals seeking treatment for some forms
of substance use disorder are more prone to use their money for purchasing specific substances than for gambling, whereas others use their
money for gambling rather than for purchasing specific substances.
Gupta and Derevensky (2004) reported that adolescent pathological
gamblers greatly prefer to use their limited available money for gambling activities, thus likely minimizing their potential for substance
abuse. Although many of these clients reported indulging in use of marijuana, alcohol, and other substances, they reported that if they spent
their money on these substances, they would have less for gambling. A
number of youth often suggest that there is nothing that replaces the
high from gambling—not sex, not drugs, not alcohol, nothing (Derevensky 2012). Although discussing the concept of an "addictive personality" is not within the scope of this chapter, there appears to be some

commonality among substance users and individuals with gambling disorder (Ernst et al. 2003; Jessor 1998; Martin et al. 2014), suggesting that the findings may be reflecting aspects of adolescent risk taking in general, poor decision-making processes, and experiential learning.

Derevensky et al. (2011) and Gupta and Derevensky (2004), through their clinical work, have long suggested that adolescents with gambling problems frequently use gambling as a coping strategy, albeit not a positive strategy, to help escape past and current problems, including daily hassles and major traumatic life events (Bergevin et al. 2006; Felsher et al. 2010). It is not surprising that given their poor or maladaptive general coping skills (Bergevin et al. 2006; Gupta and Derevensky 2004; Nower et al. 2004a), some youths turn to alcohol and drug abuse or excessive gambling as a way of coping with adversity and major life problems. Lynch et al. (2004) and Chambers and Potenza (2003) have suggested that these findings need to be considered from a neurodevelopmental framework, whereas other authors have suggested that excessive gambling should be placed within a public health framework (Messerlian and Derevensky 2005; Messerlian et al. 2005; Shaffer and Korn 2002).

A number of studies have reported that adolescents with gambling problems exhibit greater depressive symptomatology compared with adolescents who do not gamble and those who are social/occasional gamblers, with a large percentage of those with gambling problems meeting criteria for clinical depression (Gupta and Derevensky 2004). Other studies have found that children of adult problem gamblers exhibit a number of mental health, substance use, and psychosomatic problems and remain at heightened risk for long-term mental health problems, including gambling problems (Gupta and Derevensky 1998a; Jacobs et al. 1989; Lesieur and Rothschild 1989). Although minimal longitudinal data are available from adolescent studies, the data for adults indicate poor long-range mental health prospects for disordered gamblers. Nevertheless, it is important to note that similar to individuals who use substances, individuals who exhibit a gambling disorder likely will stop gambling over time (with or without therapy). However, the relapse rate remains high. In spite of the lower adult prevalence rates of gambling disorder, which suggest that adolescent problem gamblers may undergo natural recovery and no longer exhibit the clinical signs of disordered gambling, the impact of adolescent gambling and associated personal, social, familial, and legal consequences can be so catastrophic and severe that for many, their life and career trajectories are altered.

Protective Factors

Although few in number, several studies have begun to examine protective factors as a way of providing valuable information to be used in developing effective prevention programs. These studies have focused on identifying the protective and buffering factors thought to reduce the incidence of adolescent disordered gambling. Adopting Jessor's (1998) general theory of adolescent risk behaviors, which conceptualizes the interactive nature of risk and protective factors as a way of predicting the likelihood of the acquisition or maintenance of particular risky behaviors, Dickson et al. (2002) expanded the original Substance Abuse and Mental Health Services Administration model to include excessive adolescent gambling. Although some unique risk factors are associated with problem gambling compared with other adolescent high-risk and addictive behaviors, many of these risk factors have been shown to be consistent with those associated with other aberrant behaviors (e.g., drug and alcohol use and abuse, cigarette smoking, unprotected sex). In a large study with adolescent problem gamblers, Dickson et al. (2008) attempted to test whether specific protective factors common to other adolescent risky behaviors were applicable to youths experiencing gambling problems. Using multiple self-report measures, the authors concluded that poor family and school connectedness was symptomatic of adolescent problem gambling, with family cohesion playing a significant role as a protective factor.

In a series of studies, Lussier et al. (2004) and Lussier et al. (2014) examined the concept of resilience in the presence of identified risk factors as a possible protective factor for youth gambling problems and other adolescent high-risk behaviors (this was also addressed in a study of the impact of physical, sexual, and mental abuse on disordered gambling by Felsher et al. [2010]). The 2004 results revealed that adolescents perceived to be *vulnerable* (with high risk/low protective factors) had a mean gambling severity score nine times higher than that of the *resilient* group (with high risk/high protective factors), eight times higher than that of the *fortunate* group (with low risk/low protective factors), and 13 times higher than that of the *ideal* group (with low risk/high protective factors). Those youths identified as *vulnerable* were at greatest risk for experiencing gambling problems. The results further revealed that 100% of the youths classified as pathological/disordered gamblers and 87% of those classified as at risk for problem gambling (i.e., those exhibiting a number of identifiable problems but not reaching clinical criteria for pathological gambling) scored on the resilient measure as being *vulnerable*, whereas only 4.3% of youths identified as *resilient* had been classified as at-risk gamblers and none were pathological gamblers despite reporting high levels of risk exposure. These data were strongly supported by a number of more recent studies (e.g., Lussier et al. 2014; Nower et al. 2004a). There is little doubt that resilience appears to be a key protective factor (Felsher et al. 2010) and needs to be included in mental health initiatives and prevention programs.

Even though a number of individual, situational, and environmental risk and protective factors have been found to be related to youth problem gambling behaviors, it is important to emphasize that the causal links have not yet been empirically verified. Current knowledge remains limited regarding what combinations of risk and protective factors interact to increase the likelihood that specific individuals will engage in gambling excessively and regarding at what developmental period this is most critical. Similarly, understanding of those protective factors that may minimize the risk of excessive gambling remains limited. Large longitudinal and prospective studies are only beginning; they are needed to elucidate the underlying mechanism associated with a gambling disorder. It is hoped that such studies will help to discern and identify how risk and resilience interact, within and across individuals, and how these factors affect different forms of gambling.

Assessing and Measuring Gambling Severity

Despite advances in the understanding of the etiology, correlates, and risk factors associated with adolescent problem and disordered gambling, few new screening instruments assessing the severity of adolescent problem gambling have been developed. Most adolescent gambling screens have been adapted from adult instruments, using adult criteria but modifying or replacing questions to make them more age appropriate. The most common instruments include the South Oaks Gambling Screen–Revised for Adolescents (Winters et al. 1993), the DSM-IV-J (Fisher 1992) and its revision the DSM-IV–Multiple Response–Juvenile (DSM-IV-MR-J; Fisher 2000), and the Massachusetts Gambling Screen (MAGS) (Shaffer et al. 1994; Stinchfield 2010). The newest adolescent gambling screen, developed exclusively for this age population, is the Canadian Adolescent Gambling Inventory (CAGI) (Stinchfield 2010; Wiebe et al. 2007). Rather than being an adaptation of an adult instrument, the CAGI assesses adolescent gambling severity on a continuum.

Although used in only a limited number of studies to date, the CAGI was developed to measure gambling behavior itself as well as problem gambling severity and to assess gambling problems over a limited time frame (3 months, in contrast to the past-year gambling-related problems assessed by most instruments). The CAGI seeks to evaluate and identify behavior in five distinct areas: 1) types of gambling behaviors/activities in which the individual engages, 2) frequency of participation in each of these activities, 3) time spent on each of the gambling activities, 4) money wagered, and 5) severity of gambling problems.

Similar to adult assessments (the former gold standard for assessment being DSM-IV [American Psychiatric Association 1994] criteria, and the new standard being DSM-5 criteria), the clinical tools for evaluating adolescents have common underlying constructs, including both psychological factors and the negative financial and behavioral costs associated with excessive gambling (Stinchfield 2010). Commonly examined constructs include stealing money to support gambling (this item is no longer listed in the DSM-5 criteria for gambling disorder), occupational/school-related problems, disrupted relationships, chasing losses, lying or deception about one's gambling problems, disrupted familial relationships, the need to increase the frequency and amount wagered, preoccupation with gambling, and concern/criticism from others. Differences in prevalence rates as well as divergent findings among different cultural groups may be due to variability in instrumentation. As a result, both Derevensky (2012) and Stinchfield (2010) have argued that greater standardization, improved nomenclature, and the development of new instruments that are reflective of current knowledge are needed.

Treatment of Youths With Gambling Problems

Because there is no single identifiable cause for gambling problems, there is no single therapeutic approach that works for all individuals (see Richard et al. 2014 for recent advances in the treatment of disordered gambling). The fact that no universal empirically validated treatment programs have been established for problem gamblers has not deterred clinicians from employing a wide diversity of approaches.

The current treatment paradigms for adolescents and young adults have in general been based on a wide variety of theoretical approaches paralleling those used for adults. These include psychoanalytic or psychodynamic (Miller 1986; Rosenthal 1987; Rugle and Rosenthal 1994), behavioral (Blaszczynski and McConaghy 1993; Petry and Roll 2001;

Walker 1993), cognitive and cognitive-behavioral (Blaszczynski and Nower 2014; Dowling 2014; Ladouceur and Walker 1998), pharmacological (Grant et al. 2003, 2004; Hollander et al. 2005), physiological (Blaszczynski et al. 1986; Carlton and Goldstein 1987), biological/genetic (Comings 1998; DeCaria et al. 1997; Saiz 1992), addiction-based (Lesieur and Blume 1991; McCormick and Taber 1988), and self-help (Ferentzy et al. 2014) models. (For a more comprehensive overview of these models, see these reviews: Hodgins et al. 2011; Ladouceur and Shaffer 2005; Petry 2005; Potenza 2005; and Richard et al. 2014.)

There is clear evidence that most adults and adolescents learn from their mistakes. Although they sometimes exceed their preset gambling limits, in terms of time and/or money, and may suffer some short-term consequences, most eventually refrain from excessive gambling; some may stop completely, whereas others retake control of their wagering behavior and continue in moderation. In contrast, other individuals, in spite of their realization that their odds of winning are indeed limited, may be driven to increase the frequency and intensity of their gambling by their physiological needs, perceived skill and knowledge, erroneous cognitions, and/or need for escape from daily and long-term stressors and mental health issues (Derevensky 2012).

Each current treatment paradigm employs a relatively narrow focus, depending on the therapist's theoretical orientation and conceptualization of the etiology of a gambling disorder, his or her background work in the field of addictions, and whether or not the therapist believes in "controlled gambling" versus abstinence. Abbott et al. (2004) concluded that the ability to design effective treatment programs for problem/disordered gamblers has been hampered by a lack of theoretical understanding of the etiology underlying problem gambling. They also averred that although the biomedical model has dominated the treatment community in the United States, the cognitive-behavioral or social learning theory models have dominated in other countries. Few randomized psychotherapeutic comparative studies exist. The limited number of empirically based studies has resulted in a lack of consensus on what constitutes best practices or empirically validated treatment approaches for treating both adolescents and adults with gambling problems (Hodgins et al. 2011; Nathan 2001, 2005; Petry 2005; Richard et al. 2014). A universal approach to the treatment of gambling problems has been seriously questioned, given the general acceptance that disordered gamblers do not constitute a homogeneous group (Blaszczynski and Nower 2002; Derevensky et al. 2011; Gupta and Derevensky 2004; Nower and Blaszczynski 2004; Temcheff et al. 2014a).

The fact that only a small percentage of youths with severe gambling disorders perceive themselves as having a gambling problem helps account for the low turnout of adolescents who seek help for a gambling disorder (Derevensky et al. 2011; Hardoon et al. 2003). Even among adults with gambling disorders, the fact that only approximately 10% of these individuals present for treatment is a serious concern (Hodgins et al. 2011; Slutske et al. 2009). Perceived barriers to treatment seeking by people who gamble include their desire to manage the problem themselves, failure to acknowledge the problem (denial), and shame (Suurvali et al. 2010). To make matters worse, logistical travel considerations and unwillingness to acknowledge a problem to parents mean that adolescents have even more barriers to seeking treatment.

There is considerable empirical support suggesting that gambling involves a complex and dynamic interaction among ecological, psychophysiological, developmental, cognitive, and behavioral components, with environmental issues (accessibility, availability, and game type) also being important. Derevensky (2012), Derevensky et al. (2011), Gupta and Derevensky (2000, 2004), and Gupta et al. (2013) contend that considering the varying underlying reasons for gambling and the absence of empirically validated treatment programs, a dynamic interactive treatment approach needs to take into account the multiplicity of interacting factors for youths experiencing significant gambling problems. Empirical support for Jacobs' General Theory of Addictions for adolescent problem gamblers (Gupta and Derevensky 1998b) further indicates that adolescent problem and pathological gamblers exhibit evidence of abnormal physiological resting states, report significantly greater emotional distress and anxiety, have increased levels of dissociation when gambling, demonstrate erroneous cognitions when gambling (e.g., they believe that they can predict the outcome of the game even when the outcome is based purely on randomness, they report exaggerated levels of skill, they have little understanding of randomness and independence of events), display depressive symptomatology, and are more likely to have higher rates of comorbidity with other addictive behaviors. Gupta and Derevensky (2004) contend that treating and addressing gambling problems in isolation from other pressing social, physiological, developmental, cognitive, and emotional difficulties may lead to short-term success. Ultimately, however, many of these individuals will relapse, especially those people with a co-occurring substance use disorder (Ledgerwood et al. 2014).

Although treatment outcome studies have been limited, there is evidence that behavioral, cognitive, and cognitive-behavioral models may be effective, at least for adults (Ledgerwood et al. 2014). Ladouceur et al. 1994, 1998) have long argued for a cognitive-behavioral approach to treating both adults and youths with gambling problems. Underlying their approach is the assumption that pathological gamblers continue to gamble in spite of repeated losses because they maintain an unrealistic belief that losses will be recovered. This perspective assumes that it is the individual's erroneous cognitions and beliefs (i.e., a lack of understanding of the notion of independence of events, erroneous perceptions concerning the level of skill required to be successful in predicting the outcome of chance events observable in most gambling activities, and an illusion of personal control and skill) that promote persistent gambling behavior (Ladouceur and Walker 1998). Although the empirical literature examining treatment paradigms for adolescents is scant, Ladouceur et al. (1998), in a study including four adolescent male pathological gamblers who completed treatment, noted clinically significant improvements in the individuals' beliefs about the perception of control when gambling and a significant postintervention reduction in the number and severity of gambling problems. Three of the four adolescents reportedly sustained initial treatment gains and were abstinent at 6 months.

Other models employed for brief interventions using motivational interviewing and motivational enhancement have reportedly been successful with adults who have gambling disorders (Hodgins et al. 2001, 2004). Also, a growing body of research supports the use of psychopharmacology, especially in conjunction with psychotherapeutic treatment (Hodgins et al. 2011); however, no accepted psychopharmacological interventions exist for youth.

Psychopharmacology may provide a promising complementary strategy for treating adolescents experiencing significant gambling problems. The current pharmacological strategies for treating pathological gambling in adults include the use of serotonin reuptake inhibitors, mood stabilizers, and naltrexone (Grant et al. 2003), but little is known about the success of these strategies with adolescents (Grant et al. 2004). Grant et al. (2004) and Hollander et al. (2005) suggest that positive short-term effects for adults will need to be replicated with youths before any definitive conclusions can be made. Potentially promising psychopharmacological treatments for adolescent pathological gambling must await completion of controlled clinical treatment studies.

Research on the effective treatment of adolescents with gambling disorders remains limited at best. Reducing the barriers to treatment for adolescents will be necessary before best practices can be established. It may well be that some of the previously established treatment models for other mental health disorders and addictive behaviors can be applied to youths with gambling problems, given the significant comorbidity and overlapping risk factors.

The issue of natural recovery is increasingly important and requires greater attention not only because it reduces the prevalence of disordered gambling but also because it may help clinicians learn more effective treatment strategies. The treatment outcome studies for natural recovery, such as attendance at Gamblers Anonymous meetings, have been limited. Although some correlational data show positive outcomes for adults (Hodgins et al. 2011), few such programs exist for youths. In spite of adolescents being welcomed into these self-help groups, clinical experience has shown that these groups have had a limited effect for this age group. Adolescents typically report having difficulty relating to older members, and they perceive their problems as minor compared to those of the adults who have lost jobs, families, lifelong savings, and so forth. If most youths are not seeking professional treatment (as is also the case with adults), then the issue of understanding the process of natural recovery remains critical, and alternative approaches (e.g., online support) may be necessary.

Although pathological/disordered gambling is currently viewed as a continuous and progressive disorder, there is some clinical support suggesting that it may, in fact, be episodic, meaning that individuals engage excessively for a limited time, experience difficulties, and then stop for undetermined amounts of time. This construct may be viewed as binge gambling (see Gupta and Derevensky 2011 for a discussion of adolescent binge gambling).

Combinations of behavioral and drug therapies for the treatment of other addictive disorders have been demonstrated to be superior to treatment alone (Carroll 1997). Further research is necessary and matching of treatment strategies with gambler typologies must be refined (see Gupta et al. 2013) before determinations can be made as to whether or not best practices for treating adolescents with gambling problems can be realized. Nevertheless, Abbott et al. (2004), Hodgins et al. (2011), and Ledgerwood et al. (2014), when reviewing treatment outcome studies, concluded that there is evidence suggesting that individuals who have received treatment for a myriad of mental health disorders and addictions typically do better than control subjects not receiving any formal treatment. Further research in understanding the barriers to treatment for adolescents, whether or not controlled gambling or abstinence is a realistic goal, and continued work toward empirically supported treatments for youths are needed.

Summary and Future Directions

Significant progress has been made in understanding the risks and protective factors associated with adolescent problem/disordered gambling. In spite of this knowledge, ample evidence suggests that most individuals do not associate problem and disordered gambling with adolescents. As the landscape of gambling continues to change, with greater acceptability and accessibility, there is an increased need for the development of prevention initiatives. There remains a fear that the incidence of problem gambling among youths will continue to rise with ongoing exposure. This changing landscape, with a heavy emphasis on technological advances (online and mobile gambling), the increase in social casino games, and the normalization and social acceptability of gambling, represents new challenges for youths and their parents, teachers, and mental health professionals.

Adolescence is a developmental stage marked by significant physical, social, cognitive, and emotional changes. Considering that it often takes several years for a person to go from occasional or recreational gambling to a significant gambling problem, the long-term social impact on society resulting from gambling expansion will likely not be realized for some time. In a recent discussion as to whether or not online gambling should be introduced in a state with multiple casinos, one legislator remarked in an unrecorded meeting that he believed it was inappropriate to bring a casino into every home; this is especially true for underage youths.

Youth today will spend their entire lives in an environment where gambling is prolific, government supported, socially acceptable, and easily accessible in spite of some age-restricted prohibitions. Several studies examining the perspectives of parents, teachers, and mental health professionals on youth problematic behavior revealed that among 13 potentially risky adolescent behaviors, gambling was the least concerning (Campbell et al. 2011; Derevensky et al. 2014; Temcheff et al. 2014b). Until greater acknowledgment and acceptance of the potential impact of youth gambling have been realized, adolescents remain at heightened risk for developing gambling-related problems.

Derevensky (2008, 2012) has argued for more research to help identify common and unique risk and protective factors for gambling problems and other addictive behaviors; longitudinal research to examine the natural history of both regular and pathological gambling from childhood to adolescence through later adulthood; and molecular, genetic, and neuropsychological research to help understand the changes in gambling progression and to identify high-risk individuals. It is important to acknowledge that the gambling industry has begun to realize the potential negative side of gambling and has worked on developing "responsible gambling strategies." Although most of these strategies have been aimed at adults, some strategies, including age identification, have been developed for lottery vendors and online gambling. These efforts have not gone unnoticed, but more work is needed.

Other factors, including the widespread use of social media and social casino gambling and their impact, need to be examined. A variety of treatment and prevention models need to be tested and validated before best practices can be reliably established. Although the research has pointed to the importance of examining commonalities between gambling and comorbid substance use, preventive interventions targeting common risk factors may also need to be complemented by modules specific to each behavior (Vitaro et al. 2014). Youth problem/disordered gambling represents an important public health issue that needs to be addressed.

KEY POINTS

- Gambling among youth has become a socially acceptable form of entertainment.

- Between 2% and 8% of adolescents have a very serious gambling problem, and another 10%–15% are at risk for the development of a gambling problem.

- Adolescent problem gamblers often exhibit a variety of comorbid risky behaviors and mental health disorders.

- Gambling problems among adolescents is becoming an important public health issue.

- Additional research is needed to identify best practices for the prevention and treatment of gambling problems in adolescents.

References

Abbott MW, Volberg RA, Bellringer M, et al: A Review of Research on Aspects of Problem Gambling, Final Report. London, Responsibility in Gambling Trust, 2004

American Psychiatric Association: Diagnostic and Statistical Manual of Mental Disorders, 4th Edition. Washington, DC, American Psychiatric Publishing, 1994

American Psychiatric Association: Diagnostic and Statistical Manual of Mental Disorders, 5th Edition. Arlington, VA, American Psychiatric Publishing, 2013

Arndt S, Palmer J: Iowa youth gambling using the 2012 Iowa Youth Survey: who, what, where and what else? Iowa City, Iowa Consortium for Substance Abuse Research and Evaluation, 2013

Barnes GM, Welte JW, Hoffman JH, et al: Gambling and alcohol use among youth: influences of demographic, socialization, and individual factors. Addict Behav 24(6):749–767, 1999 10628510

Barnes GM, Welte JW, Hoffman JH, et al: The co-occurrence of gambling with substance use and conduct disorder among youth in the United States. Am J Addict 20(2):166–173, 2011 21314760

Bergevin T, Gupta R, Derevensky J, et al: Adolescent gambling: understanding the role of stress and coping. J Gambl Stud 22:195–208, 2006 16838102

Blaszczynski A, McConaghy N: A two to nine year treatment follow-up study of pathological gambling, in Gambling Behavior and Problem Gambling. Edited by Eadington W, Cornelius JA. Reno, NV, Institute for the Study of Gambling and Commercial Gambling, 1993, pp 215–233

Blaszczynski A, Nower L: A pathways model of problem and pathological gambling. Addiction 97(5):487–499, 2002 12033650

Blaszczynski A, Nower L: Cognitive-behavioral therapy: translating research into clinical practice in The Wiley-Blackwell Handbook of Disordered Gambling. Edited by Richard D, Blaszczynski A, Nower L. Chichester, UK, Wiley, 2014, pp 204–224

Blaszczynski A, Winter S, McConaghy N: Plasma endorphin levels in pathological gambling. Journal of Gambling Behavior 2(1):3–14, 1986

Campbell C, Derevensky J, Meerkamper E, et al: Parents' perceptions of adolescent gambling: a Canadian national study. Journal of Gambling Issues 25:36–53, 2011

Carlton P, Goldstein L: Physiological determinants of pathological gambling, in The Handbook of Pathological Gambling. Edited by Galski Y. Springfield, IL, Charles C Thomas, 1987, pp 111–135

Carroll KM: Integrating psychotherapy and pharmacotherapy to improve drug abuse outcomes. Addict Behav 22(2):233–245, 1997 9113217

Chambers RA, Potenza MN: Neurodevelopment, impulsivity, and adolescent gambling. J Gambl Stud 19(1):53–84, 2003 12635540

Comings D: The genetics of pathological gambling: the addictive effect of multiple genes. Paper presented at the National Conference on Problem Gambling, Las Vegas, NV, June 1998

Cook S, Turner N, Paglia-Boak A, et al: Ontario Youth Gambling Report: Data From the 2009 Ontario Student Drug Use and Health Survey. Toronto, ON, Canada, Problem Gambling Institute of Ontario, 2010

DeCaria C, Hollander E, Wong C: Neuropsychiatric functioning in pathological gamblers. Paper presented at the National Conference on Problem Gambling, New Orleans, LA, August 1997

Derevensky JL: Gambling behaviors and adolescent substance use disorders, in Adolescent Substance Abuse: Psychiatric Comorbidity and High-Risk Behaviors. Edited by Kaminer Y, Bukstein OG. New York, Haworth Press, 2008, pp 403–433

Derevensky JL: Teen Gambling: Understanding a Growing Epidemic. Lanham, MD, Rowman & Littlefield, 2012

Derevensky JL, Gupta R: Youth gambling problems: a new issue for school psychologists. Nova Scotia Psychologist 12(11):8–11, 1999

Derevensky JL, Gupta R: Prevalence estimates of adolescent gambling: a comparison of the SOGS-RA, DSM-IV-J, and the GA 20 questions. J Gambl Stud 16(2–3):227–251, 2000 14634314

Derevensky JL, Gupta R: Le problème de jeu touche aussi les jeunes. Psychologie Québec 18(6):23–27, 2001

Derevensky JL, Gupta R: Adolescents with gambling problems: a synopsis of our current knowledge. Journal of Gambling Issues 10, 2004a. Available at http://jgi.camh.net/doi/abs/10.4309/jgi.2004.10.3.

Derevensky JL, Gupta R: Internet gambling amongst adolescents: a growing concern. Int J Ment Health Addict 5(2):93–101, 2007

Derevensky JL, Gupta R, Della Cioppa G: A developmental perspective of gambling behavior in children and adolescents. J Gambl Stud 12(1):49–66, 1996 24233846

Derevensky JL, Gupta R, Winters K: Prevalence rates of youth gambling problems: are the current rates inflated? J Gambl Stud 19(4):405–425, 2003 14634300

Derevensky JL, Pratt LM, Hardoon KK, et al: Gambling problems and features of attention deficit hyperactivity disorder among children and adolescents. J Addict Med 1(3):165–172, 2007 21768953

Derevensky JL, Temcheff C, Gupta R: Treatment of adolescent gambling problems: more art than science? in Youth Gambling Problems: The Hidden Addiction. Edited by Derevensky J, Shek D, Merrick J. Berlin, De Gruyter, 2011, pp 167–186

Derevensky JL, St-Pierre RA, Temcheff CE, et al: Teacher awareness and attitudes regarding adolescent risky behaviours: is adolescent gambling perceived to be a problem? J Gambl Stud 30(2):435–451, 2014 23423729

Dickson LM, Derevensky JL, Gupta R: The prevention of youth gambling problems: a conceptual model. J Gambl Stud 18(2):97–159, 2002 12096450

Dickson L, Derevensky JL, Gupta R: Youth gambling problems: an examination of risk and protective factors. International Gambling Studies 8(1):25–47, 2008

Dowling N: The cognitive-behavioral treatment of female problem gambling, in The Wiley-Blackwell Handbook of Disordered Gambling. Edited by Richard D, Blaszczynski A, Nower L. Chichester, UK, Wiley, 2014, pp 225–250

Ellenbogen S, Derevensky J, Gupta R: Gender differences among adolescents with gambling-related problems. J Gambl Stud 23(2):133–143, 2007 17265189

Ernst M, Grant SJ, London ED, et al: Decision making in adolescents with behavior disorders and adults with substance abuse. Am J Psychiatry 160(1):33–40, 2003 12505799

Everard KM, Lach HW, Fisher EB, et al: Relationship of activity and social support to the functional health of older adults. J Gerontol B Psychol Sci Soc Sci 55(4):S208–S212, 2000 11584883

Felsher JR, Derevensky JL, Gupta R: Young adults with gambling problems: the impact of childhood maltreatment. Int J Ment Health Addict 8(4):545–556, 2010

Ferentzy P, Skinner W, Antze P: Understanding Gamblers Anonymous: a practitioner's guide, in The Wiley-Blackwell Handbook of Disordered Gambling. Edited by Richard D, Blaszczynski A, Nower L. Chichester, UK, Wiley, 2014, pp 251–262

Fisher S: Measuring pathological gambling in children: the case of fruit machines in the U.K. J Gambl Stud 8(3):263–285, 1992

Fisher S: Developing the DSM-IV-DSM-IV criteria to identify adolescent problem gambling in non-clinical populations. J Gambl Stud 16(2–3):253–273, 2000 14634315

Gillespie M, Gupta R, Derevensky J, et al: Adolescent problem gambling: evaluating perceived risks and benefits [Le jeu problématique chez les adolescents: perceptions des risques et des bénéfices]. Report prepared for the Fonds de recherche du Québec—Santé (FRSQ), Quebec, QC, Canada 2005

Grant J, Chamberlain SR: Gambling disorder and its relationship with substance use disorders: implications for nosological revisions and treatment. Am J Addict 2013 24102900 [Epub ahead of print]

Grant JE, Potenza MN: Tobacco use and pathological gambling. Ann Clin Psychiatry 17(4):237–241, 2005 16402757

Grant J, Kim SW, Potenza MN: Advances in the pharmacological treatment of pathological gambling. J Gambl Stud 19(1):85–109, 2003 12635541

Grant J, Chambers R, Potenza M: Adolescent problem gambling: neurodevelopment and pharmacological treatment, in Gambling Problems in Youth: Theoretical and Applied Perspectives. Edited by Derevensky J, Gupta R. New York, Kluwer Academic/Plenum, 2004, pp 81–98

Griffiths M: Fruit machine gambling: the importance of structural characteristics. J Gambl Stud 9(2):101–120, 1993

Griffiths M: Adolescent Gambling. London, Routledge, 1995

Griffiths MD, Parke J: Adolescent gambling on the internet: a review. Int J Adolesc Med Health 22(1):59–75, 2010 20491418

Griffiths M, Wood R: Adolescent Internet gambling: preliminary results of a national survey. Education and Health 25(2):23–27, 2007

Griffiths M, King D, Delfabbro P: Adolescent gambling-like experiences: are they cause for concern? Education and Health 27(2):27–30, 2009

Gupta R, Derevensky J: Familial and social influences on juvenile gambling behavior. J Gambl Stud 13(3):179–192, 1997 12913385

Gupta R, Derevensky JL: Adolescent gambling behavior: a prevalence study and examination of the correlates associated with problem gambling. J Gambl Stud 14(4):319–345, 1998a 12766444

Gupta R, Derevensky JL: An empirical examination of Jacobs' General Theory of Addictions: do adolescent gamblers fit the theory? J Gambl Stud 14(1):17–49, 1998b 12766433

Gupta R, Derevensky JL: Adolescents with gambling problems: from research to treatment. J Gambl Stud 16(2–3):315–342, 2000 14634318

Gupta R, Derevensky J: A treatment approach for adolescents with gambling problems, in Gambling Problems in Youth: Theoretical and Applied Perspectives. Edited by Derevensky J, Gupta, R. New York, Kluwer Academic/Plenum, 2004, pp 165–188

Gupta R, Derevensky J: Defining and assessing binge gambling, in Youth Gambling Problems: The Hidden Addiction. Edited by Derevensky J, Shek D, Merrick J. Berlin, De Gruyter, 2011, pp 79–97

Gupta R, Derevensky J, Ellenbogen S: Personality characteristics and risk-taking tendencies among adolescent gamblers. Can J Behav Sci 38(3):201–213, 2006

Gupta R, Nower L, Derevensky JL, et al: Problem gambling in adolescents: an examination of the Pathways Model. J Gambl Stud 29(3):575–588, 2013 22695971

Hardoon K, Derevensky J, Gupta R: Empirical measures vs. perceived gambling severity among youth: why adolescent problem gamblers fail to seek treatment. Addict Behav 28(5):933–946, 2003 12788266

Hodgins DC, Currie SR, el-Guebaly N: Motivational enhancement and self-help treatments for problem gambling. J Consult Clin Psychol 69(1):50–57, 2001 11302277

Hodgins DC, Currie S, el-Guebaly N, et al: Brief motivational treatment for problem gambling: a 24-month follow-up. Psychol Addict Behav 18(3):293–296, 2004 15482086

Hodgins DC, Stea JN, Grant JE: Gambling disorders. Lancet 378(9806):1874–1884, 2011 21600645

Hollander E, Sood E, Pallanti S, et al: Pharmacological treatments of pathological gambling. J Gambl Stud 21(1):99–110, 2005 15789195

Hope J, Havir L: You bet they're having fun! Older Americans and casino gambling. J Aging Stud 16(2):177–197, 2002

Ipsos MORI: British Survey of Children: the National Lottery and Gambling 2008–2009: Report of a Quantitative Survey. London, National Lottery Commission, 2009

Jacobs D, Marston A, Singer R, et al: Children of problem gamblers. Journal of Gambling Behavior 5(4):261–268, 1989

Jessor R (ed): New Perspectives on Adolescent Risk Behavior. Cambridge, UK, Cambridge University Press, 1998

Kaminer Y, Haberek R: Pathological gambling and substance use. J Am Acad Child Adolesc Psychiatry 43(11):1326–1327, 2004 15502590

Kaminer Y, Burleson JA, Jadamec A: Gambling behavior in adolescent substance abuse. Subst Abus 23(3):191–198, 2002 12444352

Ladouceur R, Shaffer HJ: Treating problem gamblers: working towards empirically supported treatment. J Gambl Stud 21(1):1–4, 2005 15789183

Ladouceur R, Walker M: Cognitive approach to understanding and treating pathological gambling, in Comprehensive Clinical Psychology. Edited by Bellack AS, Hersen M. New York, Pergamon, 1998, pp 588–601

Ladouceur R, Boisvert J-M, Dumont J: Cognitive-behavioral treatment for adolescent pathological gamblers. Behav Modif 18(2):230–242, 1994 8002927

Ladouceur R, Sylvain C, Letarte H, et al: Cognitive treatment of pathological gamblers. Behav Res Ther 36(12):1111–1119, 1998 9745796

Ledgerwood DM, Loree A, Lundahl LH, et al: Predictors of treatment outcome in disordered gambling, in The Wiley-Blackwell Handbook of Disordered Gambling. Edited by Richard D, Blaszczynski A, Nower L. Chichester, UK, Wiley, 2014 pp 283–305

Lesieur HR, Blume SB: Evaluation of patients treated for pathological gambling in a combined alcohol, substance abuse and pathological gambling treatment unit using the Addiction Severity Index. Br J Addict 86(8):1017–1028, 1991 1912747

Lesieur H, Rothschild J: Children of Gamblers Anonymous members. Journal of Gambling Behavior 5(4):269–281, 1989

Loroz P: Golden-age gambling: psychological benefits and self-concept dynamics in aging consumers' consumption experiences. Psychology and Marketing 21(5):323–349, 2004

Lussier I, Derevensky J, Gupta R: Youth gambling behaviour: an examination of resilience. Paper presented at the 5th National Child Welfare Symposium, Ottawa, ON, Canada, August 2004

Lussier I, Derevensky J, Gupta R, et al: Risk, compensatory, protective, and vulnerability processes influencing youth gambling problems and other high-risk behaviours. Psychol Addict Behav 28:404–413 2014

Lynch WJ, Maciejewski PK, Potenza MN: Psychiatric correlates of gambling in adolescents and young adults grouped by age at gambling onset. Arch Gen Psychiatry 61(11):1116–1122, 2004 15520359

Maccallum F, Blaszczynski A: Pathological gambling and comorbid substance use. Aust NZ J Psychiatry 36(3):411–415, 2002 12060192

Martin RJ, Usdan S, Cremeens J, et al: Disordered gambling and co morbidity of psychiatric disorders among college students: an examination of problem drinking, anxiety and depression. J Gambl Stud 30(2):321–333, 2014 23430449

McBride J, Derevensky J: Internet gambling among college students. Poster presented at the Canadian Psychological Association annual conference, Montreal, QE, Canada, June 2009a

McBride J, Derevensky J: Internet gambling behavior in a sample of online gamblers. Int J Ment Health Addict 7(1):149–167, 2009b

McBride J, Derevensky J: Internet gambling and risk-taking among students: an exploratory study. J Behav Addict 1(2):50–58, 2012

McCormick RA, Taber JI: Attributional style in pathological gamblers in treatment. J Abnorm Psychol 97(3):368–370, 1988 3192832

McGrath DS, Barrett SP: The comorbidity of tobacco smoking and gambling: a review of the literature. Drug Alcohol Rev 28(6):676–681, 2009 19930023

Messerlian C, Derevensky J: Youth gambling: a public health perspective. Journal of Gambling Issues 14:97–116, 2005

Messerlian C, Derevensky J, Gupta R: Youth gambling problems: a public health perspective. Health Promot Int 20(1):69–79, 2005 15681591

Miller W: Individual outpatient treatment of pathological gambling. Journal of Gambling Behavior 2(2):95–107, 1986

Nathan P: Best practices for the treatment of gambling disorders: too soon. Paper presented at the annual Harvard-National Centre for Responsible Gambling Conference, Las Vegas, NV, December 2001

Nathan PE: Methodological problems in research on treatments for pathological gambling. J Gambl Stud 21(1):109–116, 2005 15789196

Nower L, Blaszczynski A: A pathways approach to treating youth gamblers, in Gambling Problems in Youth: Theoretical and Applied Perspectives. Edited by Derevensky J, Gupta R. New York, Kluwer Academic/Plenum, 2004, pp 189–210

Nower L, Derevensky JL, Gupta R: The relationship of impulsivity, sensation seeking, coping, and substance use in youth gamblers. Psychol Addict Behav 18(1):49–55, 2004a 15008685

Nower L, Gupta R, Blaszczynski A, et al: Suicidality ideation and depression among youth gamblers: a preliminary examination of three studies. International Gambling Studies 4(1):69–80, 2004b

Parhami I, Mojtabai R, Rosenthal RJ, et al: Gambling and the onset of comorbid mental disorders: a longitudinal study evaluating severity and specific symptoms. J Psychiatr Pract 20(3):207–219, 2014 24847994

Parke J, Griffiths M: The role of structural characteristics in gambling, in Research and Measurement Issues in Gambling Studies. Edited by Smith D, Hodgins D, Williams R. New York, Elsevier, 2007, pp 211–243

Petry NM: Pathological Gambling: Etiology, Comorbidity, and Treatment. Washington, DC, American Psychological Association, 2005

Petry NM, Roll JM: A behavioral approach to understanding and treating pathological gambling. Semin Clin Neuropsychiatry 6(3):177–183, 2001 11447569

Petry NM, Tawfik Z: Comparison of problem-gambling and non-problem-gambling youths seeking treatment for marijuana abuse. J Am Acad Child Adolesc Psychiatry 40(11):1324–1331, 2001 11699807

Petry NM, Stinson FS, Grant BF: Comorbidity of DSM-IV pathological gambling and other psychiatric disorders: results from the National Epidemiologic Survey on Alcohol and Related Conditions. J Clin Psychiatry 66(5):564–574, 2005 15889941

Potenza MN: Advancing treatment strategies for pathological gambling. J Gambl Stud 21(1):91–100, 2005 15789194

Potenza MN, Steinberg MA, McLaughlin SD, et al: Characteristics of tobacco-smoking problem gamblers calling a gambling helpline. Am J Addict 13(5):471–493, 2004 15764425

Productivity Commission: Australia's Gambling Industries, Report No 10. Canberra, Productivity Commission, AusInfo, 1999. Available at: http://www.pc.gov.au/inquiries/completed/gambling/report. Accessed January 15, 2015

Productivity Commission: Gambling Productivity Commission Inquiry Report, Report No 50. Canberra, Productivity Commission, Australian Government, 2010

Raylu N, Oei TP: Pathological gambling: a comprehensive review. Clin Psychol Rev 22(7):1009–1061, 1999 12238245

Richard D, Blaszczynski A, Nower L (eds): The Wiley-Blackwell Handbook of Disordered Gambling. Chichester, UK, Wiley, 2014

Rosenthal R: The psychodynamics of pathological gambling: a review of the literature, in The Handbook of Pathological Gambling. Edited by Galski T. Springfield, IL, Charles C Thomas, 1987, pp 41–70

Rugle LJ, Rosenthal RJ: Transference and countertransference reactions in the psychotherapy of pathological gamblers. J Gambl Stud 10(1):43–65, 1994 24234782

Saiz J: Don't begin the game [in Spanish]. Interviu 829:24–28, 1992

Schüll N: Addiction by Design: Machine Gambling in Las Vegas. Princeton, NJ, Princeton University Press, 2012

Shaffer HJ, Hall MN: Estimating the prevalence of adolescent gambling disorders: a quantitative synthesis and guide toward standard gambling nomenclature. J Gambl Stud 12(2):193–214, 1996 24233916

Shaffer HJ, Korn DA: Gambling and related mental disorders: a public health analysis. Annu Rev Public Health 23(1):171–212, 2002 11910060

Shaffer HJ, Labrie R, Scanlan KM, et al: Pathological gambling among adolescents: Massachusetts Gambling Screen (MAGS). J Gambl Stud 10(4):339–362, 1994 24234969

Shead NW, Derevensky JL, Gupta R: Risk and protective factors associated with youth problem gambling. Int J Adolesc Med Health 22(1):39–58, 2010 20491417

Slutske WS, Blaszczynski A, Martin NG: Sex differences in the rates of recovery, treatment-seeking, and natural recovery in pathological gambling: results from an Australian community-based twin survey. Twin Res Hum Genet 12(5):425–432, 2009 19803770

Ste-Marie C, Gupta R, Derevensky J: Anxiety and social stress related to adolescent gambling behavior. International Gambling Studies 2(1):123–141, 2002

Ste-Marie C, Gupta R, Derevensky J: Anxiety and social stress related to adolescent gambling behavior and substance use. J Child Adolesc Subst Abuse 15(4):55–74, 2006

Stinchfield R: Gambling and correlates of gambling among Minnesota public school students. J Gambl Stud 16:153–173, 2000 14634311

Stinchfield R: A critical review of adolescent problem gambling assessment instruments. Int J Adolesc Med Health 22(1):77–93, 2010 20491419

Stinchfield R, Winters K: Gambling and problem gambling among youth. Ann Am Acad Pol Soc Sci 556(1):172–185, 1998

St-Pierre R, Derevensky J, Gupta R, et al: Preventing lottery ticket sales to minors: factors influencing retailers' compliance behaviour. International Gambling Studies 11(2):173–191, 2011

Suurvali H, Hodgins DC, Cunningham JA: Motivators for resolving or seeking help for gambling problems: a review of the empirical literature. J Gambl Stud 26(1):1–33, 2010 19768660

Temcheff CE, St-Pierre RA, Derevensky JL: Gambling among teens, college students and young adults, in The Wiley-Blackwell Handbook of Disordered Gambling. Edited by Richard D, Blaszczynski A, Nower L. Chichester, UK, Wiley, 2014a, pp 306–326

Temcheff CE, Derevensky JL, St-Pierre RA, et al: Beliefs and attitudes of mental health professionals with respect to gambling and other high risk behaviors in schools. Int J Ment Health Addict 12(6):716–729, 2014b

Vander Bilt J, Dodge HH, Pandav R, et al: Gambling participation and social support among older adults: a longitudinal community study. J Gambl Stud 20(4):373–389, 2004 15577273

Vitaro F, Wanner B, Ladouceur R, et al: Trajectories of gambling during adolescence. J Gambl Stud 20(1):47–69, 2004 14973397

Vitaro F, Hartl AC, Brendgen M, et al: Genetic and environmental influences on gambling and substance use in early adolescence. Behav Genet 44(4):347–355, 2014 24824822

Volberg R, Reitzes D, Boles J: Exploring the links between gambling, problem gambling, and self-esteem. Deviant Behav 18(4):321–342, 1997

Volberg RA, Gupta R, Griffiths MD, et al: An international perspective on youth gambling prevalence studies. Int J Adolesc Med Health 22(1):3–38, 2010 20491416

Walker M: Treatment strategies for problem gambling: a review of effectiveness, in Gambling Behavior and Problem Gambling. Edited by Eadington WR, Cornelius JA. Reno, University of Nevada, 1993 pp 533–566

Wardle H, Moody A, Spence S, et al: British Gambling Prevalence Survey, 2010. Report to the (UK) Gambling Commission. London, National Centre for Social Research, 2011

Wareham JD, Potenza MN: Pathological gambling and substance use disorders. Am J Drug Alcohol Abuse 36(5):242–247, 2010 20575651

Welte J, Barnes G, Wieczorek W, et al: Type of gambling and availability as risk factors for problem gambling: a Tobit regression analysis by age and gender. International Gambling Studies 7(2):183–198, 2007

Wiebe J, Wynne H, Stinchfield R, et al: The Canadian Adolescent Gambling Inventory (CAGI): Phase II Final report. Ottawa, ON, Canada, Canadian Centre on Substance Abuse, 2007

Winters KC, Stinchfield RD, Fulkerson J: Toward the development of an adolescent gambling problem severity scale. J Gambl Stud 9(1):371–386 1993

Wood RT, Griffiths MD: The acquisition, development and maintenance of lottery and scratchcard gambling in adolescence. J Adolesc 21(3):265–273, 1998 9657894

Wynne HJ, Smith GJ, Jacobs DF, et al: Adolescent Gambling and Problem Gambling in Alberta. Edmonton, AB, Canada, Alberta Alcohol and Drug Commission, 1996

Zuckerman M: Behavioral Expressions and Biosocial Bases of Sensation Seeking. New York, Cambridge University Press, 1994

CHAPTER 14

Pathological Preoccupation With the Internet

Yvonne H.C. Yau, M.Sc.

Jeffrey L. Derevensky, Ph.D.

Marc N. Potenza, M.D., Ph.D.

The Internet has permeated almost all aspects of daily functioning. Given that adolescents and young adults have typically grown up with access to computers and the Internet from early ages, they are considered to belong to the so-called digital generation. As of 2014, a staggering 97% of American adolescents reported at least occasional Internet use (Fox and Rainie 2014). Internet accessibility has undergone a major transformation in that stationary connections tied to desktops are no longer required, and "always-on" connections are available on portable devices and smartphones that move with individuals throughout the day. The adoption of related technologies has also been extraordinary; gambling, gaming, shopping, and sexual activities are among the behaviors that have been redefined by the Internet. The ready availability of the Internet coupled with a substantial increase in the amount of time spent using the Internet has raised concerns among clinicians, researchers, and the public regarding the potential for some youths (as well as older individuals) to exhibit problematic and/or pathological patterns of engagement.

Most Internet users have no serious disruptions in their psychosocial functioning. When used appropriately, the Internet may help facilitate information retrieval, provide entertainment and communication, increase social support by enabling easier connections with friends, assist in the formation of new relationships, and provide other resources. However, emerging empirical studies and numerous anecdotal media reports suggest possible links between problematic Internet use (PIU)—also commonly referred to in the literature as Internet addiction, compulsive Internet use, pathological Internet use, or Internet dependence (Block 2008; Yau et al. 2012)—and negative health consequences, such as depression, attention-deficit/hyperactivity disorder (ADHD), excessive daytime sleepiness, problematic substance use, or injuries (Ko et al. 2009a; Morris 2012; Yen et al. 2007). PIU has also been associated with negative academic consequences, including poor class attendance, lower academic performance, and even academic dismissal in extreme cases (Chen and Tzeng 2010; Kubey et al. 2001). Although the digital generation may have advantages over older adults because of the former's early development of Internet skills and experiences, this population may also be at greater risk for the development of PIU. Although PIU has received increased research attention in recent years, how best to define and categorize PIU remains debated. Currently, diagnostic criteria are not uniformly accepted, and the use of varied instruments and thresholds to define PIU has complicated interpretations of findings and comparisons across studies.

Epidemiology

A systematic review of PIU prevalence among U.S. youth found that studies reported vastly different rates, ranging from 0% to 26.3% (Moreno et al. 2011). Research involving European youth has also yielded varying prevalence rates, although considerably lower, ranging from 1.5% to 8.2% (Johansson and Götestam 2004; Kormas et al. 2011; Pallanti et al. 2006; Siomos et al. 2008; Zboralski et al. 2009). In Asia, findings indicate even higher variations in PIU prevalence among adolescents, ranging from 2.4% to 37.9% (Cao and Su 2007; Deng et al. 2007; Kim et al. 2006; Park et al. 2008). It is unclear whether these large variations in the reported prevalence estimates of PIU among youth could be due to cultural differences, differences in methodologies or cohort characteristics, year of data collection, varying PIU taxonomies in the studies performed, and/or other factors. Nevertheless, these preliminary prevalence estimates tell a cautionary tale and highlight the need for a better understanding of PIU.

Features and Diagnosis

Efforts toward developing diagnostic criteria for PIU began in the 1990s, and several conceptual models have since been proposed. Young (1998) proposed that PIU be conceptualized as an impulse-control disorder. She adapted the DSM-IV (American Psychiatric Association 1994) criteria for pathological gambling—a condition categorized at that time as an impulse-control disorder—and created the Young's Diagnostic Questionnaire (Young 1999). Briefly, the proposed criteria included 1) a maladaptive preoccupation with Internet use characterized by either an irresistible use or use that is excessive and longer than planned, 2) clinically significant distress or impairment, and 3) an absence of other Axis I disorders (Shapira et al. 2003; Young 1998). These criteria were subsequently adopted by multiple other researchers investigating PIU (Bakken et al. 2009; Dowling and Quirk 2009), but they were not formally included in DSM-IV.

PIU has also been proposed to represent a "behavioral addiction" (Przepiorka et al. 2014). Researchers have posited that certain behaviors may prompt neurobiological responses that influence feelings of pleasure and reward in a manner similar to psychoactive substances, with some neurobiological studies lending credence to this proposal (Yau et al. 2015). Much like substance-related addictions, behavioral addictions are characterized by failures to resist impulses, appetitive drives or cravings, compulsive performance of behaviors, and diminished control over engagement in behaviors despite adverse consequences (Potenza 2006). Furthermore, over time, individuals may experience less pleasure from the behavior (Grant et al. 2006) and require a higher intensity and/or frequency to achieve the same effects (Blanco et al. 2001; Grant et al. 2006), akin to tolerance (Block 2008).

In DSM-5 (American Psychiatric Association 2013), a new diagnostic class is included: substance-related and addictive disorders. Pathological gambling, termed *gambling disorder* in DSM-5, was reassigned to this class based on similarities between substance use and gambling disorders (Potenza 2006). This reclassification reflects the idea that addiction is not exclusive to substance use and can manifest in pathological engagement with non-substance-related behaviors. Although PIU was also considered for inclusion in this DSM-5 diagnostic class, the Substance-Related Disorders Work Group concluded that there is currently a lack of empirical evidence and documentation of the adverse consequences to support this move. However, a related condition—namely, Internet gaming disorder (IGD)—was included in Section III among the conditions in need of further study. The work group chose and worded the IGD criteria to parallel some substance use and gambling disorder criteria but also took into account that the expression of Internet gaming may differ from these disorders. The proposed diagnostic criteria for IGD (American Psychiatric Association 2013) include nine items (Box 14–1), and the diagnostic threshold was set at meeting five or more inclusionary criteria.

Box 14–1.   Proposed Criteria for Internet Gaming Disorder

Persistent and recurrent use of the Internet to engage in games, often with other players, leading to clinically significant impairment or distress as indicated by five (or more) of the following in a 12-month period:

1. Preoccupation with Internet games. (The individual thinks about previous gaming activity or anticipates playing the next game; Internet gaming becomes the dominant activity in daily life.)
   Note: This disorder is distinct from Internet gambling, which is included under gambling disorder.
2. Withdrawal symptoms when Internet gaming is taken away. (These symptoms are typically described as irritability, anxiety, or sadness, but there are no physical signs of pharmacological withdrawal.)
3. Tolerance—the need to spend increasing amounts of time engaged in Internet games.
4. Unsuccessful attempts to control the participation in Internet games.
5. Loss of interests in previous hobbies and entertainment as a result of, and with the exception of, Internet games.
6. Continued excessive use of Internet games despite knowledge of psychosocial problems.
7. Has deceived family members, therapists, or others regarding the amount of Internet gaming.
8. Use of Internet games to escape or relieve a negative mood (e.g., feelings of helplessness, guilt, anxiety).
9. Has jeopardized or lost a significant relationship, job, or educational or career opportunity because of participation in Internet games.

Note: Only nongambling Internet games are included in this disorder. Use of the Internet for required activities in a business or profession is not included; nor is the disorder intended to include other recreational or social Internet use. Similarly, sexual Internet sites are excluded.

Specify current severity:

   Internet gaming disorder can be mild, moderate, or severe depending on the degree of disruption of normal activities. Individuals with less severe Internet gaming disorder may exhibit fewer symptoms and less disruption of their lives. Those with severe Internet gaming disorder will have more hours spent on the computer and more severe loss of relationships or career or school opportunities.

By listing IGD in Section III of DSM-5, the American Psychiatric Association aims to encourage research to determine whether the condition should be included in future editions as a recognizable disorder. It should be noted that IGD focuses specifically on Internet *gaming* (not gambling) and not other forms of Internet use. Whether these proposed criteria may be adapted to accurately assess PIU more broadly remains unclear. Additionally, it is currently not clear how IGD, PIU, or another Internet-related diagnostic entity might be considered in the forthcoming 11th edition of the World Health Organization's *International Classification of Diseases*. Regardless, the similarities and differences between IGD and PIU have yet to be systematically examined and warrant additional study.

Course of Problem Internet Use and Relationship With SUDs

Non-Internet addiction–related problems may occur in conjunction with PIU. Individuals with PIU are more likely to report higher rates of substance use, problematic alcohol use, and problematic gambling (Weinstein and Lejoyeux 2010). A recent study found that college students with co-occurring PIU and substance use disorders/behaviors reported higher levels of negative consequences/life events, less academic success, and higher levels of psychological distress than students reporting either problematic Internet or substance use but not both (Eckhoff 2013). Moreover, preliminary data suggest that PIU may serve as a predictor variable for substance use in adolescents (Fisoun et al. 2012).

The high co-occurrence between PIU and substance use disorders (SUDs) may be explained by shared phenomenological characteristics. A recent review of 17 prevalence-estimate studies suggests that adolescents expressing PIU or substance use behaviors display common characteristics, including high novelty-seeking behavior and low reward dependence (Ko et al. 2012). Similar to individuals with SUDs (e.g., Kotov et al. 2010; Ruiz et al. 2008; Sargent et al. 2010; Verdejo-García et al. 2008), individuals expressing PIU have been noted to display impulsivity (Cao et al. 2007), excessive risk-taking behavior (Wood et al. 2004), low self-esteem (Niemz et al. 2005; Young and Rogers 1998), and disadvantageous decision making (Sun et al. 2009).

Although PIU may have significant overlaps with other mental health disorders, there may also be characteristics unique to PIU. For example, in contrast to the observed low harm avoidance among adolescents with various SUDs, adolescents with PIU tend to report high harm avoidance (Ko et al. 2006). This finding may reflect key differences between problematic engagements with the Internet and substance use and help to explain why the Internet may be particularly appealing to certain individuals.

Etiology and Clinical Course

PIU appears to be comorbid with multiple psychiatric conditions and premorbid symptoms in addition to SUDs. In adolescents, PIU has been reported to be comorbid with depression (Ha et al. 2007), ADHD, social anxiety disorder (Ko et al. 2009a; Tokunaga and Rains 2010), schizophrenia, obsessive-compulsive disorder (Ha et al. 2006), and aggression (Ko et al. 2009b).

There is debate regarding whether PIU may represent a primary disorder that contributes to the development of other disorders or whether PIU may represent a secondary disorder preceded by or merely concomitant with other disorders. Several short-term longitudinal studies have been conducted in Asia, where the incidence of PIU is reportedly high. In Taiwan, a 2-year study investigating 2,162 adolescents ages 11–13 years found that ADHD and hostility preceded PIU development and represented potential risk factors for both males and females (Ko et al. 2009a). Depression and social phobia were reported as potential risk factors only among girls. In China, adolescents ages 13–18 years endorsing PIU items on Young's Diagnostic Questionnaire were 2.5 times more likely to have developed depressive symptoms at a 9-month follow-up than were those who did not endorse any items (Lam and Peng 2010). Similar findings were reported for problematic video game playing among primary school students (average age of 9 years) and secondary school students (average age of 13 years) in Singapore (Gentile et al. 2011). Depression, as well as anxiety and social phobia, became worse at the end of a 2-year period if children or adolescents developed problematic video game playing during this period. Interestingly, these features may improve when individuals stop exhibiting problematic gaming behaviors. This study, however, did not differentiate between online and offline gaming. For IGD specifically, a prospective study of adolescents ages 13–16 in the Netherlands found that those individuals reporting IGD generally scored higher on measures of depression, loneliness, social anxiety, and negative self-esteem at multiple points within a 1-year time frame. At the end of this 1-year period, adolescents with IGD scored higher on the depression scale than did heavy online gamers who did not express IGD (Van Rooij et al. 2011).

Few studies have examined PIU in the context of age and development. Cross-sectional studies indicate that adolescents tend to report higher levels of PIU and IGD than adults (Yau et al. 2012), suggesting that there may be decreases in PIU prevalence with age. However, a 2-year study of Canadian adolescents ages 14–16 years found that there was no change over that time period in the prevalence of Internet use, although a decrease in the frequency of video game playing was observed over time among both genders (Willoughby 2008). Further studies are needed before definitive conclusions can be drawn.

Prevention and Treatment Interventions

The clinical evaluation of patients with PIU should include a careful assessment of Internet use behaviors and possible co-occurring conditions, all of which should be taken into account when selecting optimal treatment strategies. Although it is unclear whether Internet-related problems may stem from other diagnoses (e.g., a patient presenting with depression symptoms starting to lead a "virtual" life to boost self-esteem at the expense of offline interactions and duties) or predispose individuals to the other disorders (e.g., a patient becoming depressed in the setting of experiencing consequences relating to excessive Internet use), treatment for PIU may help address problems underlying multiple conditions and improve overall psychosocial well-being.

Although PIU remains a controversial topic, there has been a demand for treatment for individuals with this problem. Some interventions have involved "boot camp"–style programs specializing in the treatment of PIU (King et al. 2011; Young 2012). Programs may promote abstinence models and incorporate aspects of family therapy and social skills training into treatment. Strategies may include improving face-to-face communication and helping family members appropriately monitor Internet use. However, details of such therapeutic programs and the empirical support for the efficacies of the treatments they employ are not entirely clear (Griffiths 2007; Weinstein and Lejoyeux 2010). There is also some preliminary evidence for the usefulness of group and multimodal counseling as well as motivational interviewing (Kim et al. 2008; Orzack et al. 2006), although further investigation is needed to determine the efficacy of each approach.

In terms of pharmacological treatments, several studies have shown that selective serotonin reuptake inhibitors (SSRIs) may be beneficial for treating PIU. A case study has reported the successful use of quetiapine (a medication primarily used in the treatment of schizophrenia or bipolar disorder) in combination with citalopram (an SSRI) in alleviating symptoms in a 23-year-old patient presenting with PIU (Atmaca 2007). This improvement was maintained at a 4-month follow-up. Another SSRI, escitalopram, has also been reported as being efficacious in treating 19 patients with PIU symptoms (Dell'Osso et al. 2008). During the 10-week treatment program, patients showed significant improvements in global functioning and reduction in time spent online. Following the 10-week period, participants were blindly randomly assigned to either continued escitalopram treatment or placebo for an additional 9 weeks. The two groups did not demonstrate significant differences at the end of this second phase, and the positive effects initially achieved in the first 10 weeks were maintained among all patients, raising questions about the role of the medication in the recovery process.

Of psychotherapeutic approaches, cognitive-behavioral therapy (CBT) has arguably received the most empirical investigation. The largest study to date investigated 114 adults expressing PIU who received CBT interventions, including keeping a daily log of Internet activity, learning time management skills, restructuring cognitive distortions, and engaging in other activities (Young 2007). Following treatment completion, participants showed significant improvements, which were maintained at a 6-month follow-up. CBT has also demonstrated efficacy in treating PIU symptoms in adolescents. In one study, 56 adolescents ages 12–17 years were randomly assigned to an active treatment group or a clinical control group (Du et al. 2010). Participants in the treatment group received eight CBT sessions, whereas the control group received no intervention. Although Internet use was found to have decreased in both groups, those in the treatment group displayed improved time management skills and performed better on various emotional, cognitive, and behavioral assessments.

Pharmacological and psychotherapeutic interventions specific to PIU have yet to receive adequate testing in large, rigorous studies. More randomized controlled trials are needed for both pharmacological and psychotherapeutic interventions. Improvements in research study designs, such as blinding procedures, would provide important information regarding the extent to which clinical changes are related to the intervention being studied.

Summary and Future Directions

Internet use has radically changed many lives, arguably more so than any other technology of this era, yet comparatively little is known about its effects on individuals' psychological functioning, mental health, and well-being. PIU remains ill defined, and the lack of a standard set of diagnostic criteria is a major impediment to advancing this area of study and clinical care. Although research about the effects of PIU is still in its infancy, preliminary evidence has highlighted potential harms of excessive Internet use, particularly for today's youth. Going forward, more research is needed on the prognosis of PIU, the temporal relationships between psychiatric disorders and PIU, mechanisms of comorbidity, and more subtle psychological changes that may occur with PIU over time. Parents, educators, and clinicians would be well advised to monitor the impact of excessive Internet use by youth.

KEY POINTS

- Problematic Internet use (PIU) is a serious concern with a significant public health impact.

- Formal diagnostic criteria for PIU have yet to be established.

- Emerging evidence suggests similarities between PIU and substance use disorders, although differences also exist.

- Preliminary findings suggest that some treatments (e.g., cognitive-behavioral therapy) may be efficacious in treating PIU.

- An improved understanding of the prognosis of PIU will enhance clinicians' ability to recognize, prevent, and treat more effectively.

References

American Psychiatric Association: Diagnostic and Statistical Manual of Mental Disorders, 4th Edition. Washington, DC, American Psychiatric Association, 1994

American Psychiatric Association: Diagnostic and Statistical Manual of Mental Disorders, 5th Edition. Arlington, VA, American Psychiatric Association, 2013

Atmaca M: A case of problematic Internet use successfully treated with an SSRI-antipsychotic combination. Prog Neuropsychopharmacol Biol Psychiatry 31(4):961–962, 2007 17321659

Bakken IJ, Wenzel HG, Götestam KG, et al: Internet addiction among Norwegian adults: a stratified probability sample study. Scand J Psychol 50(2):121–127, 2009 18826420

Blanco C, Moreyra P, Nunes EV, et al: Pathological gambling: addiction or compulsion? Semin Clin Neuropsychiatry 6(3):167–176, 2001 11447568

Block JJ: Issues for DSM-V: Internet addiction. Am J Psychiatry 165(3):306–307, 2008 18316427

Cao F, Su L: Internet addiction among Chinese adolescents: prevalence and psychological features. Child Care Health Dev 33(3):275–281, 2007 17439441

Cao F, Su L, Liu T, et al: The relationship between impulsivity and Internet addiction in a sample of Chinese adolescents. Eur Psychiatry 22(7):466–471, 2007 17765486

Chen SY, Tzeng JY: College female and male heavy Internet users' profiles of practices and their academic grades and psychosocial adjustment. Cyberpsychol Behav Soc Netw 13(3):257–262, 2010 20557244

Dell'Osso B, Hadley S, Allen A, et al: Escitalopram in the treatment of impulsive-compulsive Internet usage disorder: an open-label trial followed by a double-blind discontinuation phase. J Clin Psychiatry 69(3):452–456, 2008 18312057

Deng YX, Hu M, Hu GQ, et al: An investigation on the prevalence of Internet addiction disorder in middle school students of Hunan province [in Chinese]. Zhonghua Liu Xing Bing Xue Za Zhi 28(5):445–448, 2007 17877171

Dowling NA, Quirk KL: Screening for Internet dependence: do the proposed diagnostic criteria differentiate normal from dependent Internet use? Cyberpsychol Behav 12(1):21–27, 2009 19196045

Du YS, Jiang W, Vance A: Longer term effect of randomized, controlled group cognitive behavioural therapy for Internet addiction in adolescent students in Shanghai. Aust NZJ Psychiatry 44(2):129–134, 2010 20113301

Eckhoff M: Impact of harm avoidance, novelty seeking and reward dependence on Internet addiction and substance abuse in college students. Unpublished doctoral dissertation, New York, New School University, 2013

Fisoun V, Floros G, Siomos K, et al: Internet addiction as an important predictor in early detection of adolescent drug use experience—implications for research and practice. J Addict Med 6(1):77–84, 2012 22227578

Fox S, Rainie L: The Web at 25 in the U.S. Washington, DC, Pew Research Internet Project, 2014. Available at: http://www.pewinternet.org/2014/02/27/the-web-at-25-in-the-u-s/. Accessed September 20, 2014.

Gentile DA, Choo H, Liau A, et al: Pathological video game use among youths: a two-year longitudinal study. Pediatrics 127(2):e319–e329, 2011 21242221

Grant JE, Brewer JA, Potenza MN: The neurobiology of substance and behavioral addictions. CNS Spectr 11(12):924–930, 2006 17146406

Griffiths MD: Online gaming addictions: legislation or moderation? E-commerce, Law and Policy 9(9):10–11, 2007

Ha JH, Yoo HJ, Cho IH, et al: Psychiatric comorbidity assessed in Korean children and adolescents who screen positive for Internet addiction. J Clin Psychiatry 67(5):821–826, 2006 16841632

Ha JH, Kim SY, Bae SC, et al: Depression and Internet addiction in adolescents. Psychopathology 40(6):424–430, 2007 17709972

Johansson A, Götestam KG: Internet addiction: characteristics of a questionnaire and prevalence in Norwegian youth (12–18 years). Scand J Psychol 45(3):223–229, 2004 15182240

Kim EJ, Namkoong K, Ku T, et al: The relationship between online game addiction and aggression, self-control and narcissistic personality traits. Eur Psychiatry 23(3):212–218, 2008 18166402

Kim K, Ryu E, Chon MY, et al: Internet addiction in Korean adolescents and its relation to depression and suicidal ideation: a questionnaire survey. Int J Nurs Stud 43(2):185–192, 2006 16427966

King DL, Delfabbro PH, Griffiths MD, et al: Assessing clinical trials of Internet addiction treatment: a systematic review and CONSORT evaluation. Clin Psychol Rev 31(7):1110–1116, 2011 21820990

Ko CH, Yen JY, Chen CC, et al: Tridimensional personality of adolescents with Internet addiction and substance use experience. Can J Psychiatry 51(14):887–894, 2006 17249631

Ko CH, Yen JY, Chen CS, et al: Predictive values of psychiatric symptoms for Internet addiction in adolescents: a 2-year prospective study. Arch Pediatr Adolesc Med 163(10):937–943, 2009a 19805713

Ko CH, Yen JY, Liu SC, et al: The associations between aggressive behaviors and Internet addiction and online activities in adolescents. J Adolesc Health 44(6):598–605, 2009b 19465325

Ko CH, Yen JY, Yen CF, et al: The association between Internet addiction and psychiatric disorder: a review of the literature. Eur Psychiatry 27(1):1–8, 2012 22153731

Kormas G, Critselis E, Janikian M, et al: Risk factors and psychosocial characteristics of potential problematic and problematic Internet use among adolescents: a cross-sectional study. BMC Public Health 11(1):595, 2011 21794167

Kotov R, Gamez W, Schmidt F, et al: Linking "big" personality traits to anxiety, depressive, and substance use disorders: a meta-analysis. Psychol Bull 136(5):768–821, 2010 20804236

Kubey RW, Lavin MJ, Barrows JR: Internet use and collegiate academic performance decrements: early findings. J Commun 51(2):366–382, 2001

Lam LT, Peng ZW: Effect of pathological use of the Internet on adolescent mental health: a prospective study. Arch Pediatr Adolesc Med 164(10):901–906, 2010 20679157

Moreno MA, Jelenchick L, Cox E, et al: Problematic Internet use among US youth: a systematic review. Arch Pediatr Adolesc Med 165(9):797–805, 2011 21536950

Morris C: Gamer's death at Internet cafe goes unnoticed for nine hours. Yahoo News, February 3, 2012. Available at: https://games.yahoo.com/blogs/plugged-in/gamer-death-goes-unnoticed-nine-hours-internet-cafe-184733181.html. Accessed June 30, 2014.

Niemz K, Griffiths M, Banyard P: Prevalence of pathological Internet use among university students and correlations with self-esteem, the General Health Questionnaire (GHQ), and disinhibition. Cyberpsychol Behav 8(6):562–570, 2005 16332167

Orzack MH, Voluse AC, Wolf D, et al: An ongoing study of group treatment for men involved in problematic Internet-enabled sexual behavior. Cyberpsychol Behav 9(3):348–360, 2006 16780403

Pallanti S, Bernardi S, Quercioli L: The Shorter PROMIS Questionnaire and the Internet Addiction Scale in the assessment of multiple addictions in a high-school population: prevalence and related disability. CNS Spectr 11(12):966–974, 2006 17146410

Park SK, Kim JY, Cho CB: Prevalence of Internet addiction and correlations with family factors among South Korean adolescents. Adolescence 43(172):895–909, 2008 19149152

Potenza MN: Should addictive disorders include non-substance-related conditions? Addiction 101(1 suppl 1):142–151, 2006 16930171

Przepiorka AM, Blachnio A, Miziak B, et al: Clinical approaches to treatment of Internet addiction. Pharmacol Rep 66(2):187–191, 2014 24911068

Ruiz MA, Pincus AL, Schinka JA: Externalizing pathology and the Five-Factor Model: a meta-analysis of personality traits associated with antisocial personality disorder, substance use disorder, and their co-occurrence. J Pers Disord 22(4):365–388, 2008 18684050

Sargent JD, Tanski S, Stoolmiller M, et al: Using sensation seeking to target adolescents for substance use interventions. Addiction 105(3):506–514, 2010 20402995

Shapira NA, Lessig MC, Goldsmith TD, et al: Problematic Internet use: proposed classification and diagnostic criteria. Depress Anxiety 17(4):207–216, 2003 12820176

Siomos KE, Dafouli ED, Braimiotis DA, et al: Internet addiction among Greek adolescent students. Cyberpsychol Behav 11(6):653–657, 2008

Sun DL, Chen Z-J, Ma N, et al: Decision-making and prepotent response inhibition functions in excessive Internet users. CNS Spectr 14(2):75–81, 2009 19238122

Tokunaga RS, Rains SA: An evaluation of two characterizations of the relationships between problematic Internet use, time spent using the Internet, and psychosocial problems. Hum Commun Res 36(4):512–545, 2010

Van Rooij AJ, Schoenmakers TM, Vermulst AA, et al: Online video game addiction: identification of addicted adolescent gamers. Addiction 106(1):205–212, 2011 20840209

Verdejo-García A, Lawrence AJ, Clark L: Impulsivity as a vulnerability marker for substance-use disorders: review of findings from high-risk research, problem gamblers and genetic association studies. Neurosci Biobehav Rev 32(4):777–810, 2008 18295884

Weinstein A, Lejoyeux M: Internet addiction or excessive Internet use. Am J Drug Alcohol Abuse 36(5):277–283, 2010 20545603

Willoughby T: A short-term longitudinal study of Internet and computer game use by adolescent boys and girls: prevalence, frequency of use, and psychosocial predictors. Dev Psychol 44(1):195–204, 2008 18194017

Wood RTA, Gupta R, Derevensky JL, et al: Video game playing and gambling in adolescents: common risk factors. J Child Adolesc Subst Abuse 14(1):77–100, 2004

Yau YHC, Crowley MJ, Mayes LC, et al: Are Internet use and video-game-playing addictive behaviors? Biological, clinical and public health implications for youths and adults. Minerva Psichiatr 53(3):153–170, 2012 24288435

Yau Y, Leeman RF, Potenza MN: Biological underpinnings of behavioral addictions and management implications, in The Textbook of Addiction Treatment: International Perspectives. Edited by el-Guebaly N, Galanter M, Carra G. New York, Springer, 2015, pp 1411–1442

Yen JY, Ko CH, Yen CF, et al: The comorbid psychiatric symptoms of Internet addiction: attention deficit and hyperactivity disorder (ADHD), depression, social phobia, and hostility. J Adolesc Health 41(1):93–98, 2007 17577539

Young KS: Internet addiction: the emergence of a new clinical disorder. Cyberpsychol Behav 1(3):237–244, 1998

Young KS: Internet addiction: symptoms, evaluation and treatment, in Innovations in Clinical Practice: A Source Book, Vol 17. Edited by VandeCreek L, Jackson T. Sarasota, FL, Professional Resource Press, 1999, pp 19–31

Young KS: Cognitive behavior therapy with Internet addicts: treatment outcomes and implications. Cyberpsychol Behav 10(5):671–679, 2007 17927535

Young KS: Assessment and treatment of problem Internet use, in The Oxford Handbook of Impulse Control Disorders. Edited by Grant JE, Potenza MN. New York, Oxford University Press, 2012, pp 389–397

Young KS, Rogers RC: The relationship between depression and Internet addiction. Cyberpsychol Behav 1(1):25–28, 1998

Zboralski K, Orzechowska A, Talarowska M, et al: The prevalence of computer and Internet addiction among pupils. Postepy Hig Med Dosw (Online) 63:8–12, 2009 19252459

Index

Page numbers printed in **boldface** type refer to tables or figures.

Generalized anxiety disorder (GAD),
  (continued)
  shared vulnerabilities, 182
  SUD comorbidity with, 181–182
Genetics
  bipolar disorder and, 162–163
  bulimia nervosa and, 293–294
  conduct disorder and, 84
  eating disorders and, 287
  as risk factor for SUDs, 6
  schizophrenia and, 260–261
Global Appraisal of Individual
  Needs (GAIN), 53, 54, 212
Global Assessment of Functioning
  (GAF) scale, 254
Great Smoky Mountains Study,
  135–137, 139
Group therapy. *See also* Family
  behavior therapy
  CBT and, 58–59
  iatrogenic effects of, 94
Growing Up Today Study, 289

Hamilton Anxiety Rating Scale
  (HARS), 184, **188**
HAP (Hilson Adolescent Profile), 55
HARS (Hamilton Anxiety Rating
  Scale), 184, **188**
Harvard Trauma Questionnaire
  (HTQ), 213
Hilson Adolescent Profile (HAP), 55
Hopelessness Scale for Children,
  243
HTQ (Harvard Trauma Question-
  naire), 213
Hyperactivity, 104

I-CBT (integrated cognitive-behavioral
  therapy), 244–245
IGD (Internet gaming disorder),
  339–341
Impulsivity, 104
Inattention, 104
Infancy

caregiver-infant relationship, 8
stress during, 7–8
SUD liability and clinical outcome, 7–8
Integrated care
  barriers to, 22–24, 38–41
  clinical practice approaches,
    38–40
  in depressive disorders, 138
  development of the workforce,
    30–32, 40
  diagnostic approaches to, 24–27
    specificity versus sensitivity
    and, 24–25
  economic incentives, 41
  expanding treatment capacity,
    40–41
  organizational and financial
    incentives for, 35–38
  primary care and, 41
  treatment matching and place-
    ment strategies, 32–35
  of the treatment team, 30
Integrated cognitive-behavioral
  therapy (I-CBT), 244–245
Interdisciplinary treatment, for
  schizophrenia, 268–270
Internet, 337–349
Internet gaming disorder (IGD),
  339–341
  DSM-5 proposed criteria for,
    340–341
Interpersonal therapy (IPT), for eating
  disorders, 296
Interventions
  brief, 56–57
  brief motivational, 59–61
Interviews
  Adolescent Diagnostic Interview,
    54
  diagnostic, 54, 141–142
  motivational, 93
  opportunistic, 267–268
  problem-focused, 54–55